Advanced Structured Materials

Volume 249

Common engineering materials are reaching their limits in many applications, and new developments are required to meet the increasing demands on engineering materials. The performance of materials can be improved by combining different materials to achieve better properties than with a single constituent, or by shaping the material or constituents into a specific structure. The interaction between material and structure can occur at different length scales, such as the micro, meso, or macro scale, and offers potential applications in very different fields.

This book series addresses the fundamental relationships between materials and their structure on overall properties (e.g., mechanical, thermal, chemical, electrical, or magnetic properties, etc.). Experimental data and procedures are presented, as well as methods for modeling structures and materials using numerical and analytical approaches. In addition, the series shows how these materials engineering and design processes are implemented and how new technologies can be used to optimize materials and processes.

Advanced Structured Materials is indexed in Google Scholar and Scopus.

Andreas Öchsner
Editor

Progress in Biomaterials and Biomedical Engineering

Springer

Editor
Andreas Öchsner
Faculty of Mechanical and Systems Engineering
Esslingen University of Applied Sciences
Esslingen am Neckar, Baden-Württemberg
Germany

ISSN 1869-8433 ISSN 1869-8441 (electronic)
Advanced Structured Materials
ISBN 978-3-032-13550-6 ISBN 978-3-032-13551-3 (eBook)
https://doi.org/10.1007/978-3-032-13551-3

This Springer imprint is published by the registered company Springer Nature Switzerland AG
The registered company address is: Gewerbestrasse 11, 6330 Cham, Switzerland

Contents

Chapter 1
Biomechanical Evaluation on 3D Printing PMMA Plates Proposals, for Upper Head and Mandible

Carolina Alvarado-Moreno, Juan Alfonso Beltrán-Fernández, Mauricio González-Rebattú, and Alejandro Tonatiu Velázquez-Sánchez

Abstract Based on digital acquisition, the main objective of this study is to demonstrate the endurance of different proposals for mandibular and cranial reconstruction, as well as the advantages of using 3D printing technology in biomedicine. Using high-resolution thermoplastic 3D printers, the bone was reconstructed and fixed. Finally, each proposal underwent mechanical evaluation, and optical results detecting internal stress were presented as an additional advantage of using thermoplastic materials.

Keywords Mandible · Cranium · PMMA · Compression · 3D printing technology

C. Alvarado-Moreno (✉) · J. A. Beltrán-Fernández (✉) · M. González-Rebattú · A. T. Velázquez-Sánchez
Instituto Politécnico Nacional—Escuela Superior de Ingeniería Mecánica y Eléctrica—Sección de Estudios de Posgrado e Investigación Edificio 5, 2do Piso, Unidad Profesional Adolfo López Mateos "Zacatenco" Col. Lindavista, Mexico City, Mexico
e-mail: calvaradom1800@alumno.ipn.mx

J. A. Beltrán-Fernández
e-mail: jbeltran@ipn.mx

M. González-Rebattú
e-mail: mauriciorebattu@yahoo.com.mx

A. T. Velázquez-Sánchez
e-mail: atvelazquezs@ipn.mx

M. González-Rebattú
Hospital Regional "1 de Octubre" del ISSSTE, Av Instituto Politécnico Nacional 1669, Revolución IMSS, Gustavo A. Madero, Mexico City, Mexico

Centro de Investigación y Laboratorio de Biomecánica, Carmen #18, Chimalistac, San Ángel, Mexico City, Mexico

A. Öchsner (ed.), *Progress in Biomaterials and Biomedical Engineering*, Advanced Structured Materials 249, https://doi.org/10.1007/978-3-032-13551-3_1

1.1 Introduction

Three-dimensional photo-curing printing technology transforms a digital model into a solid 3D object by slicing and printing an array of polygons known as stereolithography (STL). This method was first described in 1983 and patented in 1986 by Charles Hull, with its first commercial introduction in 1987. The first printer model used a laser to cure photopolymer in a pool of liquid resin selectively. Still, it had the disadvantage of requiring constant refilling of the resin tank, which was not cost-effective. Moreover, acquiring the printer involved very high costs (Kovalenko and Garan 2017, Smith et al. 2021).

Nowadays the printer costs are more approachable, but it is still expensive depending on the size of the printing area. Additionally, there are some improvements to promote investment in a printer such as software availability, resin developments, and authorized third parties to open the international market (Coasey 2024).

In 3D printing with resin, the main technologies are stereolithography (SLA), digital light processing (DLP), and liquid crystal display (LCD). Typically, 3D printer resins sensitive to UV wavelength are used. Photopolymer solutions consist of three elements: monomers, photo-initiators, and blockers, which create different levels of radiation penetration and consequently affect layer thickness, making the properties of the resins vary from one to another (Kovalenko and Garan 2017).

The equipment used in this study was the LCD 3D printing technology, a recent system derived from SLA printing. It employs a screen that applies an electric field to the liquid crystal, causing a change in its molecular arrangement. This results in some molecules blocking the light while others remain transparent, curing the photosensitive resin (Guido et al. 2023).

Processes for generating 3D printing layers include vector, rasterization, or mask approaches. In terms of time, mask processing is the most efficient due to the exposure of the entire layer simultaneously. LCD printing uses the mask process (Guido et al. 2023).

All patient data originated from a picture archiving and communication system (PACS), meaning that all X-ray and computed tomography medical images were stored in a digital database that could be shared across other medical areas such as biomechanical clinical research. Using medical image information, the reconstruction of the area was performed with a CAD software and tools. For the qualitative test, the printer and its parameters are described in the methodology.

1.2 Methodology

For each reconstruction case, a 3D model of the damaged bone was generated from a standard DICOM file using SCAN-IP© (Synopsys Inc. 1986) (Fig. 1.1). Additionally, the CAD program SpaceClaim© (Swanson Analysis Systems 2025) was used to design different plate proposals, as shown in Fig. 1.2. With the final design saved as an STL file, the next step was slicing.

The printing process was performed through photopolymerization (light-induced polymerization) using the HALOT-ONE© Creality© UV printer (Shenzhen Creality 3D Technology Co. Ltd. 2025a) (Fig. 1.3). The HALOT-BOX© software (Shenzhen Creality 3D Technology Co. Ltd. 2025b) (Table 1.1) allows users to generate automatic or customized supports. These tools help calibrate the stereolithography file

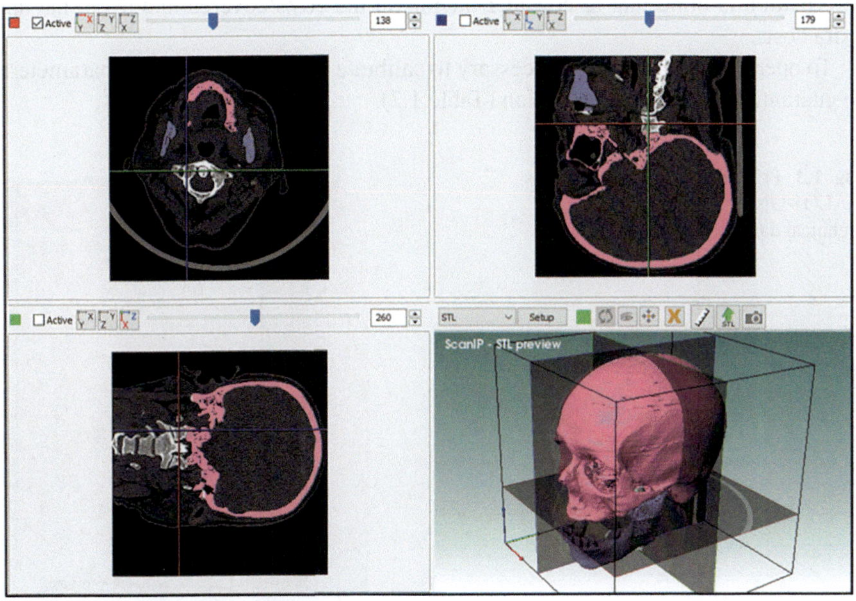

Fig. 1.1 SCAN-IP© processing image

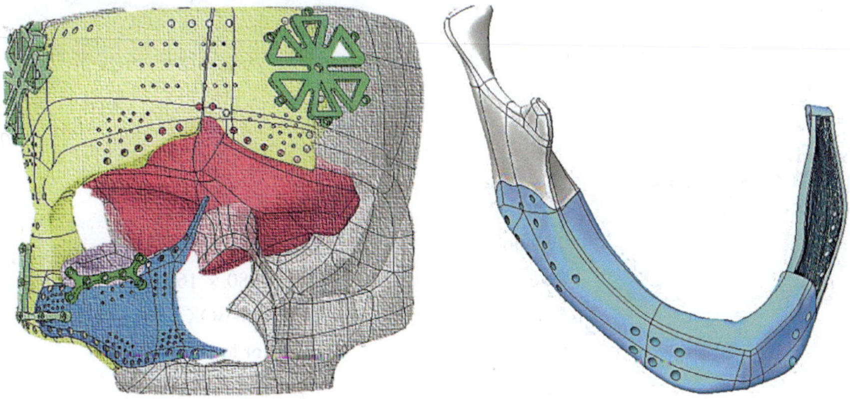

Fig. 1.2 Reconstructions design for the biomechanical analysis

and correctly position the designs in the working area, ensuring that the figures do not exceed the printing limits and thereby avoiding partial or complete printing failures.

In addition, on the slicing program, a preview file is obtained completely parameterized for printing on the HALOT-ONE© machine (Fig. 1.4), in case that is required a modification.

The slicing software can estimate the duration of 3D printing and an estimation of the amount of material required. This is important to keep in mind, because the 3D figures obtained include support which means more resin and more time. This information is important to consider having all the costs covered and avoid having extra costs.

To operate the printer, it is necessary to calibrate the printing material parameters to guarantee a correct reproduction (Table 1.2).

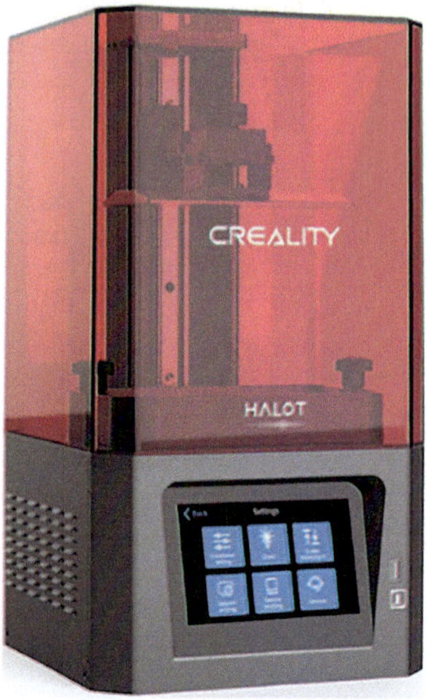

Fig. 1.3 Printer HALOT-ONE© with its technical data sheet

Table 1.1 Printer HALOT-ONE© (Swanson Analysis Systems 2025)

Manufacturer	Creality
Material	Photopolymers
Technology	Photopolymerization
Size	127 × 80 × 160 mm
Software	HALOT-BOX
Connectivity	USB or local
Resolution	0.05 mm

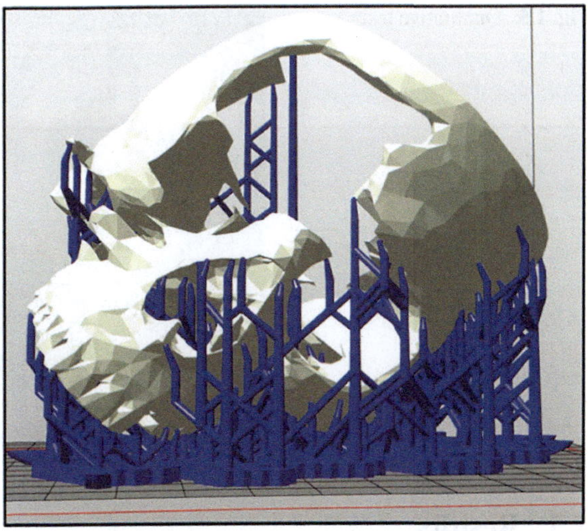

Fig. 1.4 Slicing prosthesis with the generated support

Table 1.2 Printing parameters (Shenzhen Creality 3D Technology Co. Ltd. 2025b)

Initial exposure	40 s
Exposure time by layers	3.0 s
Printing speed	1 mm/s
Delay in turning off the light beam	4 s
Layer's growth	6 mm
Base immersion	Every two layers

Due to its high mechanical properties, high-quality photo-initiators, strong scratch resistance, and photosensitivity, an ABS-like photopolymer resin (UV wavelength 405 nm–Clear Blue) was used in this study

Finally, for the qualitative compression test, the samples were positioned so that the applied force was vertical. Other additional observations that this qualitative test must meet according to the D695–23 Standard Test Method for Compressive Properties of Rigid Plastics are that there must be two fixed parallel points on an apparatus that can: apply different pressures and show the force applied.

To identify these requirements, the analysis was conducted using an INTERFACE Polariscope, model SSM-AJ Series 60 (Fig. 1.5).

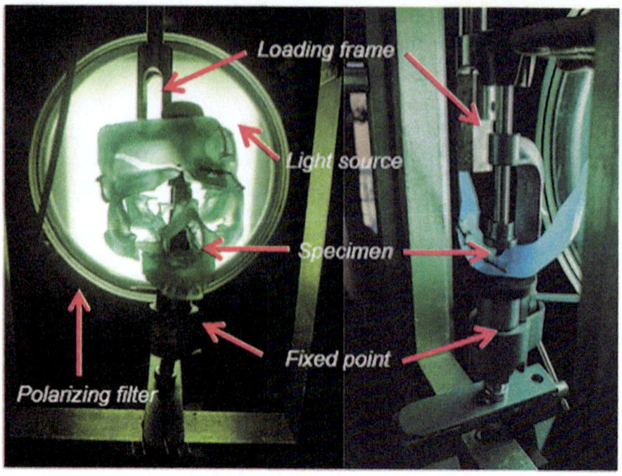

Fig. 1.5 Qualitative test

1.3 Results

In each of the models created, a maximum laminate of 0.05 mm was used. Depending on the type of resolution, the printing time and volume of material increase. To obtain several workpieces for photosensitive evaluation (Fig. 1.6), a total of 94 h 06 min were invested, as shown in Table 1.3.

For the demonstration of complex stress states, photosensitive polymer models were used under a constant mechanical load, showing a double optical refraction effect. Each test had different maximum force values applied, as shown in Table 1.4.

1.4 Discussion

With the technology applied, the time for each print (Table 1.3) is useful to estimate the production time required to obtain high qualitative samples (Fig. 1.6), and the inversion of capital that will be necessary.

Additionally, the properties of the photosensitive resins play a key role during the qualitative test on the compressive method applied on the implants. As claimed by the user manual for HALOT-ONE© without changing the properties of the solution and with the printers' parameters mentioned in Table 1.2, the mechanical properties of the models were 1.86–2.645 MPa (Shenzhen Creality 3D Technology Co. Ltd. 2025c) (Young's modulus).

Finally, the analysis with an INTERFACE Polariscope, model SSM-AJ Series 60, was used for quantitative measurement and demonstration of complex stress states. The system displays a range of colors when viewed under polarized light. They also indicate where no meaningful force was observed in the joints (Table 1.4), which is useful for the verification in:

(a) The reconstruction of the cranial vault.

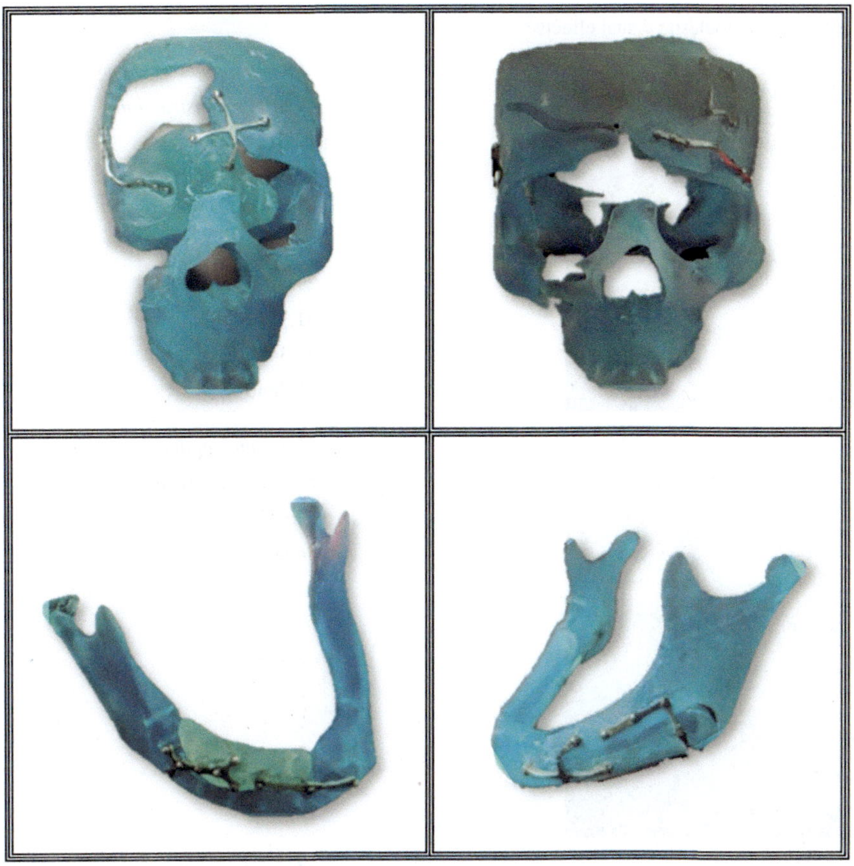

Fig. 1.6 Printing PMMA plates proposals, for upper head and mandible—3D-printed PMMA plate proposals for the upper skull and mandible

Table 1.3 Printing time for each implant

Implants	Printing time	Acrylic volume	Number of prints
Skull	12 hr. 20 min	395 ml	3
Cranial reconstruction prototype 1	4 hr. 17 min	140 ml	3
Cranial reconstruction prototype 2	4 hr. 23 min	140 ml	3
Mandible	8 hr. 04 min	225 ml	3
Lower jaw reconstruction prototypes 3 and 4	2 hr. 22 min	< 140 ml	3
Total printing time: 94 h 06 min		*Total resin consumption:* 3120 ml	

Table 1.4 Photoelastic visual effects

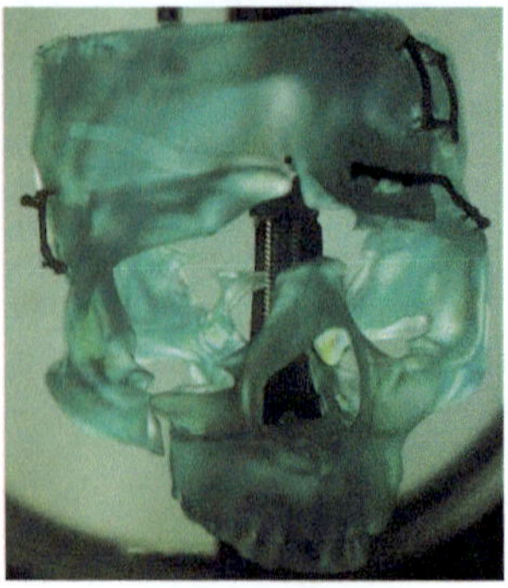	*Maximum applied force (N)*
	Cranial reconstruction 1
	19.6133
	21.5746
	22.5553
	27.4586
	29.4199
	31.3813
	33.3426
	36.2846
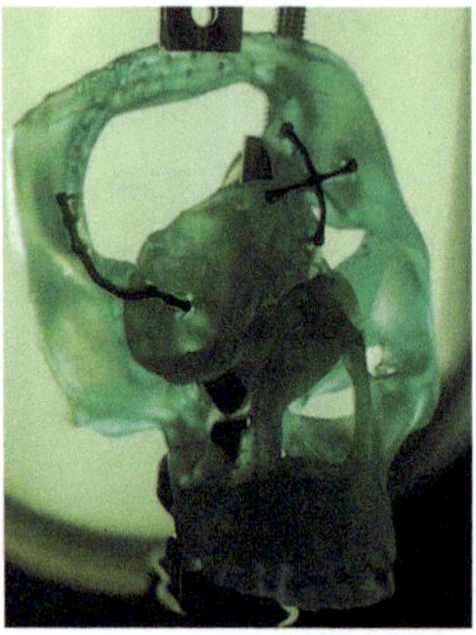	*Maximum applied force (N)*
	Cranial reconstruction 2
	2.942
	4.9033
	5.884
	6.8647
	8.826
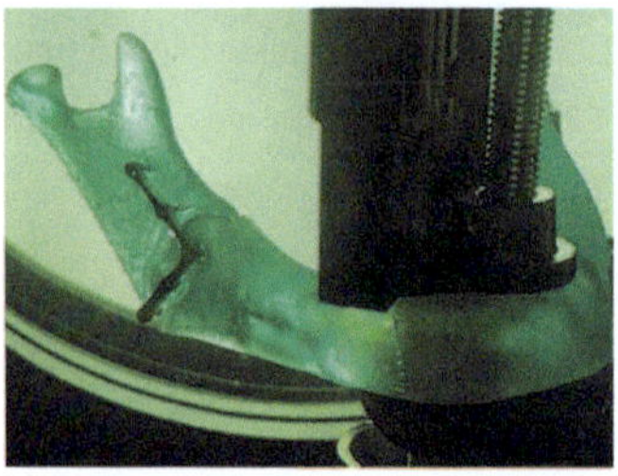	*Maximum applied force (N)*
	Lower jaw reconstruction 1
	8.826
	14.71
	15.6906
	18.6326
	19.6133

(continued)

Table 1.4 (continued)

	20.594
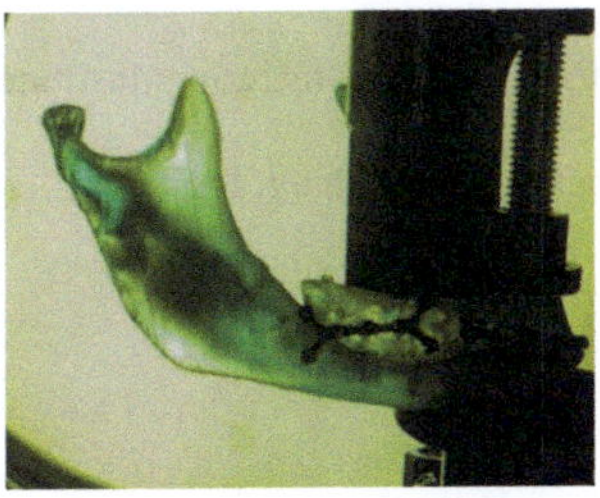	*Maximum applied force (N)*
	Lower jaw reconstruction 2
	8.826
	7.8453
	10.7873
	13.7293
	15.6906

(b) The restoration of the continuity of the lower jaw, where there is not viewed a meaningfully force in the joints where the implant is located, and naturally the pressure is on the coronoid and condylar process.

1.5 Conclusion

The present study demonstrates that the implants, under qualitative testing, did not present critical failure and maintained their structural integrity. Furthermore, with 3D resin prototypes, it is possible to test implants with high resolution and a greater number of details without increasing costs or performing unnecessary procedures that could result in failure. Additionally, the approach increases production capacity.

Acknowledgement The authors gratefully acknowledge the support of national institutions, including the *Secretaría de Ciencia, Humanidades, Tecnología e Innovación* (SECIHTI), *Instituto Politécnico Nacional* (IPN), and the *Comisión de Operación y Fomento de Actividades Académicas del Instituto Politécnico Nacional* (COFAA), which supported this research. Special thanks are extended to the *Hospital 1° de Octubre* for its contributions during the research and to the *Centro de Investigación y Laboratorio de Biomecánica*, which continues to actively advance healthcare research.

References

Coasey K (2024) Characterization of UV curing resins for photo-curing 3D printing. TA Instruments. https://www.linkedin.com/posts/ta-instruments_characterization-of-uv-curing-resins-for-activity-7189724941418737665-qCJw#:~:text=Characterization%20of%20UV%20Curing%20resins,Curing%203D%20Printing%20%7C%20TA%20Instruments

Guido C, González MA, et al. (2023) Validación de la tecnología de impresión 3D por LCD para la fabricación de microcanales. Rev Iberoam Cienc 10(4)

Kovalenko I, Garan M (2017) Effect of UV radiation by projectors on 3D printing. MATEC 88. https://doi.org/10.1051/matecconf/20178801001

Shenzhen Creality 3D Technology Co. Ltd. (2025a) 3D printer. Shenhen, China

Shenzhen Creality 3D Technology Co. Ltd. (2025b) Software halot box. Shenhen. https://wiki.creality.com/en/halot-series/halot-play/user-manual. Accessed 15 Apr 2025
Shenzhen Creality 3D Technology Co. Ltd. (2025c) 3D printer user manual. Shenhen. https://wiki.creality.com/en/halot-series/halot-play/user-manual. Accessed 16 Apr 2025
Smith Z, Davis A, Dan H (2021) The past, present and future of additive manufacturing. Institute of Packing Professionals. 3D printing. 3D printing webinar
Swanson Analysis Systems (2025) Software SpaceClaim. Ansys, Inc., Canonsburg, PA
Synopsys Inc. (1986) Software Scan IP (portable version 2013). Exeter

Chapter 2
Complex and Functional Biological Model Design of the Knee Applying a Numerical Analysis to the Bending Movement

Jorge Albero Gomez-Niebla, Guillermo Urriolagoitia-Sosa, Beatriz Romero-Ángeles, Jonathan Rodolfo Guereca-Ibarra, Santiago Barrañón-Salmón, Iván Alejandro López-Zumarán, Miguel Martinez-Mondragon, Edder Jair Rodríguez-Granados, Miguel Angel García-Laguna, and Guillermo Manuel Urriolagoitia-Calderón

Abstract The investigation begins by utilizing biomodeling to elucidate the behavior of structural elements within the human body, with potential applications for technological and scientific advancements. The development of numerical simulations of biological human components is then applied to interpret the mechanical behavior in various service actions that may occur in everyday life (Lohfeld et al.

J. A. Gomez-Niebla · G. Urriolagoitia-Sosa · B. Romero-Ángeles · J. R. Guereca-Ibarra (✉) · S. Barrañón-Salmón · I. A. López-Zumarán · M. Martinez-Mondragon · E. J. Rodríguez-Granados · M. A. García-Laguna · G. M. Urriolagoitia-Calderón
Instituto Politécnico Nacional, Escuela Superior de Ingeniería Mecánica y Eléctrica, Sección de Estudios de Posgrado e Investigación, Unidad Profesional Adolfo López Mateos, Zacatenco, Mexico City, Mexico
e-mail: guerecatic@gmail.com

J. A. Gomez-Niebla
e-mail: george7gomez@gmail.com

G. Urriolagoitia-Sosa
e-mail: guiurri@hotmail.com

B. Romero-Ángeles
e-mail: bromeroa@ipn.mx

S. Barrañón-Salmón
e-mail: santibarrasalmon@gmail.com

I. A. López-Zumarán
e-mail: ivan.zumaran@utd.edu.mx

M. Martinez-Mondragon
e-mail: mikejobipn@gmail.com

E. J. Rodríguez-Granados
e-mail: erodriguezg2005@alumno.ipn.mx

A. Öchsner (ed.), *Progress in Biomaterials and Biomedical Engineering*, Advanced Structured Materials 249, https://doi.org/10.1007/978-3-032-13551-3_2

in Ann Biomed Eng 33(10):1295–1311, 2005). This work is a detailed examination of the biomechanical behavior of the knee's structural complex during bending. The structural and mechanical assessment is achieved by using a numerical simulation of the knee articulation's movement as a basis for a three-dimensional model of the middle joint of the lower limb. The methodology developed utilizes computed tomography technology and a segmentation process applied to images from a DICOM file (Marquet-Rivera et al. in BioMed Res Int 2021(1), 2021; Serrato-Pedrosa et al. in Prothesis 6(3):429–456, 2024a), resulting in a three-dimensional, complex numerical model (Martínez-Mondragon et al. in Materials 15(21):7843, 2022) that is divided into a finite number of elements (Serrato-Pedrosa et al. in Appl Sci 14(4):1650, 2024b) for using the finite element method. This analysis aims to understand the mechanics of the knee joint's bending. As a result, we can visually observe the behavior of the different soft components of the joint structure. The results of this analysis were not only positive but also favorable, demonstrating correct articular movement and a healthy structure. This analysis provides a numerical demonstration of human knee flexion. It identifies areas where knee injuries are likely to occur, offering a promising outlook for the potential applications of this research.

Keywords Biomechanics · Hyperelasticity · Knee mechanics · Numerical simulation

2.1 Introduction

Anatomy as a study of body structures indicates the geometry, location, and topography of body components (Biga et al. 2010). This study allows us to know the structures where the vital activities of the being are performed, separating the body into different areas for specific analysis, such as joints, calling this science as arthrology (Vargas-Domínguez and Palacios-Álvares 2017). In addition, it is possible to find from the head, neck, trunk, and upper and lower limbs (arms and legs) (Moore et al. 2013), where one can study more specifically the members that one wants to analyze, this being the case of the analysis of the knee as a joint structure of the lower limb. The knee is a structural element with joint characteristics, which comprises a large number of elements with different tasks, each one of them, in charge of fulfilling a function as a whole that allows the mobility of the lower limb. This is part of a daily movement for the individual, the area responsible for different tasks such as body support, mobility for displacement and stability, so each of the components is important for the structure to continue to function in the best way. Thus, throughout this project the investigation of each of the components of the knee is performed,

M. A. García-Laguna
e-mail: obkmpe@gmail.com

G. M. Urriolagoitia-Calderón
e-mail: gurriolagoitiac@ipn.mx

reducing the number of these to the most structurally important, as well as the development of a three-dimensional modeling of the joint to analyze numerically, using the finite element method (FEM), visualizing in a graphical way the behavior of the components in a bending movement, giving guideline to be able to make all kinds of analysis involving this body area, seeking to reach results approximate to reality, also using the mechanical properties of the components to analyze the point where you can get to suffer an injury.

Methodology

Description of the components that make up the articular structure.

The knee, as a joint structure, contains different elements that serve distinct functions. Each of these components is responsible for maintaining stability in the bones involved, as well as allowing and restricting various movements. Therefore, evaluating each of these components is crucial to understanding their specific operation within the joint. The various components of the knee are listed below.

- Femur: The longest and strongest bone in the body that connects the hip to the knee, responsible for shaping the leg and structuring the various muscles in the area (Panesso-Natera et al. 2008).
- Tibia: Long bone located in the lower area of the lower limb, parallel to the fibula and useful as a support for the mass of the individual and structural for the muscles (Panesso-Natera et al. 2008).
- Fibula: Bone with which one of the lateral ligaments connects, parallel to the tibia that helps the stability of the knee, avoiding displacements (Bickels et al. 2007).
- Patella: Bone that provides joint protection as well as being a fundamental part of the knee extensor mechanism (Panesso-Natera et al. 2008).
- Meniscus: Fundamental structure in the functioning of the knee, in charge of transmitting the load and avoiding stress generated on the articular cartilage, secondary in shock absorption, stability, nutrition, and joint lubrication (Fox et al. 2011, 2014).
- Lateral ligaments: Bands of tissue located in the lateral and medial area of the joint that connect the bones that make up the joint.
- Medial collateral ligament: Ligament that provides support to prevent the knee from valgus (Seering et al. 1980).
- Lateral collateral ligament: Ligament providing support to prevent the knee from varus (Seering et al. 1980).
- Cruciate ligaments: Bands of tissue located inside the joint responsible for stabilizing the knee.
- Anterior cruciate ligament: Key ligament in the articular structure of the knee, resisting the translation of the tibia and the rotational load generated in flexion (Duthon et al. 2006; Panesso-Natera et al. 2008).
- Posterior cruciate ligament: It is the largest and strongest ligament of the joint, besides being the primary stabilizer (Beynnon et al. 1997; Panesso-Natera et al. 2008; Pache et al. 2018).

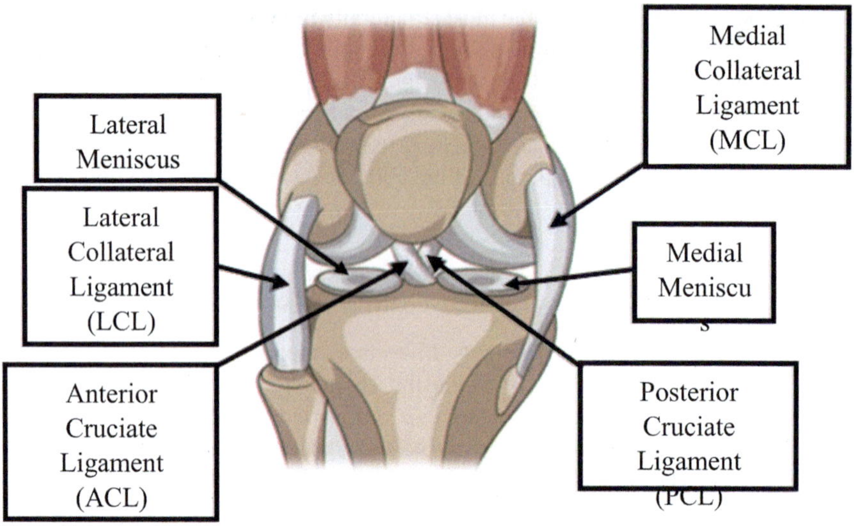

Fig. 2.1 Location of the different soft components of the knee joint structure

The location of each of the previously mentioned soft components is illustrated in Fig. 2.1, which utilizes this visual tool to understand the location of the soft components better and facilitate detailed modeling based on a CT scan.

2.2 Development of a Joint Biomodeling System for the Analysis

The procedure to reach a biomodeling system consists first of obtaining medical images from an imaging study, such as magnetic resonance imaging (MRI) or computed tomography (CT), and ultrasound (US) (Santos et al. 2011). Then importing the image files to a computer program specialized in image segmentation, processing the two-dimensional images and then converting them into a three-dimensional model. This leads to the construction of voxels from pixels, using the Materialise MIMICS® tool (Shin et al. 2015), where it is possible to see the exported images in three different anatomical planes, being these coronal, axial, and sagittal, in addition to a three-dimensional representation of the segmented modeling of the areas of interest according to the model to be made in the different color layers (Fig. 2.2).

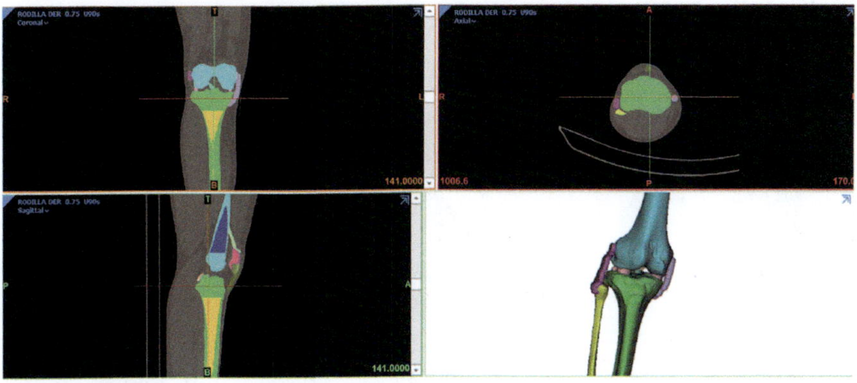

Fig. 2.2 Segmentation of the different components for the elaboration of the three-dimensional model of the knee

2.3 Numerical Analysis of the Structural Complex

Once the three-dimensional anatomical model of the desired area for the study has been obtained, a first result is exported to a new computer program. This is the software Materialise 3-Matic, where it is possible to correct errors caused in the segmentation, in addition to discretizing the model in a finite number of the same proportions (Serrato-Pedrosa et al. 2024a, b), and then the three-dimensional model of the knee, created from a CT scan is taken to a computer program for its structural static analysis, where the finite element method (FEM) is used. For this step, to each of the components hyperelastic mechanical properties are assigned (García et al. 2003; Marquet-Rivera et al. 2021; Taracido-López 2019) being this the Ogden first order used to simulate how the ligaments movement is, in order to arrive at the application of loads to analyze the mechanical behavior of the components involved, respecting the free body diagram shown in Fig. 2.3.

For the application of the movement, it was necessary to define the bone that leads the mobility of the joint, introducing an extra coordinate axis where the movement would be represented, bending in this case the z-axis, this independent of the coordinates of the articular body. This action will provoke that the selected bone (femur) moves in a 90° flexion, showing the behavior of the different biocomponents in the knee structure.

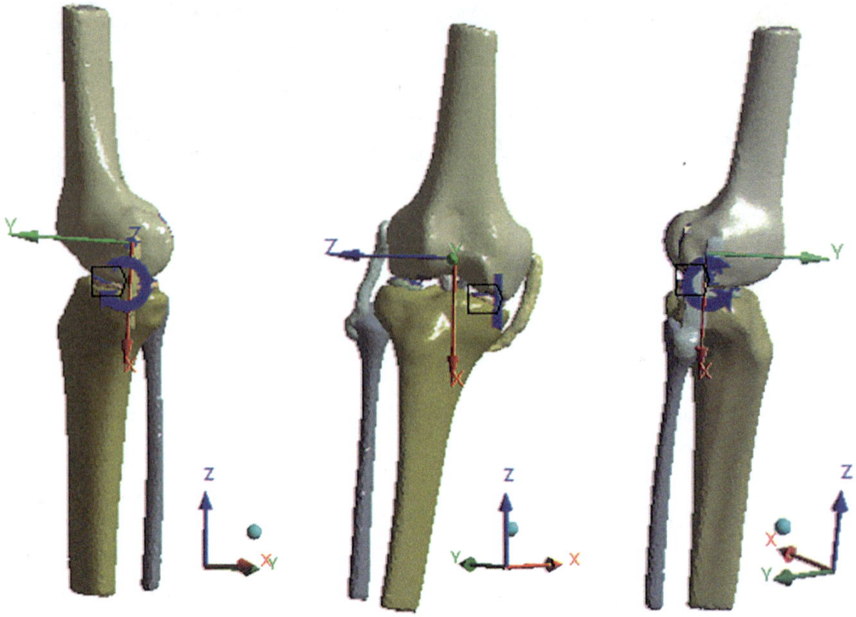

Fig. 2.3 Free body diagram of the joint complex for FEM analysis

2.4 Results

According to the bending analysis performed, it is possible to visually observe the behavior of each component during bending, while also presenting the numerical data generated during the analysis. This is illustrated in Fig. 2.4, which shows the results of the displacements in A and the stresses generated in the B components.

Through this simple analysis, we demonstrate how the knee complex joint functions when subjected to this movement, highlighting the components that are likely to be injured if we increase the applied force.

2.5 Discussion

The numerical analysis data show how each ligament behaves during bending. The analysis also highlights areas where stress concentrates. This information helps identify the regions most likely to be injured during flexion. As a result, we are prompted to pay closer attention to this joint region in future analyses.

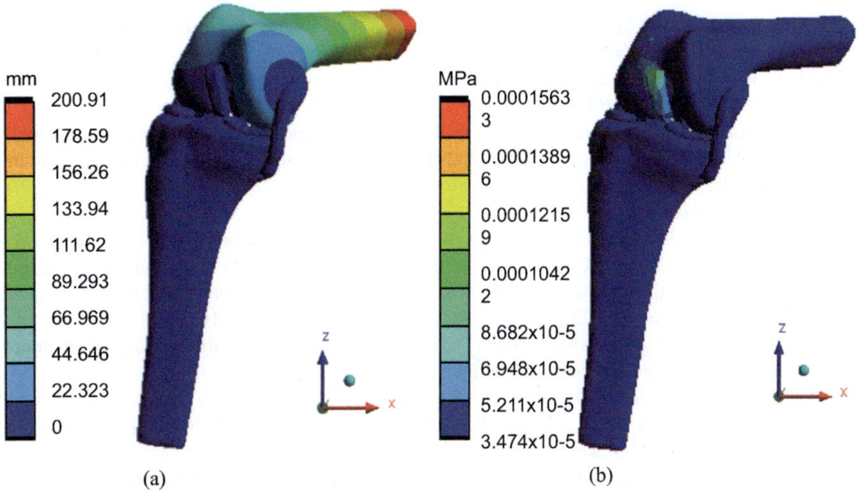

Fig. 2.4 Numerical results of the bending analysis. **a** Displacement (mm), **b** equivalent stress (MPa)

Acknowledgments The authors would like to thank the support and training institutions, the Instituto Politécnico Nacional (IPN) and the Secretaría de Investigación y Posgrado (SIP), as well as the organizers of the ACEX 2025 congress.

References

Beynnon BD, Johnson RJ, Fleming BC, Peura GD, Renstrom PA, Nichols CE, Pope MH (1997) The effect of functional knee bracing on the anterior cruciate ligament in the weightbearing and nonweightbearing knee. Am J Sports Med 25(3):353–359. https://doi.org/10.1177/036354659702500314

Bickels J, Kollender Y, Pritsch T, Meller I, Malawer MM (2007) Knee stability after resection of the proximal fibula. Clin Orthop Relat Res 1(454):198–201. https://doi.org/10.1097/01.blo.0000238781.19692.16

Biga LM, Dawson S, Harwell A, Hopkins KJ, LeMaster M, Matern P, Morrison-Graham K, Quick D, Runyeon J (2010) Anatomy & Physiology. Oregon State University, pp 5–10

Duthon VB, Barea C, Abrassart S, Fasel JH, Fritschy D, Ménétrey J (2006) Anatomy of the anterior cruciate ligament. Knee Surg Sports Traumatol Arthrosc 14(3):204–213. https://doi.org/10.1007/s00167-005-0679-9

Fox AJS, Bedi A, Rodeo SA (2011) The basic science of human knee menisci: structure, composition, and function. Sports Health 4(4):340–351. https://doi.org/10.1177/1941738111429419

Fox AJ, Wanivenhaus F, Burge AJ, Warren RF, Rodeo SA (2014) The human meniscus: a review of anatomy, function, injury, and advances in treatment. Clin Anat 28(2):269–287. https://doi.org/10.1002/ca.22456

García JM, Gómez PH, López XP, González NB, Mur FG, Soleda JB (2003) Cicatrización del Tendón Rotuliano Tras la Extensión de su Tercio Central. Estudio Experimental en el Conejo,

Revista Española de Cirugía Ortopédica y Traumatología 47(2):141–145. https://doi.org/10.1016/S1888-4415(03)76087-1

Lohfeld S, Barron V, McHugh PE (2005) Biomodels of bone: a review. Ann Biomed Eng 33(10):1295–1311. https://doi.org/10.1007/s10439-005-5873-x

Martínez-Mondragon M, Urriolagoitia-Sosa G, Romero-Ángeles B, Martínez-Reyes J, Gallegos-Funes FJ, Urriolagoitia-Calderón GM (2022) Numerical analysis of zirconium and titanium implants under the effect of critical masticatory load. Materials 15(21):7843. https://doi.org/10.3390/ma15217843

Marquet-Rivera RA, Urriolagoitia-Sosa G, Hernández-Vázquez RA, Romero-Ángeles B, Mastache-Miranda OA, Urriolagoitia-Calderón GM (2021) High biofidelity 3D biomodel reconstruction from soft and hard tissues (knee), FEM, and 3D printing: a three-dimensional methodological proposal. Biomed Res Int 2021(1). https://doi.org/10.1155/2021/6688164

Moore KL, Dailey AF, Agur AMR (2013) Anatomía de superficie de los huesos del miembro inferior. In: Anatomía con orientación clínica. E. Wolters Kluwer, pp 572–575

Santos M, Bastião L, Costa C, Silva A, Rocha N (2011) DICOM and clinical data mining in a small hospital PACS: a pilot study. Int Conf ENTERprise Inf Syst 221:254–263. https://doi.org/10.1007/978-3-642-24352-3_27

Seering WP, Piziali RL, Nagel DA, Schurman DJ (1980) The function of the primary ligaments of the knee in varus-valgus and axial rotation. J Biomech 13(9):785–794. https://doi.org/10.1016/0021-9290(80)90240-7

Serrato-Pedrosa JA, Urriolagoitia-Sosa G, Romero-Ángeles B, Carrasco-Hernández F, Gallegos-Funes FJ, Trejo-Enriquez A, Carbajal-López A, Gomez-Niebla JA, Correa-Corona MI, Urriolagoitia-Calderón GM (2024a) Numerical analysis of the plantar pressure points during the stance phases for the design of a 3D-printable patient-specific insole. PRO 6(3):429–456. https://doi.org/10.3390/prosthesis6030032

Serrato-Pedrosa JA, Urriolagoitia-Sosa G, Romero-Ángeles B, Urriolagoitia-Calderón GM, Cruz-López S, Urriolagoitia-Luna A, Carbajal-López DE, Guereca-Ibarra JR, Murillo-Aleman G (2024b) Biomechanical evaluation of plantar pressure distribution towards a customized 3D orthotic device: a methodological case study through a finite element analysis approach. Appl Sci 14(4):1650. https://doi.org/10.3390/app14041650

Shin DS, Lee S, Park HS, Lee SB, Chung MS (2015) Segmentation and surface reconstruction of a cadaver heart on mimics software. Folia Morphol (Warsz) 74(3):372–377. https://doi.org/10.5603/FM.2015.0056

Pache S, Aman ZS, Kennedy M, Nakama GY, Moatshe G, Ziegler C, LaPrade RF (2018) Posterior cruciate ligament: current concepts review. Arch Bone Joint Surg 6(1):8–18

Panesso-Natera MC, Trillos-Chacon MC, Tolosa-Guzman IA (2008) Componentes articulares de la rodilla. In: Biomecánica Clínica de la Rodilla, E. Universidad del Rosario, pp 8–15

Taracido-López I (2019) Modelización de Ligamentos como Elementos Finitos y Estudio de su Comportamiento en una Rodilla Humana. Universidade da Coruña, Escola Politécnica Superior

Vargas-Domínguez A, Palacios-Álvares VP (2017) Concepto de salud y enfermedad. In Ciencias de la Salud, E. Patria, pp 7–16

Chapter 3
Advances in Carotid Artery Studies from a Mechanical Point of View; Mechanical Properties, Fluid Analysis, and Finite Element Method

Jonathan Rodolfo Guereca-Ibarra, Guillermo Urriolagoitia-Sosa, Beatriz Romero-Ángeles, Jorge Alberto Gomez-Niebla, Felix de Jesus Mar-Luna, Yonathan Yael Rojas-Castrejon, Gabriela Ramirez-Sanchez, Brayan Díaz-Roldán, Irvin Mondragón-Hernández, and Guillermo Manuel Urriolagoitia-Calderón

Abstract The main objective of this study is to highlight recent advances in the biomechanical analysis of the carotid artery. This artery plays a critical role in supplying blood to the brain and face but is vulnerable to atherosclerosis—an

---

J. R. Guereca-Ibarra · G. Urriolagoitia-Sosa · B. Romero-Ángeles · J. A. Gomez-Niebla (✉) · F. de J. Mar-Luna · Y. Y. Rojas-Castrejon · G. Ramirez-Sanchez · B. Díaz-Roldán · I. Mondragón-Hernández · G. M. Urriolagoitia-Calderón
Instituto Politécnico Nacional, Escuela Superior de Ingeniería Mecánica y Eléctrica, Sección de Estudios de Posgrado e Investigación, Unidad Profesional Adolfo López Mateos, Zacatenco, Edificio 5, 2do Piso, Col. Lindavista, Alcaldía Gustavo A. Madero, Mexico City, Mexico
e-mail: george7gomez@gmail.com

J. R. Guereca-Ibarra
e-mail: guerecatic@gmail.com

B. Romero-Ángeles
e-mail: BROMEROA@ipn.mx

F. de J. Mar-Luna
e-mail: felix.mar@utd.edu.mx

Y. Y. Rojas-Castrejon
e-mail: yrojasc1300@alumno.ipn.mx

G. Ramirez-Sanchez
e-mail: iqgramirezsanchez@gmail.com

B. Díaz-Roldán
e-mail: bdiazr1501@alumno.ipn.mx

I. Mondragón-Hernández
e-mail: irvinmondra01@gmail.com

A. Öchsner (ed.), *Progress in Biomaterials and Biomedical Engineering*, Advanced Structured Materials 249, https://doi.org/10.1007/978-3-032-13551-3_3

obstruction caused by the accumulation of lipid particles over time. Such blockages can lead to serious health risks, including stroke. Treatment typically involves medication or the insertion of stents to restore blood flow. While the mechanical properties of the carotid artery have historically received limited attention, recent studies have made significant progress using the finite element method (FEM). This computational method, often based on medical imaging such as CT or MRI, allows researchers to model and analyze the artery's structural and hemodynamic behavior under pathological conditions. Numerical results obtained through FEM have shown strong agreement with clinical data, confirming their reliability in simulating disease scenarios. Additionally, research has demonstrated that altered blood flow due to vascular diseases can deform the artery's geometry, further impeding circulation. Advances in modeling techniques have not only improved our understanding of carotid artery biomechanics but also contributed new tools for clinical evaluation and treatment planning.

Keywords Carotid artery · Fluids analysis · Finite element analysis · Mechanical properties

3.1 Introduction

The structure of the human body is composed of multiple systems that make it work the way it does; one of these systems is the cardiovascular system which is composed of the heart, blood vessels, and blood. The blood vessels are divided into veins, arteries, and capillaries (Álvarez-Uría et al. 2009; Latarjet 2005). For several decades, there has been an interest in studying the cardiovascular system from the mechanical point of view and one of the main points of research has been the arteries. One of the arteries that is usually studied in multiple species due to its geometry is the carotid artery, as this is a bifurcation that can be affected in various ways so that studies of this can be extended to meet different cases of study (Cabrera et al. 2013).

3.2 Anatomy of Carotid Artery

The carotid arteries emerge from two distinct points. The left carotid artery originates from the aorta, while the right carotid artery originates from the brachiocephalic trunk. Each artery consists of a single artery that is referred to as common (common carotid artery, CCA) and then reaches the bifurcation where it divides into its two parts: internal carotid artery (ICA) and external carotid artery (ECA) as shown in Fig. 3.1; (Latarjet 2005; Micheau and Hoa 2025).

The carotid bifurcation is where blockages often occur and can cause disease due to the change in blood pressure and the amount of blood that is transported to the brain and main arterioles. This area can be highly affected by cardiovascular diseases

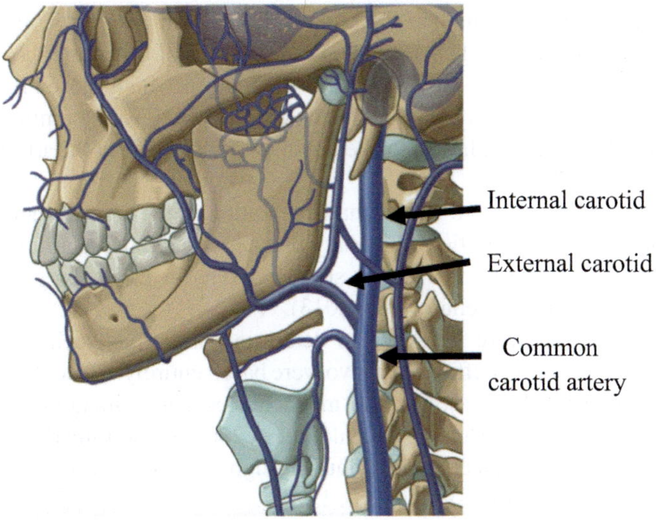

Fig. 3.1 Anatomical Location of the Carotid artery (Micheau and Hoa 2025)

Fig. 3.2 Obstruction on artery due to atherosclerosis

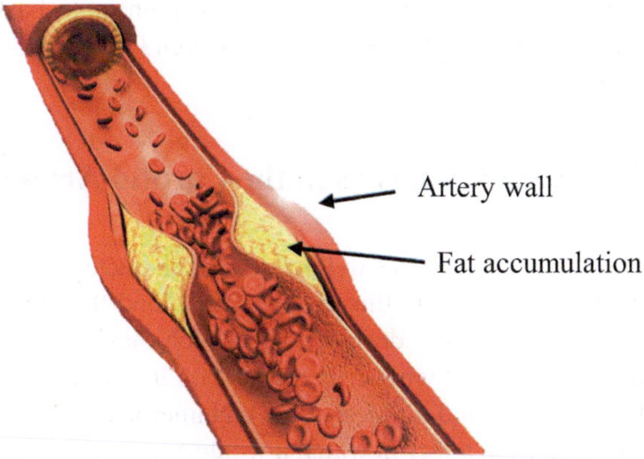

due to the accumulation of lipids in the blood as shown in Fig. 3.2; (Gaidai et al. 2023).

3.3 Characterization of the Carotid Artery

In order to perform mechanical studies on arteries, as well as other biological components, experiments were carried out for the characterization of the arterial tissue. For the most part, many of the experiments performed to obtain results were based on animal biological tissue (Abe et al. 1996). At the same time, experiments have been performed to characterize human or animal soft tissue in two ways: in vivo and in dissections (Patel et al. 1961; Sedlin 1965). Both ways of obtaining data have been carried out for years, being the innovation the way in which these are performed because, in several cases, imaging has been very important for obtaining these data, as well as for the understanding of the behavior of the structure of the arteries (Wilson and Robinson 1982).

Research not only focused on the characterization of the arteries themselves, but also on obtaining the properties of the fatty plaques formed in the arteries. The tests to obtain these were based on different species due to the complexity of doing it in people or in dissections (Heiland et al. 2013).

The methods that were first used to determine properties such as elongation, elasticity, and Poisson's coefficient in vivo were based entirely on seeing the behavior of the arteries through ultrasound and magnetic resonance imaging, but this was changing as technology advanced (Greenleaf et al. 2003; Wilson and Robinson 1982). The methodology used to acquire the data through dissections was done mainly by stress testing or adaptations of this (Cox 1975).

In recent years, studies to obtain the mechanical properties of both the artery and the fatty plaques generated in it continue to develop for different reasons, ranging from innovating the way in which they can be performed, updating data due to the biological composition of each person or to have an objective understanding according to the objective of the research (Wang et al. 2024).

3.4 Fluids Analysis in the Carotid Artery

Carotid artery analysis did not stop at characterization alone. One of the important points to understand this artery is the blood flow that travels through it, so several investigations were developed in which they sought to understand how the liquid traveled in it and what effects it had on the structure of the artery as can be seen in Fig. 3.3; (Ku and Giddens 1983). Numerous investigations focused on performing simulations in a way in which it would encounter some type of obstruction or change in geometry that could affect the hemodynamics on the artery. These studies encompass a range of scenarios, from healthy arteries to arteries that present additional complications apart from obstructions, but also aneurysms, cancerous masses, variations in blood density, obstruction by calcification, and narrowing of the arteries due to stenosis (Ku et al. 1985; Simon et al. 1973; Perktold et al. 1988).

The analysis of fluids in the arteries has not ceased to be studied, mainly because of the cases that may arise. Arteries offer a wide range of case studies in which different investigations can be derived either by the change of geometry between each person, changes due to some pathology or blood pressure (Lopes et al. 2020; Xu et al. 2023). Arteries exhibit significant variations in terms of structural composition, blood flow velocity, and pressure. These differences have enabled the development of diverse investigative approaches tailored to specific arterial types. In the case of the carotid artery, research has predominantly concentrated on its bifurcation and the

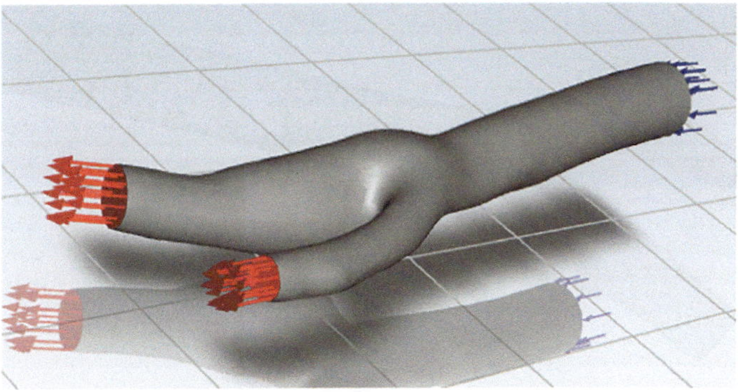

Fig. 3.3 Direction of the flow through the artery

subsequent division into arterioles, which facilitate the distribution of blood flow in multiple directions (Curcio et al. 2023).

3.5 Finite Element Method Applied in Arteries Analysis

The finite element method (FEM) has long been employed in the analysis of arterial behavior, serving as a fundamental tool for solving the mathematical models proposed in numerous studies as seen in Fig. 3.4; (Ku and Liepsch 1986; Wiederhielm et al. 1968). With advancements in computational technologies and simulation software, these analyses have evolved, enabling the development of more sophisticated and detailed models. This progression has made it possible to investigate arterial behavior under increasingly complex physiological and pathological conditions. Modern FEM-based simulations allow for the examination of how arteries respond to various diseases, including stenosis, aneurysms, and atherosclerosis, as well as changes in structural properties of the arterial wall and the rheological characteristics of blood. Such analyses provide crucial insights into the mechanical behavior of vascular tissues and contribute to the development of more effective diagnostic tools and treatment strategies.

The application of the finite element method has significantly enhanced the understanding of arterial structural behavior under a wide range of physiological and pathological conditions. The specific conditions analyzed vary across studies and may include differences in material properties of the arterial wall, flow direction, turbulence intensity, and rheological characteristics of the blood, among other factors (Costa-Sousa et al. 2012). FEM has proven to be a powerful and versatile computational tool, offering a more accurate and reliable approach to simulating the mechanical response of arteries. Its use has led to improved predictive models that contribute to a deeper comprehension of vascular biomechanics and facilitate the development of more effective clinical interventions (Guimaraes-Valentim et al. 2023).

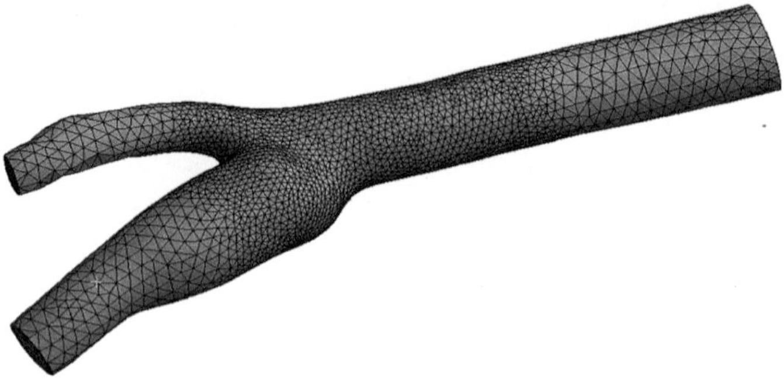

Fig. 3.4 Discretized carotid artery

3.6 Results

Many of the advances made in the area of biomechanics have been due to the research carried out in the past decades, and with it came a better understanding of the components of the human body mechanically.

The analyses seen throughout the review give a better understanding of how these have evolved and changed to suit each of the case studies they had. From the normal analysis of the structure, to how blood flow can change its behavior through obstructions. Each of the analyses offers insights and results that will help future research.

3.7 Conclusion

Arteries proved to be of great interest due to the possibilities they provide for mechanical analysis. Structural and fluid analysis have been the main focus of studies. Analyses evolved by adding obstructions or changes in the structure of the arteries that made considerable changes in the results of the analyses.

It is concluded that the advances that have been made in mechanical analysis of arteries have given a much better understanding of how arteries behave and how analyses can be carried out to acquire results that are accurate and can be considered as truthful in the effect of arterial geometry and blood flow.

Acknowledgments The authors thank to the Instituto Politécnico Nacional, the Secretaria de Investigacion y Posgrado, and SECIHTI for the given support for the presentation of this investigation.

References

Abe H, Hayashi K, Sato M (1996) Data book on mechanical properties of living cells, tissues, and organs, 1th edn. Springer, Tokyo, pp 65862–65867

Álvarez-Uría TMJ, Sáiz-Ayala A, Fernández-Rey C, Santamarta-Liébana E (2009) Agenesia unilateral de la arteria carótida interna. Angiologia 61(4):213–217

Cabrera MS, Oomens CWJ, Bouten CVC, Bogers AJJC, Hoerstrup SP, Baaijens FPT (2013) Mechanical analysis of ovine and pediatric pulmonary artery for heart valve stent design. J Biomech 46:2075–2081. https://doi.org/10.1016/j.jbiomech.2013.04.020

Costa-Sousa L, Castro CF, Conceicao-António C (2012) Blood flow simulation and applications. Technologies for medical sciences (eds). Lecture notes in computational vision and biomechanics, Springer, vol 1, pp 67–86. https://doi.org/10.1007/978-94-007-4068-6_4

Cox RH (1975) Anisotropic properties of the canine carotid artery in vitro. J Biomech 8(5):293–300. https://doi.org/10.1016/0021-9290(75)90081-0

Curcio N, Rosato A, Mazzacaro D, Nano G, Conti M, Matrone G (2023) 3D patient-specific modeling and structural finite element analysis of atherosclerotic carotid artery based on computed tomography angiography. Sci Rep 13(19911):1–15. https://doi.org/10.1038/s41598-023-46949-5

Gaidai O, Cao Y, Loginov S (2023) Global cardiovascular diseases death rate prediction. Curr Probl Cardiol 48(5). https://doi.org/10.1016/j.cpcardiol.2023.101622

Greenleaf JF, Fatemi M, Insana M (2003) Selected methods for imaging elastic properties of biological tissues. Annu Rev Biomed Eng 5(1):57–78. https://doi.org/10.1146/annurev.bioeng.5.040202.121623

Guimaraes-Valentim MX, Franceschini-Zinani FS, Elsner da Fonseca C, Pacheco-Wermunth D (2023) Systematic review on the application of computational fluid dynamics as a tool for the design of coronary artery stents. Beni-Suef Univ J Basic Appl Sci 12(49). https://doi.org/10.1186/s43088-023-00382-9

Heiland VM, Forsell C, Roy J, Hedin U, Gasser TC (2013) Identification of carotid plaque tissue properties using an experimental-numerical approach. J Mech Behav Biomed Mater 27:226–238. https://doi.org/10.1016/j.jmbbm.2013.05.001

Ku DN, Giddens DP (1983) Pulsatile flow in a model carotid bifurcation arteriosclerosis. Off J Am Hear Assoc 3(1):31–39

Ku DN, Giddens DP, Phillips DJ, Strandness DE (1985) Hemodynamics of the normal human carotid bifurcation; in vitro and in vivo studies. Ultrasound Med Biol 11(1): 13–26. https://doi.org/10.1016/0301 5629(85)90003-1

Ku DN, Liepsch D (1986) The effects on non-Newtonian viscoelasticity and wall elasticity on flow at 900 bifurcation. Biorheology 23(4):359–370. https://doi.org/10.3233/BIR-1986-23405

Latarjet RL (2005) Anatomía humana. 4a edición, Tomo 2, Editorial Medica panamericana (eds). pp 991–1011

Lopes D, Puga H, Teixeira J, Lima R (2020) Blood flow simulations in patient-specific geometries of the carotid artery; a systematic review. J Biomech 111. https://doi.org/10.1016/j.jbiomech.2020.110019

Micheau A, Hoa D (2008) e-Anatomy Atlas, ISSN 2534-5079. https://doi.org/10.37019/e-anatomy

Patel DJ, Mallos AJ, y Fry DL (1961) Aortic mechanics in the living dog. J Appl Physiol 16(2):293–299. https://doi.org/10.1152/jappl.1961.16.2.293

Perktold K, Kenner T, Hilbert D, Spork B, Florian H (1988) Numerical blood flow analysis; arterial bifurcation with a saccular aneurysm. Basic Res Cardiol 83:24–31. https://doi.org/10.1007/BF01907101

Sedlin ED (1965) A rheologic model for cortical bone; a study of the physical properties of human femoral samples. Acta Orthop Scand 36(83):1–77. https://doi.org/10.3109/ort.1965.36.suppl-83.01

Simon BR, Kobayashi AS, Wiederhielm CA, Strandness DE (1973) Deformation of the arterial vasa vasorum at normal and hypertensive arterial pressure. J Biomech 6(4):349–359. https://doi.org/10.1016/0021-9290(73)90095-X

Wang J, Yu F, Zhang M, Lu J, Qian Z (2024) A 3D framework for segmentation of carotid artery vessel wall and identification of plaque compositions in multi-sequence MR images. Comput Med Imaging Graph 116. https://doi.org/10.1016/j.compmedimag.2024.102402

Wiederhielm CA, Kobayashi AS, Stromberg GG, Woo SLY (1968) Structural response of relaxed and constricted arterioles. J Biomech 1(4):259–270. https://doi.org/10.1016/0021-9290(68)90021-3

Wilson LS, Robinson DE (1982) Ultrasonic measurement of small displacements and deformations of tissue. Ultrason Imag 4(1):71–82. https://doi.org/10.1016/0161-7346(82)90006-2

Xu S, Wang F, Mai P, Peng Y, Shu X, Nie R, Zhang R (2023) Mechanism analysis of vascular calcification based on fluid dynamics. Diagnostics 13(2362):1–19. https://doi.org/10.3390/diagnostics13162632

Chapter 4
Auxiliar Prototype for Emergency Rooms in Hospitals

Daniel Villaseñor-Chávez, Laura Guadalupe Carbajal-Figueroa, Emiliano Montoya-Gutierrez, Giran Erekose González-Villalobos, Alejandra Armenta-Molina, and Luis Héctor Hernández-Gomez

Abstract This paper reports the design and construction of a portable prototype to streamline triage, a crucial procedure in the evaluation and classification of patients according to the severity of the medical condition and the urgency of the care required in emergency rooms. The device facilitates the acquisition of vital signs. It allows a quick and reliable assessment. The prototype has three sensors to perform vital sign measurements: a pulse oximetry module, a thermistor, and a heart rate detector. These sensors allow the measurement of heart rate, oxygenation level, and temperature. A Bluetooth communication module is also incorporated to transmit data wirelessly through the serial communication through the COM ports of a computer. The information is logged in a database. It can be visualized in real-time through a graphical interface developed in Phyton. A preliminary assessment of the patient's condition is provided. The importance of this research lies in the development of a low-cost,

D. Villaseñor-Chávez · E. Montoya-Gutierrez · G. E. González-Villalobos
Universidad Nacional Rosario Castellanos, Unidad Azcapotzalco, Dirección de Asuntos Académicos, Licenciatura en Ingeniería en Control y Automatización, Ciudad de México, Mexico
e-mail: villasenor.daniel606@rcastellanos.cdmx.gob.mx

E. Montoya-Gutierrez
e-mail: emilianomontoyagutierrez@gmail.com

G. E. González-Villalobos
e-mail: gibrangonzalezvillalobos@gmail.com

L. G. Carbajal-Figueroa (✉)
Universidad Nacional Rosario Castellanos, Unidad Magdalena Contreras, Dirección de Asuntos Académicos, Licenciatura en Ingeniería en Control y Automatización, Ciudad de México, Mexico
e-mail: laura.carbajal@rcastellanos.cdmx.gob.mx

A. Armenta-Molina · L. H. Hernández-Gomez
Escuela Superior de Ingeniería Mecánica y Eléctrica Sección de Estudios de Posgrado e Investigación, Instituto Politécnico Nacional, Ciudad de México, Mexico
e-mail: aarmentamo@ipn.mx

L. H. Hernández-Gomez
e-mail: lhhernandez@ipn.mx

A. Öchsner (ed.), *Progress in Biomaterials and Biomedical Engineering*, Advanced Structured Materials 249, https://doi.org/10.1007/978-3-032-13551-3_4

portable device. It provides a preliminary evaluation which will speed up the delays experienced by emergency rooms in triaging patients.

Keywords Triage · Pulse oximetry · Thermistor · Interface

4.1 Introduction

Triage is a fundamental process in emergency departments that allows patients to be classified according to the severity of their condition. It prioritizes medical care for those who are in critical condition. Several studies have evaluated the efficiency and effectiveness of triage in different hospitals and regions in Mexico. Some studies have found that 73% of emergency service patients undergo triage, and 51% are classified as qualified emergencies (Instituto Mexicano del Seguro Social 2018a). However, it has also been observed that a considerable percentage of patients are classified as unqualified emergencies. This suggests that these could be improved in the triage process (Instituto Mexicano del Seguro Social 2018b).

Patients with medical care in emergency services are another important aspect that has been evaluated in Mexico. A study conducted at the General Hospital of Zone 89 in Jalisco found that most patients are satisfied with the care received (Vizcaíno et al. 2019). However, it is essential to improve the quality of care and reduce waiting times in emergency departments. In conclusion, the triage evaluation in Mexico is a relevant topic that requires further research. Although some studies have been conducted on the subject, it is necessary to continue generating scientific evidence to identify areas of opportunity and improve the efficiency and effectiveness of the triage process in emergency services of our country.

Hinson et al. mention that most patients who passed away after the encountering the emergency department, or who are seriously ill are not designated correctly in triage. This tells us that reliability in triage assessment must be improved to correct identify at risk patients. Studies in European countries have concluded that remote monitoring of vital signs supports medical staff and has the potential to reduce the time to detect deteriorating patients (Hinson et al. 2018; Posthuma et al. 2020; Zachariasse et al. 2019). According to the above, not only is it important to correctly classify the urgency, but also to effectively obtain the vital signs.

Some research regarding these triage prototypes that have been developed focuses on the evaluation of patient's vital signs to determine the emergency. For example, Siiria, E., Johansson and Nygeren J. (2025) developed a prototype that measures the patients' vital signs and uses them to determine their level of urgency. This prototype consists of an instrumentation module that evaluates vital signs. This data is stored and processed with a web interface. A wireless communication module is required (Siira et al. 2025). The results of the tests carried out with the prototype are promising and suggest that it could be a valuable tool for medical personnel in decision-making during triage. Other prototypes are focused on creating automated triage systems that improve the accuracy and efficiency of the process. Torenza,

Oliveira and Cavanzana (2025) developed a prototype of an automated triage system for hospital emergencies. It is based on a fuzzy model of triage data for the Venezuelan health sector and the hospital triage process of the Venezuelan Society of Emergency and Disaster Medicine (SVMED). This system has four modules: implementation of the fuzzy relational schema, FSQL client module, medical consultation module, and data and results capture module (Torezan et al. 2025).

In addition to the mentioned prototypes, mobile triage applications aimed at the community have also been developed. Rodríguez-Villamizar and Rincón-Sánchez (2022) created a mobile application. It allows users to know the right time to go to emergency services based on their symptoms. The application seeks to educate the population on the correct use of medical emergencies and reduce saturation in care centers (Ivanov and Todorova 2025).

4.2 Statement of the Problem

In Mexico, emergency services have a growing demand for medical attention. They have generated challenges regarding the efficiency and quality of triage. However, in practice, triage can be affected by several factors such as a lack of trained personnel, work overload, inadequate technological tools, and variability in triage criteria of classification.

According to data from the 2018 National Survey of Confidence and Satisfaction for Emergency Service Users (ENCONSA), 68% of emergencies attended in Mexico were "qualified" and 32% "unqualified" (Orta Peña 2021). This suggests that a considerable number of patients may not get timely and appropriate care based on severity. These data highlight the need to improve the triage process in Mexico, as inadequate triage can have negative consequences for patients, such as delays in medical care, misclassification, and an increased risk of complications and mortality. Based on these statistics, a device is proposed. The objective is to reduce waiting times in emergency rooms. The proposed prototype consists of three sensors implemented in an embedded system. It evaluates the vital signs of patients and determines the level of urgency. Its interface stores and processes the parameters recorded by the device.

4.3 Materials and Method

Figure 4.1 illustrates the methodology proposed for this purpose.

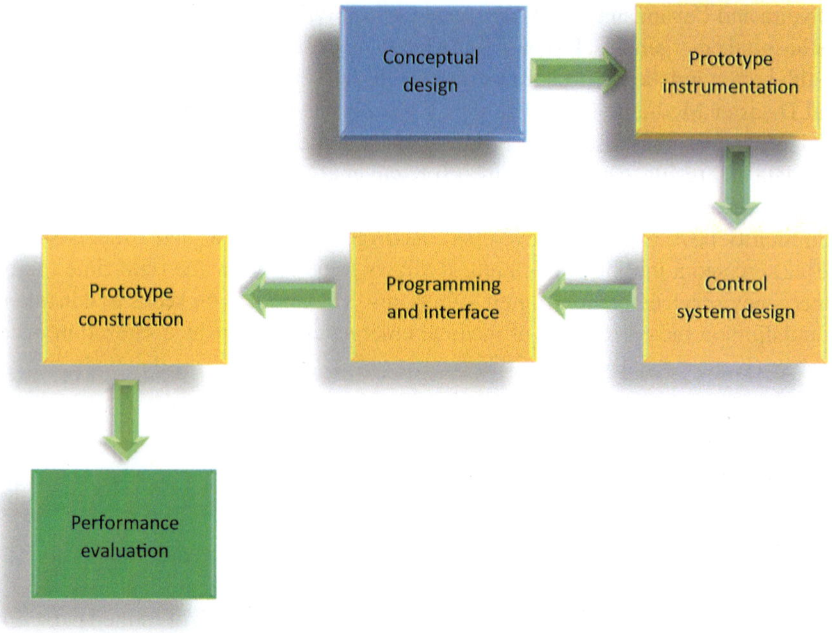

Fig. 4.1 Proposed methodology

4.3.1 *Conceptual Design*

The conceptual design is shown in Fig. 4.2. It has a heart rate sensor, a blood oxygen sensor, a temperature sensor, visual and auditory alert indicators, as well as the prototype's wireless communication and battery.

The prototype was proposed to be placed on the inner part of the patient's forearm. According with Chaurand et al., the measure of the forearm-wrist distance for the Mexican anthropometry is 22.6 cm (Chaurand et al. 2007). For this reason, the prototype was designed with the dimensions $20 \times 7 \times 5$ cm (Fig. 4.3).

4.3.2 *Prototype Instrumentation*

The KY-039 heart rate detector module was selected. It is an optical heart rate sensor that uses an infrared LED and a phototransistor to detect the finger pulse. It operates with a voltage of 3.3–5 V. Its output is analog, and it weighs 2 g. It is ideal for creating a lightweight prototype (Fig. 4.4) (Andreoni et al. 2025; Muharram et al. 2025).

The KY-013 NTC thermistor is a low-cost, easy-access, and wide-range analog temperature sensor. It is connected to a 10 kΩ resistor in a voltage divider circuit. When the temperature changes, the thermistor's resistance changes, which in turn

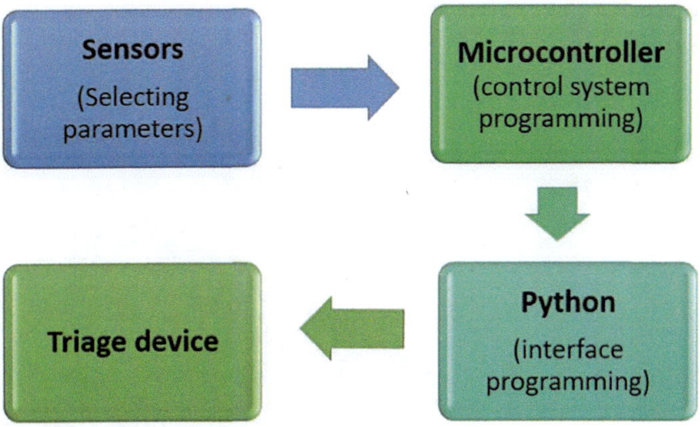

Fig. 4.2 Conceptual design of the prototype

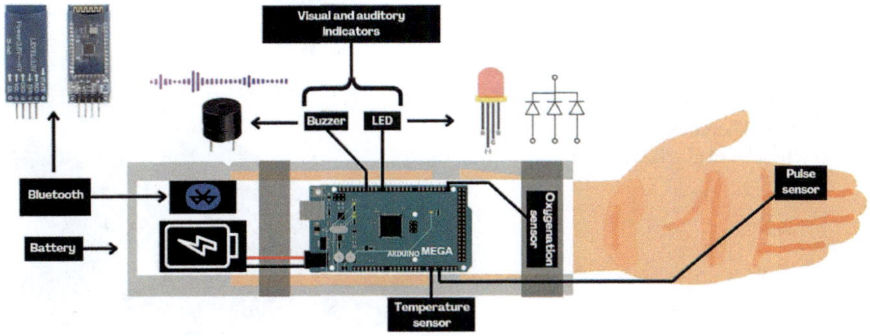

Fig. 4.3 Prototype design

changes the circuit voltage. A microcontroller measures the voltage to determine the temperature Fig. 4.5.

The last sensor selected was the MAX 30102 pulse oximeter module. It emits red and infrared light toward tissue. It is usually fixed on the patient's index finger. The amount of light absorbed and reflected varies depending on the amount of blood flowing through the tissue and the oxygen saturation of the blood. Photodetectors measure this variation and convert it into electrical signals. These signals are processed to calculate $Sp0_2$ Fig. 4.6 (Lin et al. 2025; Lee et al. 2025).

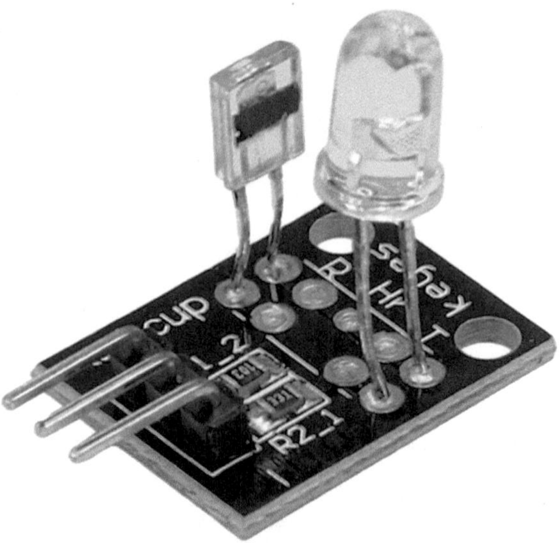

Fig. 4.4 KY-039 heart rate detector module

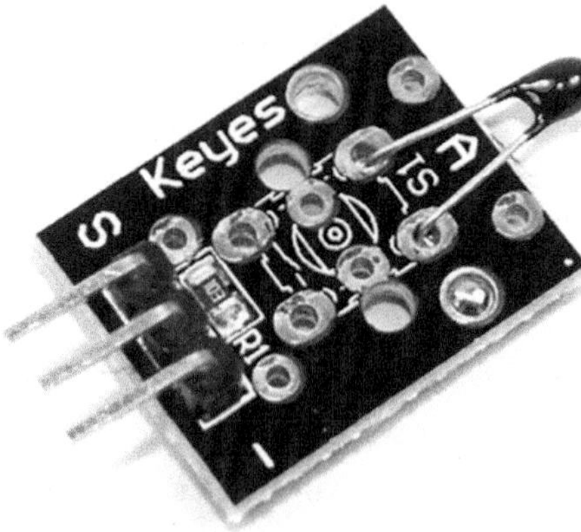

Fig. 4.5 KY-013 NTC thermistor (Kukharchuk et al. 2023; Tsebesebe et al. 2025)

4.3.3 Control System Design

The vital signs measuring device was designed using Tinkercad®. Figure 4.7 shows the electronic diagram used for this prototype.

The control circuit was designed around the ATmega2560 microcontroller. It was selected for its extensive I/O capabilities and compatibility with the Arduino platform. Programming was performed using the Arduino development environment, taking advantage of the ATmega2560 attributes. It includes 54 digital I/O pins (14 of which can generate PWM signals), 16 analog inputs, 4 UART serial ports, and a USB interface for power and communication. This configuration has great flexibility for controlling various components and peripherals in the circuit, as illustrated in Fig. 4.8.

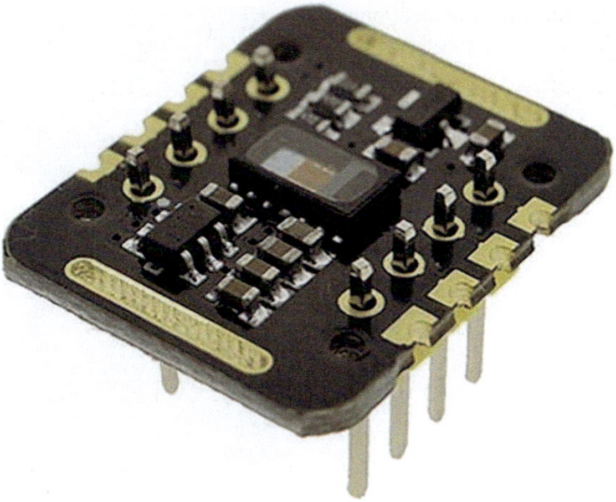

Fig. 4.6 MAX 30102 pulse oximeter module

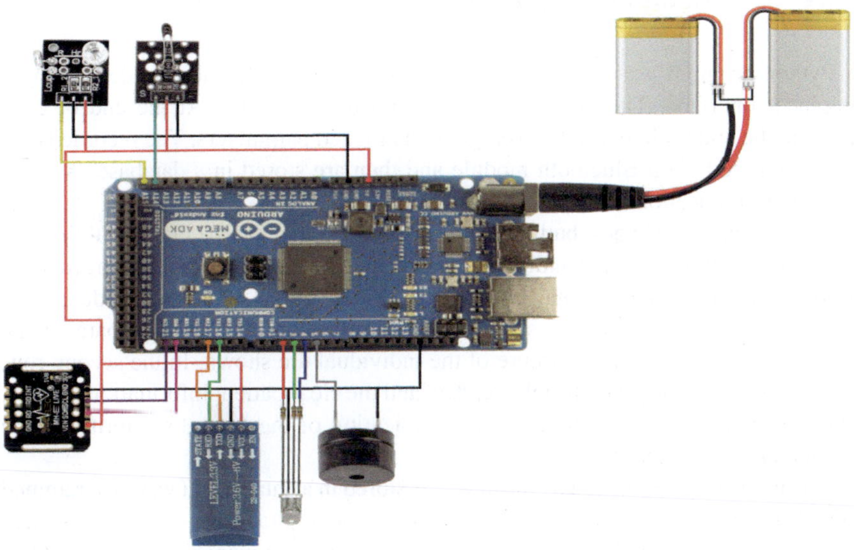

Fig. 4.7 Microcontroller ATmega 2560 connected to the peripheral sensors

The interface was developed for a computer equipment with a Core i5-8265U,16 GB DDR4 RAM, 256 GB SSD, and Windows 10 Pro.

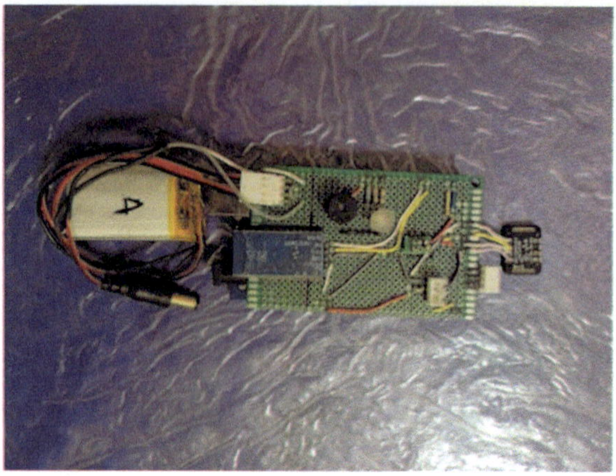

Fig. 4.8 Physical electronic circuit

4.3.4 Algorithm Development

A Python program was converted into an easy-to-use application by developing a graphical interface. The vital signs are recorded every 90 s. At the end of each interval, the code calculates the average of the logged parameters. The recorded data are transmitted via a Bluetooth module and then are stored in a database. A serial COM port connection is used (Fig. 4.9).

Text, geometric shapes, buttons, indicators, inter alia, can be created in the user interface. Additionally, the indicators and legends are created and changed. It is following the information obtained by the system. Figure 4.10 shows the developed interface. In the first row, the social security affiliation, oxygenation parameters, pulses per minute, and temperature of the individual are shown. In the second row, from left to right, there are the table update and the clear patient information buttons. The patient's admission date and the classification of the patient's priority can be included in the database.

The information obtained by the device is stored in a database. It was programmed in SQLite3. In a case of interest, the patient's emergency status needs to be consulted; it will be interconnected with the Python programming language to collect data from the sensors. This architecture that conforms this database to storing patient's vital sign information is divided into three tables "Person," "Patient," and "Vital_signs."

The first table named "Person" works like the social security number registry (NSS), where the patient's personal information, such as name, age, sex, and medical history is stored. The second table ("Patient") stores the patient's number and the emergency priority. Finally, table 3 ("Vital_signs") will store the data that were collected by the device on the patient's vital signs Fig. 4.11.

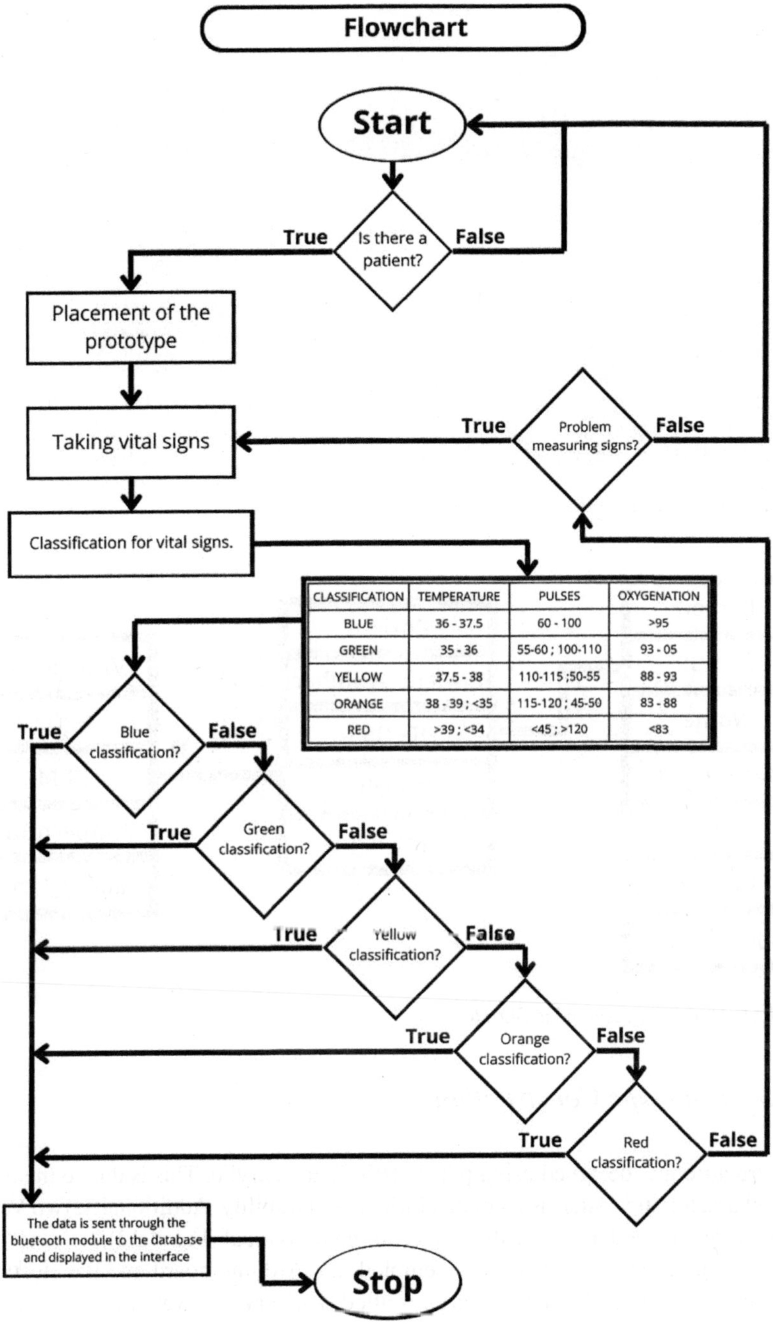

Fig. 4.9 Python flowchart

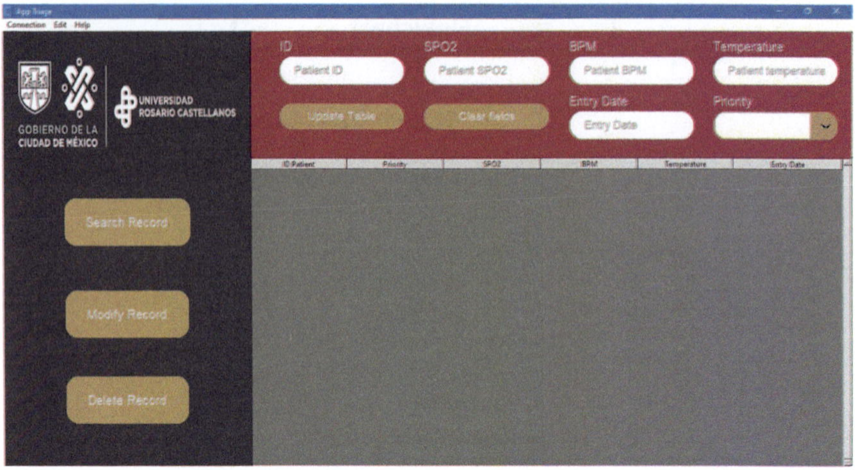

Fig. 4.10 Developed interface

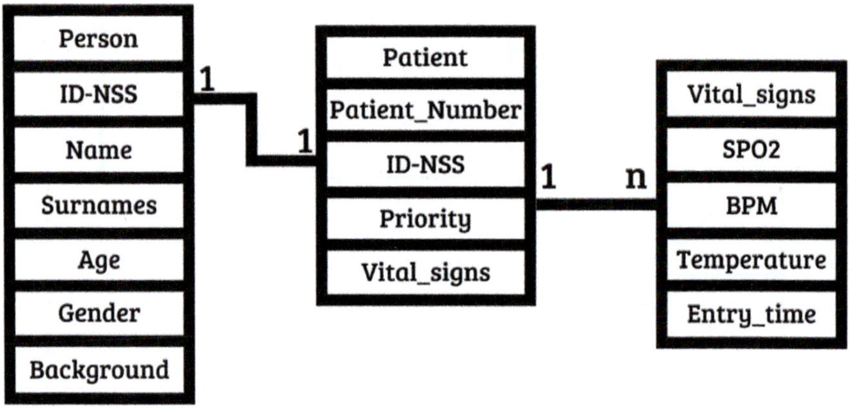

Fig. 4.11 Data base designed in SQLite3

4.3.5 Prototype Construction

The structure was designed using plastic (PVC) and acrylic. This is due to the material's characteristics, such as its malleability and durability. Additionally, two Velcro straps were attached to secure the device to the individual (Fig. 4.12).

Once the base of the device is assembled, the Arduino board and the electronic components, such as the sensors, are installed. An acrylic cover was placed on the top of the device (Fig. 4.13).

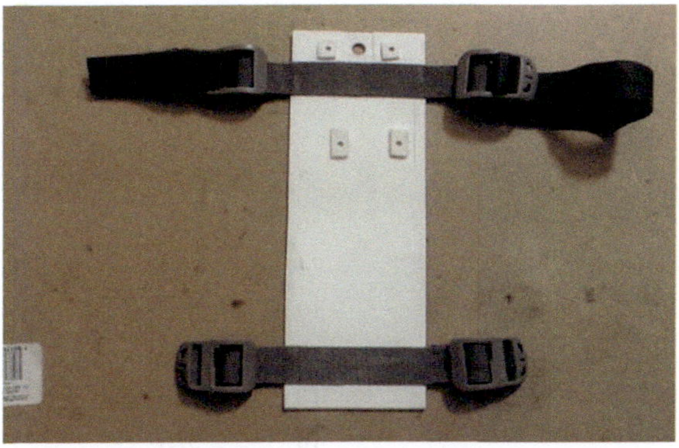

Fig. 4.12 Base of the device

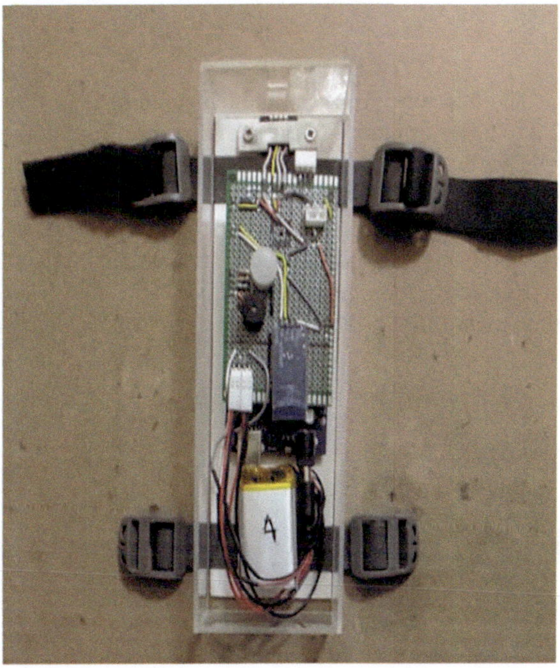

Fig. 4.13 Assembly of the electronic circuit

4.4 Results

Tests were conducted on 10 individuals with different characteristics, like age, gender, height, weight, and medical condition. The method selected was randomized to try to generalize or replicate the different types of patients that may arrive in the emergency room. The first test was performed with the temperature sensor and compared with a commercial thermometer to obtain the difference in accuracy between the two devices. The acquired data are shown in Table 4.1.

Table 4.1 Tests of the prototype and the commercial thermometer

Commercial thermometer		Thermistor NCT KY-013	
Age	Temperature (°C)	Age	Temperature (°C)
19	37	19	36.8
33	37.3	33	37.1
40	36.7	40	35.9
24	36.2	24	36
19	37.1	19	39.7
19	37.3	19	37
18	36.8	18	36
18	37.7	18	36.8
18	36.7	18	36
17	36.8	17	36.5

The difference between the temperature sensor and the commercial device was 2.25%. The similarity of the data obtained from both devices is evident (Fig. 4.14).

The divergence between the oxygen sensor of the prototype and the commercial was below 0.2127% (Fig. 4.15).

The difference between the prototype's heart rate sensor and the commercial one was 17.7%. The data obtained in the test can be seen in Fig. 4.16.

Regarding the interface, intuitive data acquisition was obtained, allowing real-time monitoring of patient parameters such as temperature, oxygenation, and pulse

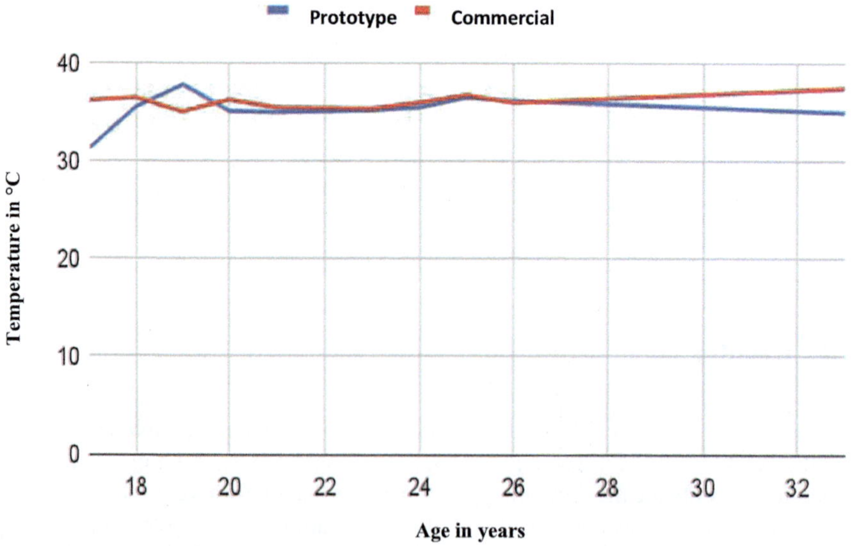

Fig. 4.14 Comparison between the temperature prototype sensor and commercial one

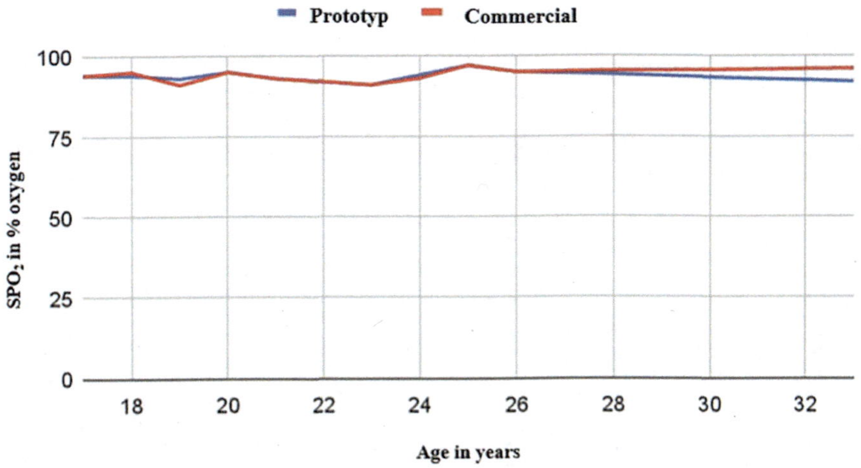

Fig. 4.15 Prototype and commercial oxygenation sensor

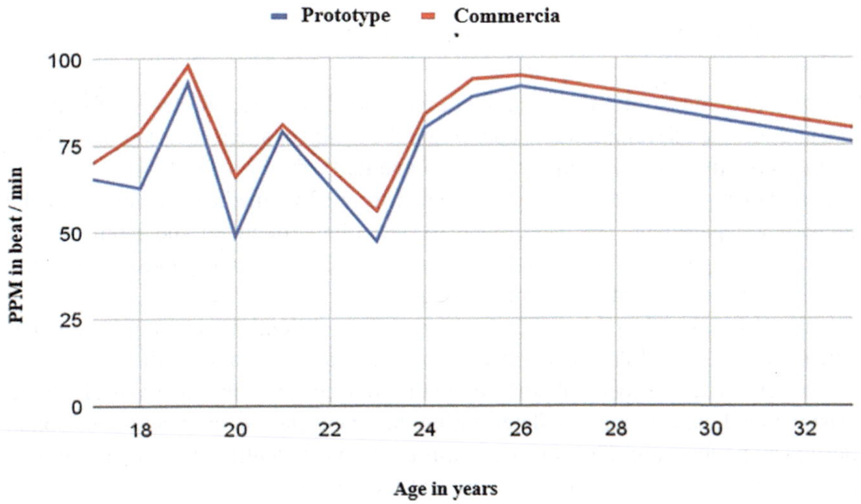

Fig. 4.16 Prototype's and commercial PPM sensor

rate. In addition, it allows patients to be searched by triage priority, as well as to be deleted from the database or their records modified. These features will help hospital personal streamline the time it takes to take vital signs (Fig. 4.17).

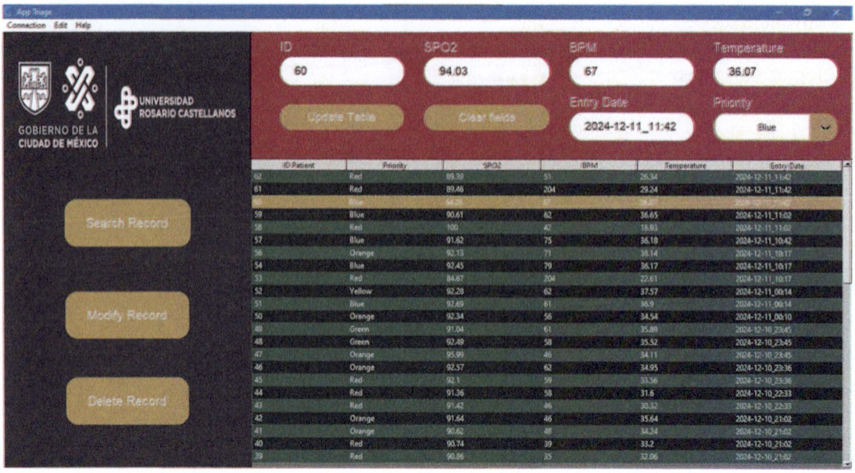

Fig. 4.17 Graphical interface completed

4.5 Conclusions

This project demonstrates the potential of embedded systems, wireless communication, and software development to address public health challenges in Mexico. These healthcare institutions have an increasing demand.

This paper presents a prototype designed to support medical personnel in the emergency department. The objective is to streamline effectively the acquisition of multiple vital signs simultaneously and thereby make the evaluation and classification of patients more efficient according to triage.

It allows for a quick and reliable acquisition of the patient's temperature, oxygenation, and pulse rate. This data along with the personal information will be displayed on an interface that is available on a computer device. This interface is designed to assist the medical personnel in determining the triage classification and to establish subsequent patient care. The purpose of this device is to identify the patient's clinical status within the first 5 minutes of arrival at the emergency room. Additionaly, the aim is to prevent the confusion of symptoms with a true emergency. In this way, patients who do not have a real emergency be referred to family medicine clinic doctors and avoid lengthy wait timer. It also aims to prevent high concentrations of people in the emergency room. The prototype features an interface supported by a database where records can be created, searched, modified, and deleted for a great patient control.

On the other hand, it is a low-cost, portable device, easy to handle, comfortable, and of the necessary size for use by most adults. This facilitates its implementation in places with limited resources. Finally, this research lays a solid foundation to future research and development in the field of auxiliary devices for triage, which could include measuring other vital signs and even specialize them in diabetic patient care.

Acknowledgements The authors gratefully acknowledge the grant awarded by the Universidad Nacional Rosario Castellanos and the support given by the Instituto Politécnico Nacional for the development of this research.

References

Andreoni G, Santangelo A, Sannicandro R, Nizardo Chailly A (2025) Health pods for automated triage improve efficiency and satisfaction in nurses and patients. Appl Sci 15(2):813. https://doi.org/10.3390/app15020813

Chaurand RÁ, León LRP, Muñoz ELG: Dimensiones antropométricas de población latinoamericana: México, Cuba, Colombia, Chile. Research Gate (PDF) Dimensiones antropométricas de la población latinoamericana: México, Cuba, Colombia, Chile/R. Avila Chaurand, L.R. Prado León, E.L. González Muñoz. (2007). Accessed 20 Nov 2024

Hinson JS, Martinez DA, Cabral S, George K, Whalen M, Hansoti B, Levin S (2018) Triage performance in emergency medicine: a systematic review. Annals Of Emergency Med 74(1):140–152. https://doi.org/10.1016/j.annemergmed.2018.09.022

Instituto Mexicano del Seguro Social (2018a) Revista Médica del IMSS, México

Instituto Mexicano del Seguro Social (2018b) Encuesta Nacional de Confianza y Satisfacción para usuarios del Servicio de Urgencias. ENCONSA, México

Ivanov G, Todorova M (2025) Design and evaluation of AI-driven triage Systems for Improving Emergency Department Workflow and Patient Outcomes. J of Emerging Cloud Tech and Cross-Platform Int Paradigms 9(4):1–14

Kukharchuk RP, Vakaliuk TA, Zaika OV, Riabko AV, Medvediev MG (2023) Implementation of STEM learning technology in the process of calibrating an NTC thermistor and developing an electronic thermometer based on it. In CTE workshop proceedings, vol 10, pp 251–264. https://doi.org/10.55056/cte.560

Lee SG, Yu KJ, Won SM, Yoo JY (2025) Advanced approaches to decoupled sensory signal monitoring in human interface systems. Int J of Extreme Manufacturing 7(4):042003. https://iopscience.iop.org/article/10.1088/2631-7990/adbc4e/meta#:~:text=10.1088/2631%2D7990/adbc4e

Lin J, Chen H, Ling Q, Shen Q, Luo S, Akhtar A, Chen D (2025) Respiratory rate monitoring based on all-fiber strain-induced humidity sensor. Opt Laser Technol 181:111840. https://doi.org/10.1016/j.optlastec.2024.111840

Muharram NA, Pratama BA, Indarto P (2025) Development of IoT-based pulse rate detection bracelet for volleyball endurance training. Retos: nuevas tendencias en educación física, deporte y recreación 65:931–940. https://doi.org/10.47197/retos.v65.109938

Orta Peña RI (2021) Prevalencia de la calidad y satisfacción percibida por usuarias a través del instrumento ENCOSA en los diferentes servicios de Ginecología y Obstetricia del Hospital Central Dr. Ignacio Morones Prieto en el año 2020. https://repositorioinstitucional.uaslp.mx/xmlui/handle/i/7883. Accessed 16 Oct 2024

Posthuma L, Downey C, Visscher M, Ghazali D, Joshi M, Ashrafian H, Khan S, Darzi A, Goldstone J, Preckel B (2020) Remote wireless vital signs monitoring on the ward for early detection of deteriorating patients: a case series. Int J Of Nursing Studies 104:103515. https://doi.org/10.1016/j.ijnurstu.2019.103515

Siira E, Johansson H, Nygren J (2025) Mapping and summarizing the research on AI Systems for Automating Medical History Taking and Triage: scoping review. J Med Internet Res 27:e53741. https://doi.org/10.2196/53741

Torezan SV, de Oliveira KS, Fontes CER, Fagundes MAV, Cavazana WC (2025) Instrumento de triagem em cirurgias de urgência. Revista Eletrônica Acervo Saúde 25:e17581–e17581

Tsebesebe NT, Mpofu K, Sivarasu S, Mthunzi-Kufa P (2025) Arduino-based devices in healthcare and environmental monitoring. Discov Internet Things 5(1):1–31. https://doi.org/10.1007/s43926-025-00139-z

Vizcaíno Ad J, Vizcaíno Marín V d P, Fregoso Jasso GS (2019) Análisis de la satisfacción de pacientes del servicio de urgencias en un hospital público de Jalisco. Horizonte Sanitario 18(1):27–36. https://doi.org/10.19136/hs.a18n1.2103

Zachariasse JM, Van Der Hagen V, Seiger N, Mackway-Jones K, Van Veen M, Moll HA (2019) Performance of triage systems in emergency care: a systematic review and meta-analysis. BMJ Open 9(5):e026471. https://doi.org/10.1136/bmjopen-2018-026471

Chapter 5
Design of a Rehabilitation System for a Wrist According to the Mexican Phenotype

Mauricio Aarón Pérez-Romero, Alejandra Armenta-Molina, Adrián Esteban Mejía-García, and Monica Montserrath Valdez-Mata

Abstract This paper reports the conceptual design and simulation of a low-cost wrist rehabilitator prototype. It is based on the Mexican phenotype. The movements of a healthy wrist are replicated. It is semi-automatic with two degrees of freedom. Flexion extension is within the range between 0° and 115°, and abduction-adduction is in a range between − 18° and 60°. The active movements of the wrist are reproduced. A user interface records the motion and speed parameters of the joint. The control algorithm, that regulates the movements of the prototype, was implemented in a low-cost ESP32 microcontroller through Arduino IDE code. In addition, it can generate circumduction movement. A data recording system collects and displays the working space following the kinematics of the movements generated for rehabilitation.

Keywords Wrist rehabilitation · Flexion extension · Abduction-adduction · Control algorithm

---

M. A. Pérez-Romero · A. E. Mejía-García · M. M. Valdez-Mata
Departamento de Ingeniería en Control y Automatización, Escuela Superior de Ingeniería Mecánica y Eléctrica Unidad Zacatenco, Instituto Politécnico Nacional, Ciudad de México, México
e-mail: maperezro@ipn.mx

A. E. Mejía-García
e-mail: aemejiag@ipn.mx

M. M. Valdez-Mata
e-mail: mvaldezma@ipn.mx

A. Armenta-Molina (✉)
Sección de Estudios de Posgrado e Investigación, Escuela Superior de Ingeniería Mecánica y Eléctrica Unidad Zacatenco, Instituto Politécnico Nacional, Ciudad de México, México
e-mail: aarmentamo@ipn.mx

A. Öchsner (ed.), *Progress in Biomaterials and Biomedical Engineering*, Advanced Structured Materials 249, https://doi.org/10.1007/978-3-032-13551-3_5

5.1 Introduction

According to the Report to the Federal Executive and the Congress of the Union of Mexico on the Financial Situation and Risks of IMSS (Mexican Social Security Institute, by its acronym in Spanish) 2023–2024, in 2023, over 37,000 pensions were granted for occupational disease or accident (partial or total permanent disability and compensation). An increase was observed in previous years. Likewise, during the same period, nearly 201,000 hand accidents were recorded. This translates to approximately 3.9 million lost workdays and a cost of around 37 million US dollars to the social security system.

Wrist and hand injuries are a public health issue with significant global impact, characterized by high incidence rates and considerable socioeconomic consequences. For example, a global systematic analysis based on the Global Burden of Disease Study reported an age-standardized incidence of 179 wrist and hand fractures per 100,000 people in 2017. It warned that countries with low or middle socioeconomic development levels have shown an increasing trend over the past decades (Crowe et al. 2020). Specifically, in low- and middle-income countries, occupational injuries account for up to 25% of workplace accidents, with a pronounced impact on workers engaged in manual or industrial activities (Rodríguez et al. 2024). A study conducted at a specialized center in Mexico City in 2015 shows that wrist and hand injuries accounted for 8.9% of all emergency cases. Young patients (21–30 years old) were involved frequently. Fractures, bruises, and sprains were common cases (Arroyo and Quinzaños 2021). Global and regional evidence highlights the need for rehabilitation strategies tailored to the specific anatomical and functional characteristics of the affected populations.

Once the injury has been treated and possibly after a long period of inactivity, a significant number of rehabilitation sessions are required (Hernandez and Touhiduzzaman 2022). In this context, therapies of specific tasks assisted by robots may be more effective for the long-term reduction of motor alterations in an individual. Furthermore, treatments assisted by mechanical devices can perform an objective evaluation of patient rehabilitation.

The Massachusetts Institute of Technology evaluated four veterans of war (VA). Results showed that patients who used the MIT-Manus robot for 12 weeks experienced a small but significant increase in arm function (Park et al. 2019). Another group got high-intensity therapy from a therapist, who correctly determined the number and intensity of robot movements, and showed similar improvements (Williams et al. 2001).

The universal haptic device (UHD) rehabilitates the arm or wrist with movements in two degrees of freedom (Bae et al. 2019). Training depends on the locking/unlocking of a passive universal joint. The device is actuated by mechanical platforms and component actuation (Oblak et al. 2010). In a different context, the Dulex-II is an active wrist rehabilitation exoskeleton (Bae and Moon 2012; Rätz et al. 2022). Its control allows three degrees of freedom movements for the wrist, the index finger, and a mechanism that encloses the other three fingers.

Several robotic systems have been developed for upper limb neurorehabilitation following a stroke. They offer intensive, cost-effective, and home-adaptable therapy. The arm assist robotic system, for instance, demonstrated significant improvements in motor function in a randomized study with subacute stroke patients.

The arm assist robotic system, for instance, demonstrated significant improvements in motor function in a randomized study with subacute stroke patients. It was assessed using the Fugl–Meyer (mean gain, 18.0 Vs. 7.5) and Wolf motor function test, compared to conventional arm training, with no adverse events reported (Tomić et al. 2017).

More broadly, meta-analyses show that robot-assisted therapy can significantly enhance upper limb motor recovery in chronic stroke survivors, especially when combined with routine rehabilitation (Mehrholz et al. 2018). Additionally, home-based robotic rehabilitation using portable devices like the ICone system has been used successfully. Autonomous patient training outside the clinic is possible with promising effects on motor outcomes in chronic stroke populations (Bressi et al. 2023).

Luna and coworkers report on the design of a forearm and wrist re-trainer machine (Luna-Avilés et al. 2013). This device has been used to recover the muscular residual capacity of individuals who have a disability after an accident. The anthropometrics of the Mexican phenotype were considered.

In general terms, wrist rehabilitation therapies are largely applied manually in Mexico. The evolution of therapies is not constant. The patient's recovery time is longer than expected. Of the few devices developed in Mexico, some have voluptuous mechanisms. They were not developed to be used in small clinics or homes. This is largely due to the high cost of the technology used in rehabilitation systems. These devices do not cover the degrees of freedom required for rehabilitation. They focus only on 1 or 2 for wrist rehabilitation. They mainly perform pronation-supination (of the forearm), flexion-extension, or adduction-abduction (of the wrist). On the other hand, according to the available information, some of these devices consider data acquisition.

5.2 Statement of the Problem

Orthopedic rehabilitation is widely applied in Mexico. However, specialized personnel are limited and there is a high demand. In general terms, it is performed without interaction with robotic devices. The time to observe an improvement in the patient is considerable. Therefore, the design and implementation of auxiliary systems are required to speed up rehabilitation and return the patient to daily activities. The development of a wrist rehabilitation system is proposed. The design considerations are as follows:

The rehabilitation device must reproduce wrist movements in the following ranges: flexion and extension, abduction and adduction. The device must perform wrist movements continuously. The anthropometry of the patients was considered.

The extended hand length is 18.082 cm, and its weight is 0.533 kg. The forearm and hand weight is 1.5 kg. The wrist size is 4.5 cm, and the hand width, including thumb, is 9.74 cm.

5.3 Materials and Methods

The state-of-the-art of hand and wrist rehabilitation mechanisms was evaluated initially. Based on the above, the general parameters of the mechanical design and the control of its position and speed were determined. The rehabilitation system's design, construction, testing, and performance evaluation were carried out in the final phase.

Based on the above, a device has been proposed that meets the adduction-abduction (15° to − 45°) and flexion-extension (90° to − 90°) movements. These must be performed continuously. The rehabilitation movement is developed with minimal effort for its function and recovery progress.

The prototype simulation was performed with a CAD-CAE program (SOLIDWORKS). The movement of the elements in the mechanism was modeled. However, a support structure made of IPS structural elements is required (Fig. 5.1). It was made with a structural profile that has an "I" shape with extra-wide round "S"-shaped pads. This reduces the range of motion for the flexion and extension of the wrist to 57.5° for each.

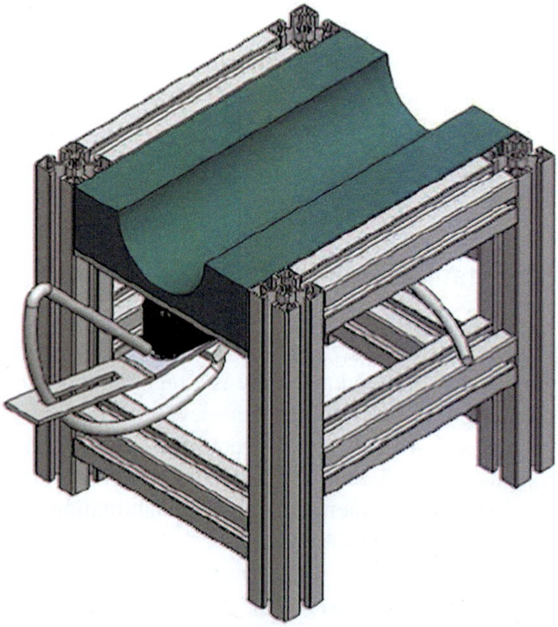

Fig. 5.1 Solid model of the wrist rehabilitation system

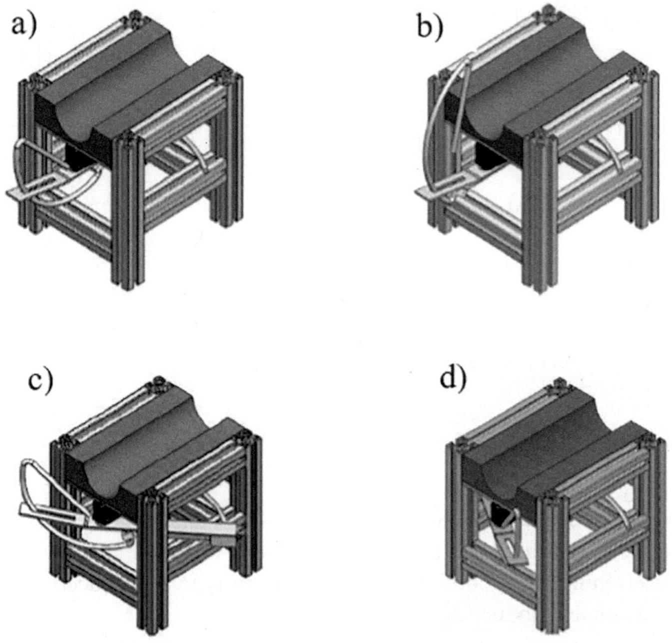

Fig. 5.2 Movements of the device: **a** adduction, **b** abduction, **c** flexion, and **d** extension

The rehabilitation mechanism has a linear actuator and a rotational actuator. These allow the system to be manipulated to reproduce the movements made by the wrist. In addition, it is possible to regulate the speed and position of these two types of motors. The adduction-abduction and flexion-extension movements performed by the device, operating with the drive of the motors, are illustrated in Fig. 5.2.

For the implementation of the system's control, an ESP32 microcontroller was used. It was programmed through the Arduino IDE platform. This device enabled the coordination of actuators with two degrees of freedom of the system: flexion-extension and abduction-adduction. ESP32 was selected due to its low cost, processing capability, and Wi-Fi connectivity, which allowed real-time data transmission to a user interface. The implemented control algorithm regulated the angular position and velocity of the motors. In addition, a data acquisition and visualization system was integrated to monitor the motion of the electric actuators and record key operational parameters. Figure 5.3 illustrates the general control system diagram.

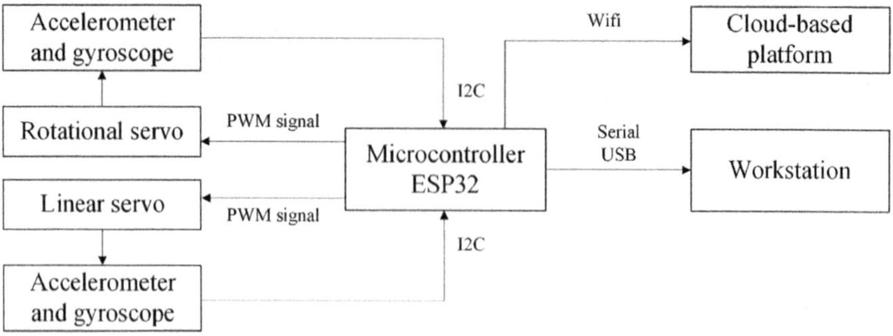

Fig. 5.3 General control system diagram

5.4 Discussion of the Results

Figure 5.4 illustrates the evolution of angular position and velocity over a complete movement cycle, in which the desired trajectory is followed at a specified speed. Angular positioning tests confirmed that the prototype reproduced the intended flexion-extension and abduction-adduction profiles.

The quantitative analysis of percent error showed a mean error below 2% across both degrees of freedom (Fig. 5.5). Peak errors remained under 3% for flexion-extension and under 7 for abduction-adduction. The effectiveness of the control algorithm implemented on the ESP32 has been confirmed.

The circumduction results demonstrated a precise performance. The circumduction trajectory traced a continuous path (Fig. 5.6). Quantitative analysis indicated a mean endpoint position error below 7 mm ($\approx$0.7% of the study radius) and a maximum peak under 10 mm. The controller's ability to coordinate both axes in a multi-planar movement is shown. Endpoint velocity exhibited variations below 3%, ensuring appropriate therapeutic dynamics for rehabilitation exercises. These findings validate the prototype's suitability for generating complete circumduction without loss of precision or data-acquisition stability.

The obtained results demonstrate that the prototype accurately meets the flexion-extension and abduction-adduction angular profiles and coordinates both axes to produce continuous, stable circumduction movements. These findings are in line with previous studies on multi-planar devices (Oblak et al. 2010). However, they surpass the reported mean error due to the optimization of the control algorithm on the ESP32. The high sampling frequency (100 Hz) and the robustness of the Wi-Fi transmission ensure real-time data availability, a crucial aspect for dynamically adjusting therapeutic protocols. However, the device's performance under variable loads or in patients with severe spasticity requires clinical validation, since the experiments were limited to laboratory conditions with healthy subjects.

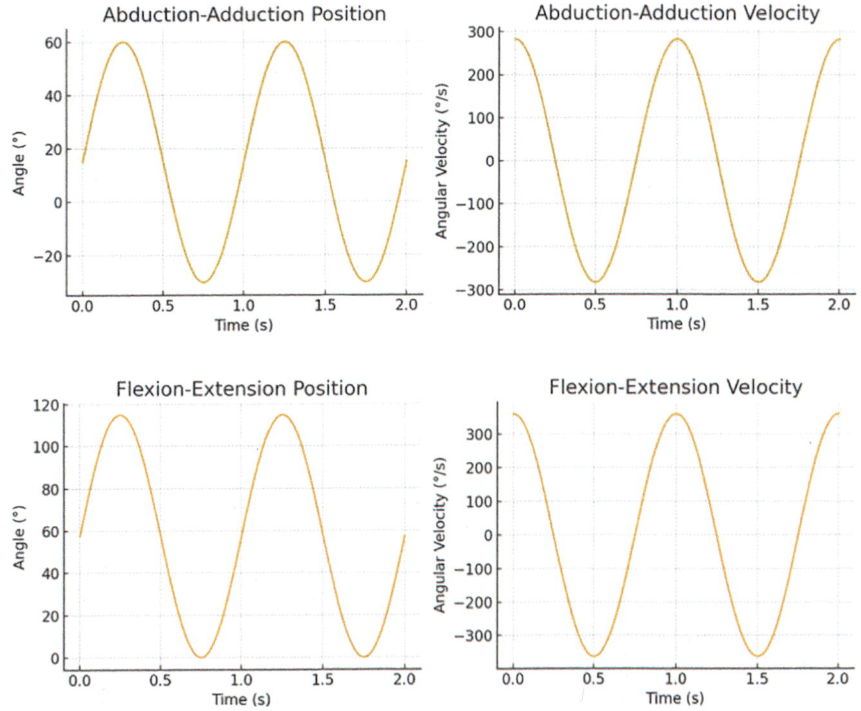

Fig. 5.4 Abduction-adduction and flexion-extension angular position and velocity

5.5 Conclusions

The functional tests of the rehabilitation system with healthy users confirmed the correct reproduction of the wrist movements. It is performed actively, and the device assists in the wrist movements.

A circumduction movement is generated when the basic wrist movements of flexion-extension and adduction-abduction are carried out together. It does not have a circular trajectory. The required space of work was developed. Although the prototype is functional, it is essential to adapt to a user-friendly interface. It is considered that this equipment can be used by therapists in the rehabilitation field.

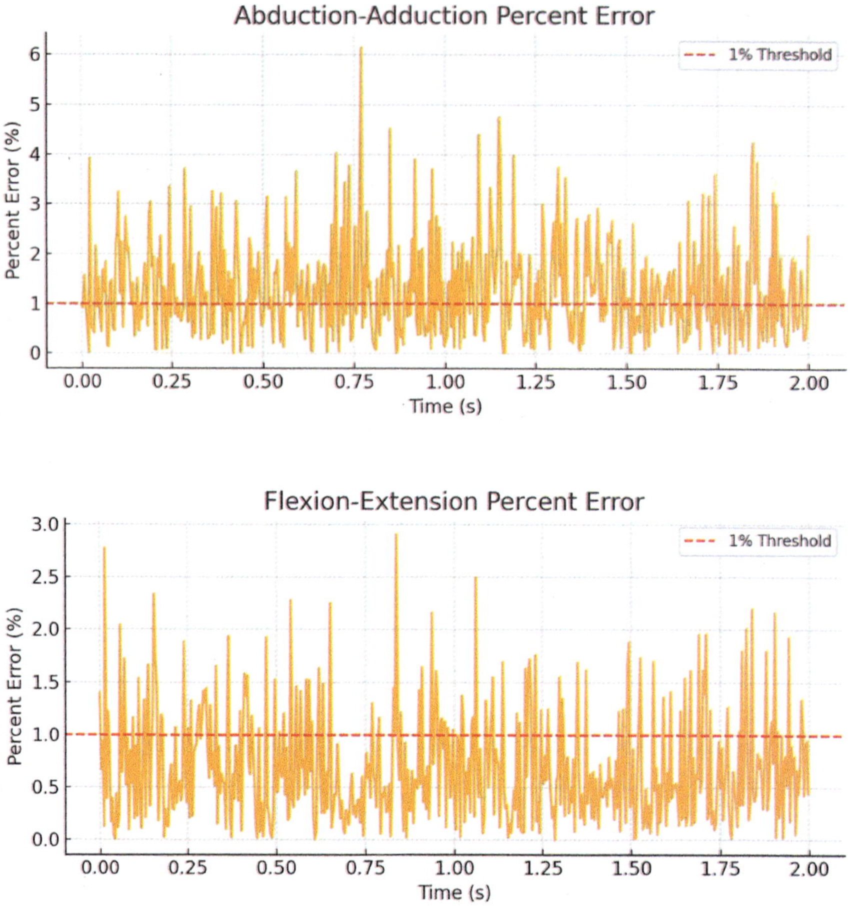

Fig. 5.5 Abduction-adduction and flexion-extension mean joint error

Fig. 5.6 Circumduction trajectory

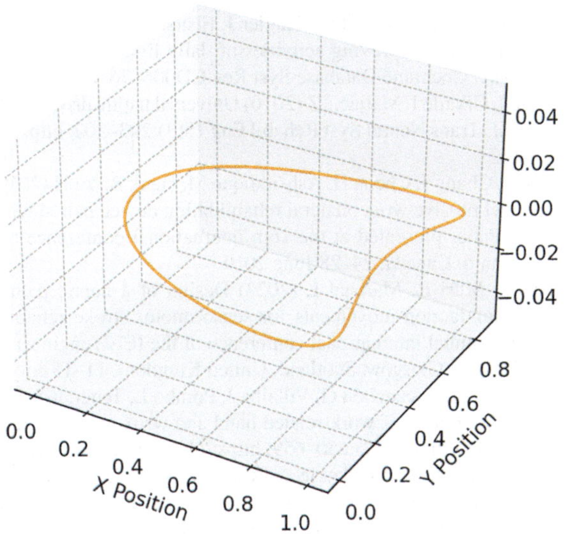

Acknowledgments The authors kindly acknowledge the grant awarded by the Instituto Politécnico Nacional and SIP for the development of this research.

References

Arroyo C, Quinzaños J (2021) Epidemiology of hand and wrist injuries treated in a reference specialty center over a year. Acta Ortop Mex 35(5):429–435. https://doi.org/10.35366/104570

Bae J, Moon I (2012) Design and control of an exoskeleton device for active wrist rehabilitation. Paper presented at the 12th international conference on control, automation and systems, Jeju, Korea (South), 17–21 October 2012

Bae J, Hwang S, Moon I (2019) Evaluation and verification of a novel wrist rehabilitation robot employing safety-related mechanism. In: Paper presented at the 16th international conference on rehabilitation robotics (ICORR), Toronto, Canada, 24–28 June 2019

Bressi F, Campagnola B, Cricenti L, Santacaterina F, Miccinilli S, Di Pino G, Fiori F, D'Alonzo M, Di Lazzaro V, Ricci L, Capone F, Pacilli A, Sterzi S, Bravi M (2023) Upper limb home-based robotic rehabilitation in chronic stroke patients: a pilot study. Front Neurorobot 17:1130770. https://doi.org/10.3389/fnbot.2023.1130770

Crowe CS, Massenburg BB, Morrison SD et al (2020) Global trends of hand and wrist trauma: a systematic analysis of fracture and digit amputation using the global burden of disease 2017 study. Inj Prev 26:i115–i124. https://doi.org/10.1136/injuryprev-2019-043495

Hernandez S, Touhiduzzaman M (2022) Wi-PT: wireless sensing based low-cost physical rehabilitation tracking. Paper presented at the IEEE International Conference on E-health Networking, Application & Services, Genoa, Italy, 17–19 October 2022

Luna-Avilés A et al (2013) Biomechanical and control design of a prototype for muscular re-training of a forearm and a wrist. In: Ochsner A, Altenbach H (eds) Advances in bio-mechanical systems and materials. Advanced structured materials, vol 40. Springer, Cham. https://doi.org/10.1007/978-3-319-00479-2_8

Mehrholz J, Pohl M, Platz T, Kugler J, Elsner B (2018) Electromechanical and robot-assisted arm training for improving activities of daily living, arm function, and arm muscle strength after stroke. Cochrane Database Syst Rev CD006876. https://doi.org/10.1002/14651858.CD006876

Oblak J, Cikajlo I, Matjačić Z (2010) Universal haptic drive: a robot for arm and wrist rehabilitation. IEEE Trans Neural Syst Rehabil Eng 18(3):293–302. https://doi.org/10.1109/TNSRE.2009.2034162

Park D, Chang J, Cheng H, Ashsiddique M, Hauk B, Yu H (2019) Development and evaluation of a novel passive wrist bilateral rehabilitation device paired with virtual reality: a feasibility study. In: Paper presented at the 16th international conference on rehabilitation robotics (ICORR), Toronto, Canada, 24–28 June 2019

Rätz R, Müri R, Marchal L (2022) Design of a haptic palmar device with thumb flexion and circumduction movements for sensorimotor stroke rehabilitation. In: Paper presented at the 44th annual international conference of the IEEE engineering in medicine and biology society (EMBC), Glasgow, Scotland, United Kingdom, 11–15 July 2022

Rodríguez A, Tocanchón G, Villalba J, Pombo L, Teherán A, Camero G, Ayala K, Acero G (2024) Epidemiology of work-related hand and wrist injuries in a referral center: a descriptive study. World Orthop 15(7):650–659. https://doi.org/10.5312/wjo.v15.i7.650

Tomić T, Savić A, Vidaković A, Rodić S, Isaković M, Rodríguez C, Keller T, Konstantinović L (2017) ArmAssist robotic system versus matched conventional therapy for poststroke upper limb rehabilitation: a randomized clinical trial. Biomed Res Int 7659893. https://doi.org/10.1155/2017/7659893

Williams D, Krebs H, Hogan N (2001) A robot for wrist rehabilitation. In: Paper presented at the 23rd annual international conference of the IEEE engineering in medicine and Biology Society, 25–28 October 2001

Chapter 6
Shoulder Joint Biomodel Analysis Ligaments Based on the Finite Element Method

Maria de la Luz Suarez-Hernandez, Guillermo Urriolagoitia-Sosa, Beatriz Romero-Ángeles, Martin Ivan Correa-Corona, Aldo Saul Laguna-Canales, Reyner Iván Yparrea-Arreola, Yaneth Rocha-Duran, Aldair Guerrero-López, Javier Gutiérrez-Simota, and Guillermo Manuel Urriolagoitia-Calderón

Abstract The shoulder joint has been particularly interesting because the joint bones do not directly contact each other; they are connected through ligaments and muscles. It is also the joint with the greatest range of motion in the human body. The ligaments, considered as statics stabilizers, are crucial in guiding joint movement while restricting excessive movement between the bones. Computational models, also known as biomodels, are designed to replicate biological tissue based on medical

M. de la Luz Suarez-Hernandez (✉) · G. Urriolagoitia-Sosa · B. Romero-Ángeles · M. I. Correa-Corona · A. S. Laguna-Canales · R. I. Yparrea-Arreola · Y. Rocha-Duran · A. Guerrero-López · J. Gutiérrez-Simota · G. M. Urriolagoitia-Calderón
Instituto Politécnico Nacional, Escuela Superior de Ingeniería Mecánica y Eléctrica, Sección de Estudios de Posgrado e Investigación Unidad Zacatenco, Ciudad de México, Mexico
e-mail: luzsuarez398@gmail.com

G. Urriolagoitia-Sosa
e-mail: guiurri@hotmail.com

B. Romero-Ángeles
e-mail: romerobeatriz97@hotmail.com

M. I. Correa-Corona
e-mail: ingenieria.ivan.95@gmail.com

A. S. Laguna-Canales
e-mail: lagunacanalesaldosaul@gmail.com

R. I. Yparrea-Arreola
e-mail: reyner.yparrea@utd.edu.mx

Y. Rocha-Duran
e-mail: rdyaneth@gmail.com

A. Guerrero-López
e-mail: aguerrerol1800@alumno.ipn.mx

J. Gutiérrez-Simota
e-mail: javiergsimota@gmail.com

A. Öchsner (ed.), *Progress in Biomaterials and Biomedical Engineering*, Advanced Structured Materials 249, https://doi.org/10.1007/978-3-032-13551-3_6

images virtually, utilizing various modeling techniques for their development. By applying biomodels in numerical simulations that use finite element method tools, researchers can study and analyze various biological tissues without compromising the physical integrity of the individual. This study aims to analyze the behavior of the shoulder ligaments during the flexion movement of the joint, utilizing a biomodel. A detailed computational biomodel of the shoulder joint has been developed using medical imaging techniques, such as tomography, which provide critical insights into the internal structures of an individual. This biomodel accurately replicates the morphology of the upper extremity, incorporating features that closely resemble the biological tissues of the joint. Key components included in the model are cancellous and cortical bones, ligaments, the articular capsule, and articular cartilage. Numerical simulations have analyzed the flexion shoulder joint movement, providing valuable knowledge about biomechanics. The results of the flexion simulation movement undergo an evaluation to determine the function of each ligament involved in this movement. The findings align clinical reports, enhancing our understanding of shoulder biomechanics and informing medical practices.

Keywords Shoulder · Biomodel · FEM · Biomechanics

6.1 Introduction

The shoulder is a joint that has complex biomechanics and is unique because there is no physical union between the bones that are part of the articulation. It consists of three primary bones: the humerus, clavicle, and scapula, and includes five subjoints: the glenohumeral, acromioclavicular, scapulothoracic, and sternoclavicular joints (Veeger and Van Der Helm 2007). This complex structure allows the shoulder a wide range of motion (Edizer 2022). The ligaments provide static stabilization of the shoulder joint, and muscles offer dynamic stabilization. Together, these components hold the bones in proper position and alignment, preventing excessive movement.

The shoulder joint performs six basic movements in three different planes of motion.

- Flexion and Extension (Sagittal Plane).

  Flexion involves moving the arm forward and upward from the body.
  Extension consists of moving the arm backward behind the body.

- Abduction and Adduction (Frontal Plane).

  Abduction occurs when you move your arm away from the side of the body.
  Adduction is the movement of bringing the arm toward or across the body.

G. M. Urriolagoitia-Calderón
e-mail: urrio332@hotmail.com

- Internal and External Rotation (Transverse Plane).

External rotation (lateral rotation) involves rotating the arm outward, away from the body.

Internal rotation (medial rotation) involves rotating the arm inward, toward the body.

6.2 Materials and Methodology

6.2.1 Computational Biomodel

Computational biomodels are defined by their capacity to accurately replicate the shape and structure of the human body with high precision. Below are the essential steps in the methodology employed for the virtual replication for the shoulder joint structures, describing the detailed processes involved in capturing the complex morphology and functionality of this pivotal anatomical region (Serrato-Pedrosa et al. 2024; Maya-Anaya et al. 2023; Corea-Corona et al. 2023).

- *Data acquisition*: A healthy female volunteer had a computer tomography (CT) scan of the upper torso on the right side, obtaining a sequence of images saved in a DICOM file, which contains the anatomical data needed for the development of the model.
- *Image processing*: The DICOM file is imported into a CAD software, in this case it was used Mimics Medical® software. A project was developed to define and delimit the structures that will be included in the virtual model. Using the tools provided by the software, a new mask is generated for each element, outlining the shape of each structure in the three planes: coronal, axial, and sagittal, as shown in Fig. 6.1b. This process results in a point cloud that represents the model. Segmentation of ligaments, cartilage, and joint capsule was performed manually, following literature guidelines based on the origins and insertions of the soft tissues in the bones (Kadi et al. 2017).
- *Generation of the virtual 3D model*: The generated structures of the model are imported into another software to correct possible errors such as cavities, overlapping triangles, and surface irregularities, as well as to develop smoothing to refine the geometry of the model (Fig. 6.1c). Materialize 3-matic® software was utilized for its tools to enhance the correction process and improve the uniformity of discretization according to the geometry of the model. This approach led to the development of a meticulous, refined virtual biomodel of the shoulder joint.
- *Solid Structure*: As illustrated in Fig. 6.1d, the solid biomodel was exported for a structural numerical analysis into a finite element method software; in this research ANSYS Workbench® was utilized.

The virtual biomodel of the shoulder joint consists of 19 structural components, including three bones (cortical and cancellous), ligaments, cartilage, the labrum, and the joint capsule (Fig. 6.2) (See Appendix Table 6.2 for the abbreviations used).

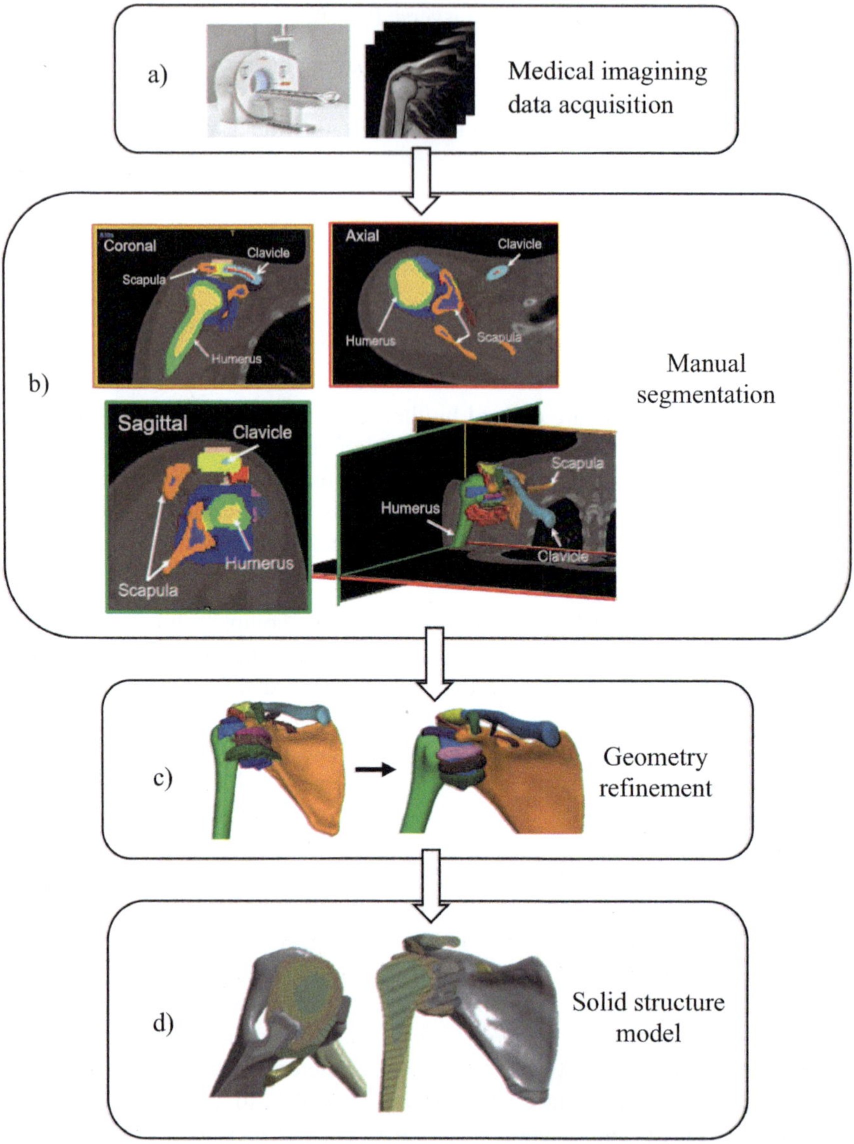

Fig. 6.1 Steps to follow for the development of the computational model (biomodel)

6.2.2 Numerical Analysis

For the numerical simulation, specific parameters were established, including the assignment of mechanical properties of biological structures, biomodel discretization, boundary conditions, and remote forces. Finite element software packages like

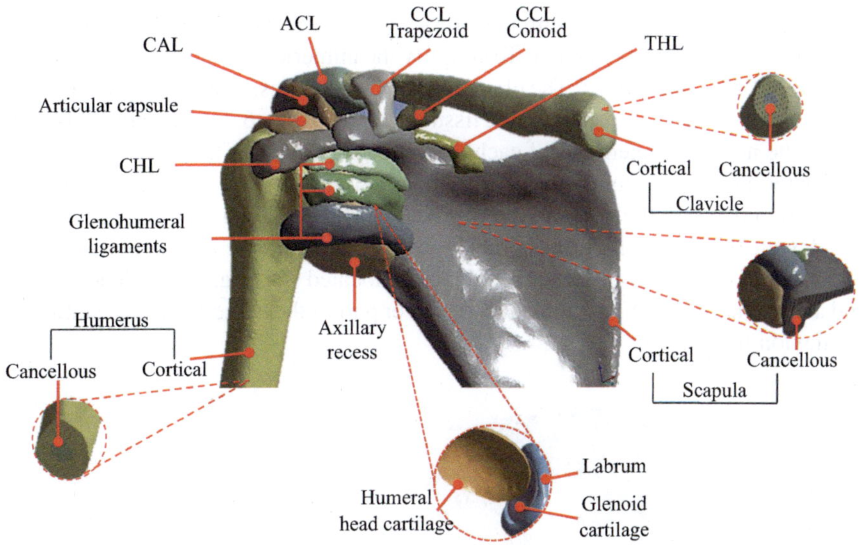

Fig. 6.2 Named structures of the shoulder joint biomodel

Abaqus and ANSYS Workbench provide essential tools for conducting numerical simulations on complex structures.

To simulate a flexion movement of the biomodel, a structural static analysis is conducted, considering linear-elastic behavior and applying isotropic mechanical properties. Since precise values for biological tissues can vary significantly due to factors such age, diet, lifestyle, and place of birth, approximate values derived from previous research were utilized. These values are summarized in Table 6.1 (Hayes et al. 1991; Castro-Abril et al. 2015; Favre et al. 2012; Mendoza-Muñoz et al. 2017; Nordin and Frankel 2004). In this study, the mechanical properties of the labrum and capsule joint are considered as equivalent to those of a ligament. This classification is essential for a concentrated analysis of the model's geometry.

The contact between cortical-cancellous bone and cortical bone-soft tissue (ligament, capsule, cartilage, and labrum) was considered *bonded*. At the same time, the contact between soft tissue (ligament-capsule, capsule-labrum, capsule-cartilage, and cartilage-cartilage) was considered *frictionless* (Maldonado et al. 2023; Zheng et al. 2020).

Table 6.1 Mechanical properties of biological tissue

Biological tissue	Young's modulus (MPa)	Poisson's ratio	Density (g/cm^3)
Cortical bone	18,000	0.3	1.9
Cancellous bone	75.5	0.3	0.43
Ligaments	62.63	0.4	-
Articular cartilage	10	0.4	-

This research aims to measure the stress, elongation, and contraction of the ligaments involved in this movement. To simplify the numerical simulation, only the soft tissues are being discretized. The elements are tetrahedrons, with a triangle length of 1 mm, due to the irregular shape of the tissue structures (Fig. 6.3). Appendix Table 6.3 shows the nodes and elements of each discretized structure of the biomodel.

For the numerical simulation, the boundary conditions are characterized by the connection between the arm and the torso at the glenohumeral joint, the junction of the clavicle and sternum at the sternoclavicular joint, and the medial border of the scapula, where various muscle attachments are located (see Fig. 6.4). A load of 50 N and a moment of 17.5 N m is added to the lower part of the humerus, which simulates the flexion movement.

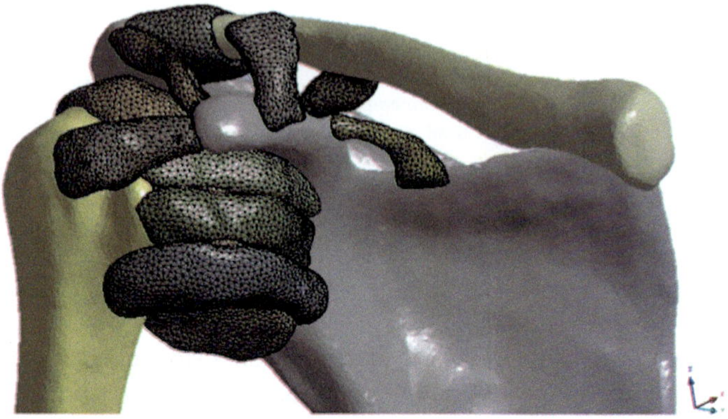

Fig. 6.3 Soft tissues discretization of the joint biomodel with in the ANSYS Workbench® software for numerical analysis

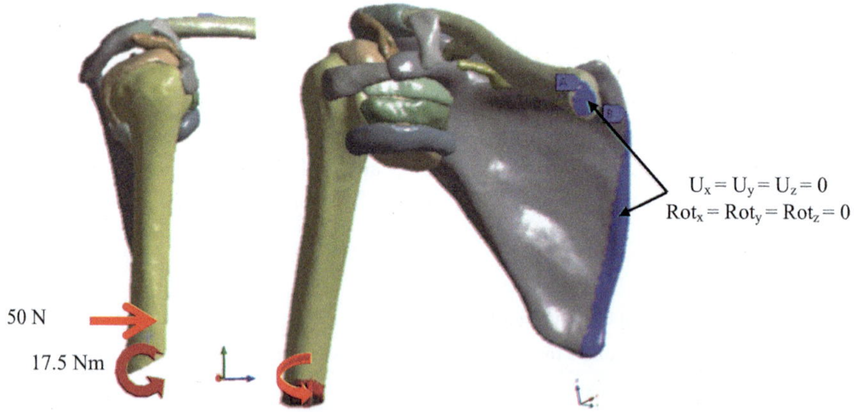

Fig. 6.4 Boundary and loading conditions. On the left, a side view of the load condition. On the right, frontal view of the boundary condition. Mark A is the representation junction of the clavicle and sternum. The mark B is the medial border of the scapula

6.3 Results

The research focuses on learning about the effects of sudden flexion movements on the static stabilizers of the shoulder. The shoulder joint numerical simulation data represents the flexion movement on the static stabilizers of the shoulder. These allow for the evaluation of the Stress, elongation, and contraction of the biological tissues.

Figure 6.5 compares the elongation and contraction results between the ligaments that provide a union between humerus and scapula (see Appendix Table 6.2 for the abbreviations used). Numerical simulations conducted on the flexion of the joint reveal that the medial ligament (1.46 mm), along with the coracohumeral ligament (1.43 mm), experiences the greatest elongation. In contrast, the articular capsule (0.17 mm) and the glenoid cartilage (0.26 mm) show the least amount of elongation. While the pIGHL (− 0.838 mm) shows negative results, it stabilized the glenohumeral joint by tightening to restrict the posterior translation of the humeral head (Fox et al. 2021).

Figure 6.6 compares the elongation and contraction results between the ligaments that provide union between scapula and clavicle. The CAL (0.579 mm) is the most elongated of these ligaments, while the ACL (0.0648 mm) is the least elongated. Therefore, it could be considered that the acromioclavicular joint exhibits minimal displacement during arm flexion, particularly when the angle is less than 90°.

Figure 6.7 shows the elongation and contraction results in soft tissues obtained from the numerical analysis simulation.

Figure 6.8 illustrates the distribution of stress along the ligaments connecting the scapula to the clavicle. The findings from the numerical simulation indicate that most of these ligaments show negative values, suggesting that they experience compressive

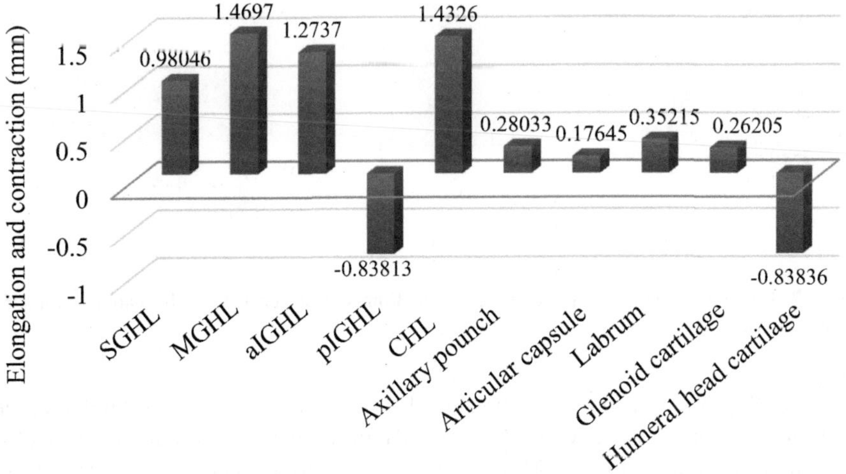

Fig. 6.5 Joining ligaments the humerus and scapula elongation and contractions results during flexion movement

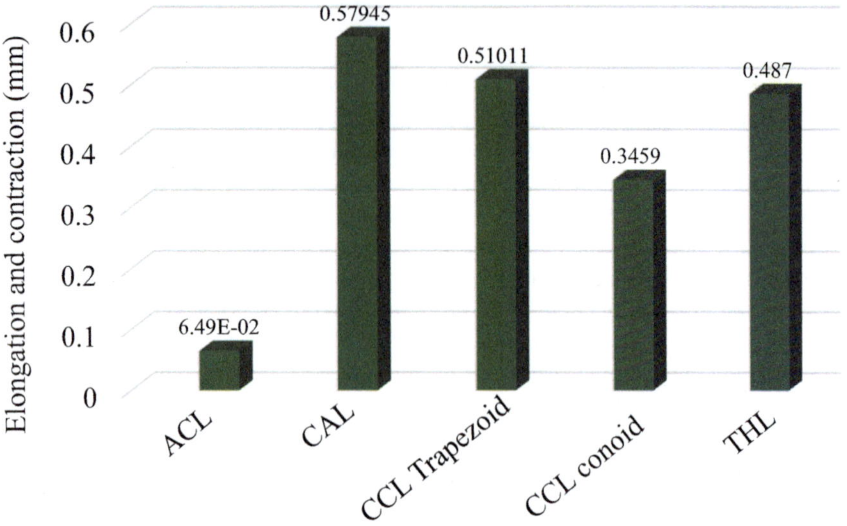

Fig. 6.6 Joining ligaments the scapula and clavicle elongation and contractions results during flexion movement

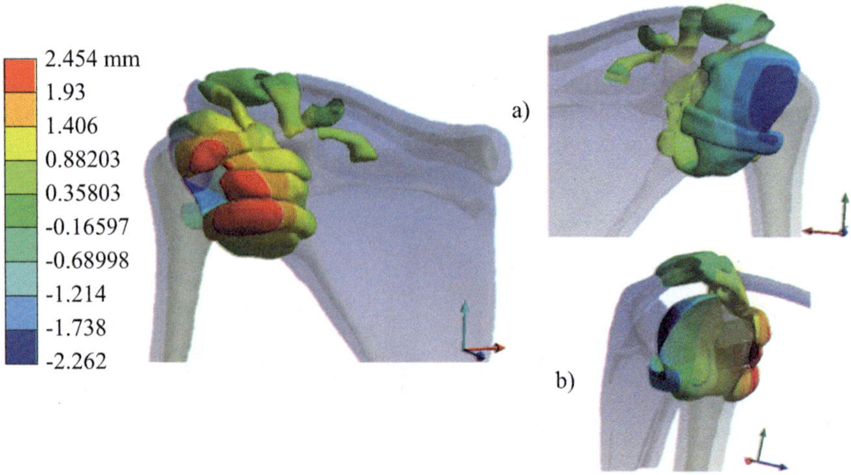

Fig. 6.7 Biomodel elongation and contraction. **a** Biomodel posterior view. **b** Scapula with soft tissue side view

stress. CHL presents a compression value of − 0.631 MPa; meanwhile MGHL has a minimum compression value of − 0.0495 MPa. In comparison, the auxiliary recesses exhibit stress values of 0.442 MPa, whereas the inferior glenoid demonstrates the lowest recorded stress value at 0.03 MPa.

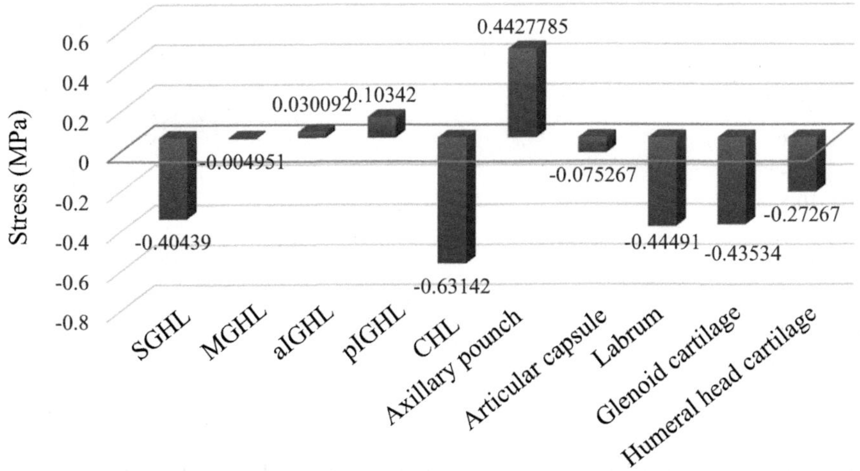

Fig. 6.8 Joining ligaments the humerus and scapula stress results during flexion movement

Figure 6.9 compares the stress results between the ligaments that provide union between scapula and clavicle. The compression results indicate that the CAL exhibited a value of − 0.44481 MPa, while the CCL trapezoid measurement showed a value of − 0.2955 MPa.

Figure 6.10 illustrates the results of stress in soft tissues and shows a range of compression stress with values between − 10.55 and − 1.145 MPa. These negative results represent a compression in ligaments while movement takes place, and it was obtained from the numerical analysis simulation.

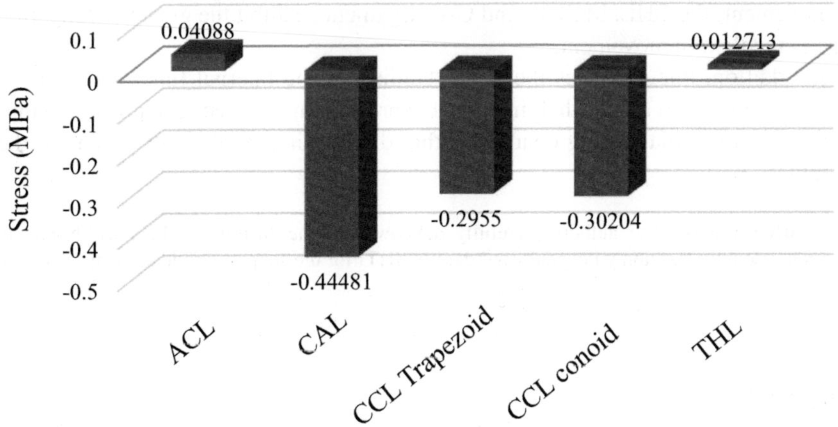

Fig. 6.9 Joining ligaments the scapula and clavicle stress results during flexion movement

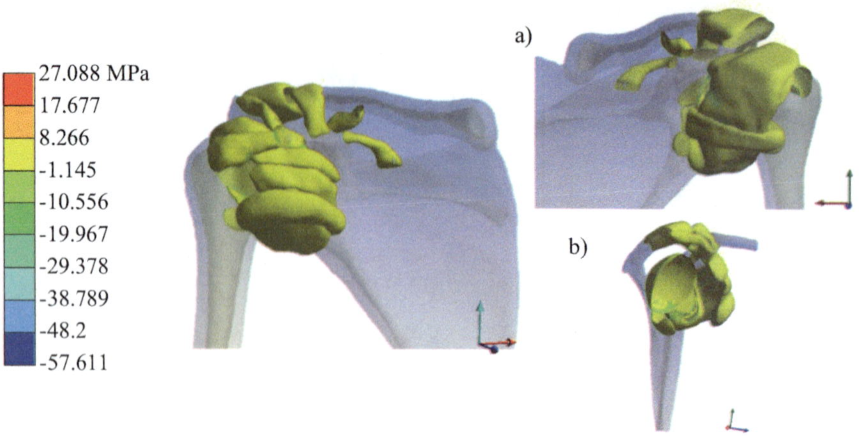

Fig. 6.10 Biomodel stress distribution. **a** Biomodel posterior view. **b** Scapula with soft tissue side view

6.4 Conclusion

Biomodels are defined by their accuracy and accurate depiction of the biological system they represent. They serve as an alternative for analyzing different biological tissues, as they avoid ethical, legal, and moral issues by not utilizing invasive methods that could hurt the patient's physical well-being, saving time, economic, and material resources. It is important for this analysis to determine the internal stress, elongation, and contractions found in the static structures of the shoulder. Therefore, taking into account the results aligned with previous literature (Fox et al. 2021), which indicated areas in the soft tissues experiencing compression and tension during the flexion movement, the regions displaying significant elongation and stress concentrations can be identified, allowing for a numerical assessment of the ligaments most engaged in movement; the CHL, MGHL, and CAL ligaments exhibit the greatest elongation during the flexion movement.

In addition, this enhances the understanding of the internal functioning of the shoulder joint's soft tissues, helping medical professionals in recognizing new symptoms that aid in diagnosing conditions that directly impact the soft tissues of the shoulder.

Acknowledgements The authors gratefully acknowledge the Instituto Politécnico Nacional, Secretaria de Investigacion y Posgrado and the SECIHTI for the support provided to this research.

Appendix

See Tables 6.2 and 6.3.

Table 6.2 Abbreviations used in this manuscript

Abbreviation	Ligament name
SGHL	Superior glenohumerla ligament
MGHL	Medial glenohumeral ligament
aIGHL	Anterior band of the inferior glenohumeral ligament
pIGHL	Posterior band of the inferior glenohumeral ligament
CHL	Coracohumeral ligament
CAL	Coracoacromial ligament
ACL	Acromioclavicular ligament
CCL	Coracoclavicular ligament
THL	Transverse humeral ligament

Table 6.3 Nodes and elements for each biomodel structure

Biological tissue	Nodes	Elements
SGHL	19,847	11,309
MGHL	17,604	10,060
aIGHL	30,476	17,864
pGHL	23,840	13,864
Articular capsule	77,645	45,152
CHLl	17,576	9416
CAL	10,097	5312
ACL	16,205	8506
CCL trapezoid	12,175	6365
CCL conoid	9043	4684
TLC	5753	2873
Labrum	17,423	9198
Glenoid cartilage	38,183	21,037
Humeral head cartilage	104,484	53,642

References

Castro-Abril HA, Ramlrez A, Silva L (2015) Modelo de elementos finitos del hombro: comparación de los esfuerzos mecánicos de un hombro sano y un hombro con síndrome del manguito rotador. Rev Invest 8(1):43–50. https://doi.org/10.29097/issn.2011-639X

Corea-Corona, MI, Urriolagoitia-Sosa G, Romero-Ángeles B, Urriolagoitia-Luna A, Maya-Anaya D, Suarez-Hemández M, de la L, Trejo-Enríquez A, Urriolagoitia-Calderón GM (2023) Application of the finite element model using modeling of a human bone system with osteoporosis for biomedical and mechanical analysis. MOJ Appl Biomech 7(1):14–15. https://doi.org/10.15406/mojabb.2023.07.00169

Edizer M (2022) Fundamentals of the shoulder. In: Huri G, Özkan M, Bilsel K (eds) Fundamentals of the shoulder. Springer, Cham. https://doi.org/10.1007/978-3-030-94702-6_1

Favre P, Senteler M, Hipp J, Scherrer S, Gerber C (2012) An integrated model of active glenohumeral stability. J Biomech 45:2248–2255. https://doi.org/10.1016/j.jbiomech.2012.06.010

Fox AJ, Fox OJ, Schär MO, Chaudhury S, Warren RF, Rodeo SA (2021) The glenohumeral ligaments: superior, middle, and inferior: anatomy, biomechanics, injury, and diagnosis. Clin Anat 34(2):283–296. https://doi.org/10.1002/ca.23717

Hayes WC, Piazza SJ, Zysset PK (1991) Biomechanics of fracture risk prediction of the hip and spine by quantitative computed tomography. Radiol Clin N Am 29(1):1–18. https://doi.org/10.1016/S0033-838902675-6

Kadi R, Milants A, Shahabpour M (2017) Shoulder anatomy and normal variants. Journal of 533 the Belgian society of. Radiology 101(Suppl 2), 3. https://doi.org/10.5334/jbr-btr.1467

Maldonado JA, Puentes DA, Quintero ID, González-Estrada OA, Villegas DF (2023) Image-based numerical analysis for isolated type II SLAP lesions in shoulder abduction and external rotation. Diagnostics 13(10):1819. https://doi.org/10.3390/diagnostics13101819

Maya-Anaya D, Urriolagoitia-Sosa G, Romero-Ángeles B, Martinez-Mondragon M, German-Carcaño JM, Correa-Corona MI, Trejo-Enriquez A, Sánchez-Cervantes A, Urriolagoitia-Luna A, Urriolagoitia-Calderón GM (2023) Numerical analysis applying the finite element method by developing a complex three-dimensional biomodel of the biological tissues of the elbow joint using computerized axial tomography. Appl Sci 13(15):8903. https://doi.org/10.3390/app13158903

Mendoza-Muñoz A, Gonzales-Angeles G, Jacobo-Garcia G, LópezAvitia R (2017) Estimation of the main properties in looking plates design for proximal humerus fracture with the finite element method and DOE. In: 2017 Global Medical Engineering Physics Exchanges/Pan American Health Care Exchanges (GMEPE/PAHCE). IEEE, 1–5, March 2017. https://doi.org/10.1109/GMEPE-PAHCE.2017.7972121

Nordin M, Frankel VH (2004) Biomecánica básica del sistema musculoesquelético. McGraw-Hill

Serrato-Pedrosa JA, Urriolagoitia-Sosa G, Romero-Ángeles B, Carrasco-Hernández F, Gallegos-Funes FJ, Trejo-Enriquez A, Carbajal-López A, Gomez-Niebla JA, Correa-Corona MI, Urriolagoitia-Calderón GM (2024) Numerical analysis of the plantar pressure points during the stance phases for the design of a 3D-printable patientspecific insole. PRO 6(3):429–456. https://doi.org/10.3390/prosthesis6030032

Veeger HEJ, Van Der Helm FCT (2007) Shoulder function: the perfect compromise between mobility and stability. J Biomech 40(10):2119–2129. https://doi.org/10.1016/j.jbiomech.2006.10.016

Zheng M, Qian Z, Zou Z, Peach C, Akrami M, Ren L (2020) Subject-specific finite element modelling of the human shoulder complex part 1; model construction and quasi-static abduction simulation. J Bionic Eng 17(6):1224–1238. https://doi.org/10.1007/s42235-020-0098-0

Chapter 7
State of the Art in Engineering Solutions for Floating Hip Cases: A Proposed Methodology for Prosthesis Design

Alfredo Carbajal-López, Juan Alfonso Beltrán-Fernández, and Elías Humberto Hermida-Ochoa

Abstract A floating hip is an ipsilateral injury affecting the pelvis, acetabulum, and the femur related to high-energy accidents. This study conducts a comprehensive literature review to analyze state-of-the-art engineering solutions for floating hip injuries, including country, gender, mechanism of injury, type of fracture, and principal treatments. There were nine studies from 1992 to 2025, and 284 patients showed cases of floating hip injuries, 189 males (67%) and 95 females (33%), with a mean age of 36.84 years. According to the literature, this pathology has three types: A, B, and C, with a predominant type B fracture in almost all cases (pelvic ring fracture associated with ipsilateral femoral fracture). This study aims to present a methodology for developing prostheses through analysis that evaluates areas of opportunity, such as computational modeling, finite element analysis, and patient-specific design considerations.

Keywords Floating hip · Fracture · Injuries · Ipsilateral · Study

---

A. Carbajal-López · J. A. Beltrán-Fernández (✉)
Sección de Estudios de Posgrado e Investigación, Escuela Superior de Ingeniería Mecánica y Eléctrica, Unidad Zacatenco, "Unidad Profesional Adolfo López Mateos", Instituto Politécnico Nacional, Ciudad de México, Mexico
e-mail: jbeltran@ipn.mx

A. Carbajal-López
e-mail: acarbajall2200@alumno.ipn.mx

E. H. Hermida-Ochoa
CILAB—Hospital Germán Díaz Lombardo, Alcaldía Álvaro Obregón, Ciudad de México, Mexico
e-mail: drelias@hermidagroup.com

A. Öchsner (ed.), *Progress in Biomaterials and Biomedical Engineering*, Advanced Structured Materials 249, https://doi.org/10.1007/978-3-032-13551-3_7

7.1 Introduction

The hip joint is located in the lower limb, as shown in Fig. 7.1, and consists of bony and soft tissues such as the femur, pelvis (ilium, ischium, and pubis), articular cartilage, and ligaments (Sen and Jha 2017; Thorp 2014). The spherical shape of the hip joint allows simultaneous movements involving the three anatomical axes (sagittal, axial, and coronal). These movements are transmitted from the femur to the pelvis or vice versa, such as abduction, adduction, extension, flexion, and circumduction, as shown in Fig. 7.2. Examples include lifting the foot or rotating the trunk while the body rests on one limb (Neumann 2010; Saputra et al. 2013).

However, these structures are affected by various pathologies involving both the femur and pelvis, as well as the surrounding soft tissues. Causes include osteoporosis, age, sex, obesity, accidents, falls, or high-impact sports.

These conditions reduce quality of life by limiting natural movements such as walking, running, or jumping, and often cause pain and discomfort. Total hip replacements allow patients to partially regain their previous lifestyle; consequently, annual

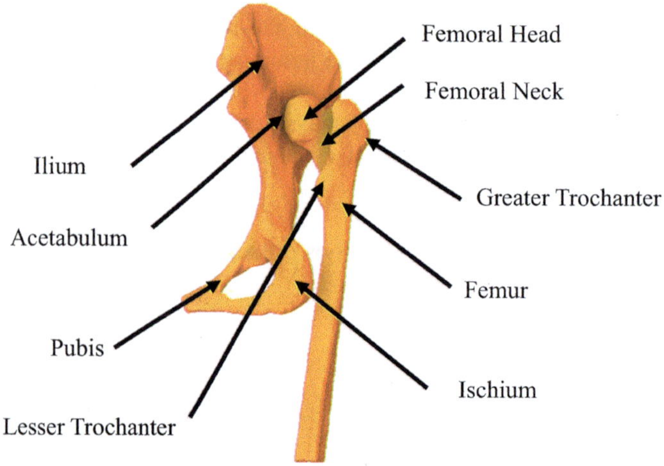

Fig. 7.1 Anatomy of the hip joint

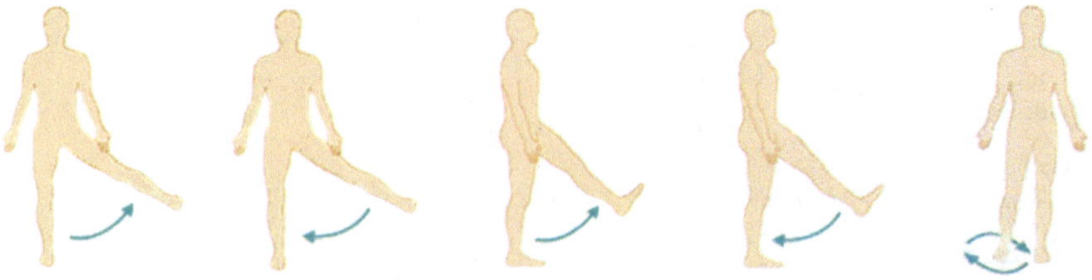

Fig. 7.2 Hip movements

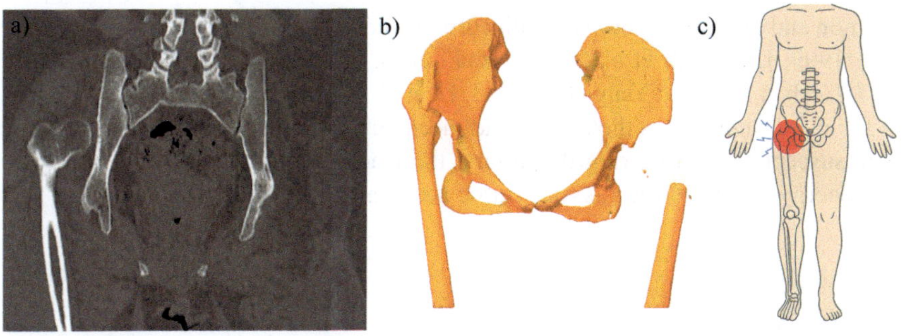

Fig. 7.3 **a** Tomography of a floating hip case. **b** Biomodel of the hip joint. **c** Location of hip injury

surgeries exceed one million worldwide (Barceló et al. 2021; Prieto-Alhambra et al. 2014; Blankenbaker and De Smet 2010; Glazebrook et al. 2008; Giordano et al. 2023; Ferguson et al. 2018).

Among these pathologies mentioned above, there are also atypical cases such as a floating hip, as shown in Fig. 7.3. This condition affects a small portion of the population, with an incidence of approximately one in ten thousand fractures (Sen and Jha 2017; Thorp 2014; Neumann 2010; Saputra et al. 2013; Barceló et al. 2021). Because different regions of the joint bones are simultaneously affected, ipsilateral fractures occur. Being uncommon, this condition presents significant challenges in biomechanics due to the limited information available in the literature. Therefore, this review aims to develop a methodology for designing customized prostheses according to the different floating hip types reported, identifying opportunities for improvement in prosthetic and implant development (Ferguson et al. 2018).

7.2 Methodology

The research began with a bibliographic compilation from the first paper in 1992 to 2025, including the type of fracture, treatments, gender, country, and mechanism of lesion (Liebergall et al. 1992; Müller et al. 1999; Liebergall et al. 2002; Suzuki et al. 2006; Burd et al. 2008; Siavashi 2017; Cech et al. 2021; Yang et al. 2023; Li et al. 2025). Table 7.1 shows this pathology's classification according to the fracture zone.

Figure 7.4 shows a demographic representation of floating hip studies. However, there is a lack of information in many countries, which means this pathology is not

Table 7.1 Floating hip types (Liebergall et al. 1992)

Type A	Acetabular fracture associated with ipsilateral femoral fracture
Type B	Pelvic ring fracture associated with ipsilateral femoral fracture
Type C	Combined pelvic and acetabular fractures with ipsilateral femoral fracture

common and difficult to compare with current studies (Liebergall et al. 1992; Müller et al. 1999; Liebergall et al. 2002; Suzuki et al. 2006; Burd et al. 2008; Siavashi 2017; Cech et al. 2021; Yang et al. 2023; Li et al. 2025).

Table 7.2 summarizes the gender and mechanism of injury of 9 studies. Men are more susceptible to suffering this injury, the leading cause of which is related to high-energy accidents such as road traffic accidents and falls from height.

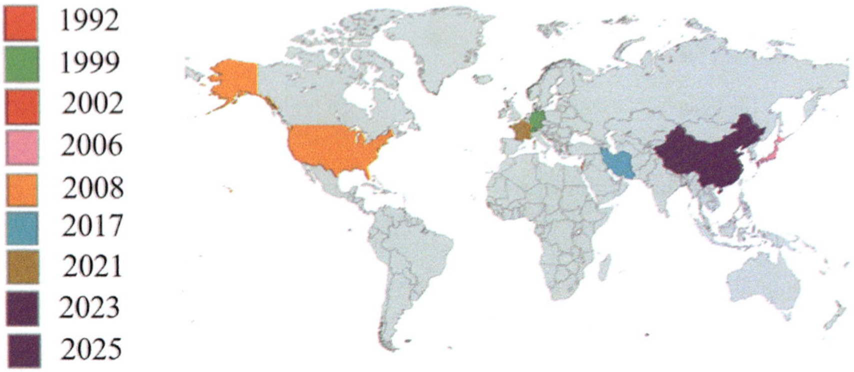

Fig. 7.4 Geographic representation of floating hip research (Liebergall et al. 1992; Müller et al. 1999; Liebergall et al. 2002; Suzuki et al. 2006; Burd et al. 2008; Siavashi 2017; Cech et al. 2021; Yang et al. 2023; Li et al. 2025)

Table 7.2 Summary of demographics and mechanisms of injury in floating hip cases (Liebergall et al. 1992; Müller et al. 1999; Liebergall et al. 2002; Suzuki et al. 2006; Burd et al. 2008; Siavashi 2017; Cech et al. 2021; Yang et al. 2023; Li et al. 2025)

Study	Demographics			Mechanism of injury		
	Male	Female	Mean age	Road traffic accident	Fall from height	Other
Liebergall et al. (1992)	12	5	33	11	6	–
Müller et al. (1999)	19	21	31	38	8	–
Liebergall et al. (2002)	16	4	33.7	16	4	–
Suzuki et al. (2006)	18	13	35.5	17	13	1
Burd et al. (2008)	36	21	33.9	52	5	–
Siavashi (2017)	6	5	42.3	–	–	11
Cech et al. (2021)	51	18	38.5	18	–	51
Yang et al. (2023)	22	6	45	15	7	6
Li et al. (2025)	9	2	38.7	6	5	–

Table 7.3 Principal treatments for floating hip (Liebergall et al. 1992; Müller et al. 1999; Liebergall et al. 2002; Suzuki et al. 2006; Burd et al. 2008; Siavashi 2017; Cech et al. 2021; Yang et al. 2023; Li et al. 2025)

Principal treatments	
1	Plate fixation
2	Intramedullary nail
3	Screw fixation
4	Dynamic compression screw
5	Extermal fixator
6	Blade-plate
7	Hemiarthroplasty
9	Non-surgical

Table 7.3 shows the main treatments for floating hips in these studies; however, there is not enough information about the design, materials, or new proposal designs.

Based on the findings, a structured methodology is proposed for developing custom prosthetic solutions to restore biomechanical stability, minimize stress shielding, and enhance functional recovery. Computational modeling, finite element analysis, and patient-specific design considerations are incorporated to ensure optimal prosthetic performance, as presented in Fig. 7.5.

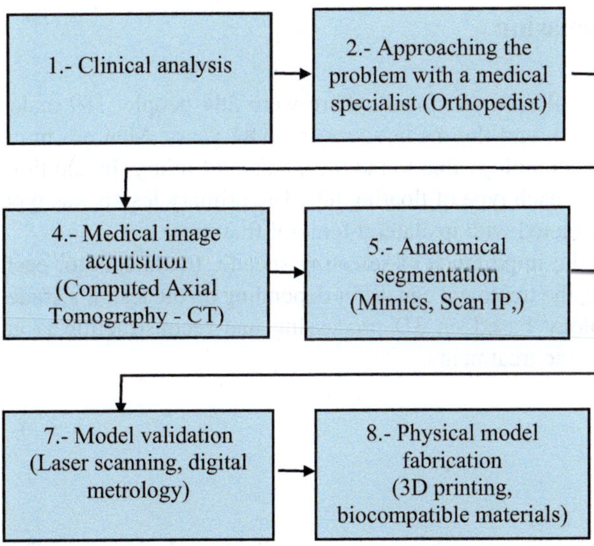

Fig. 7.5 Proposed methodology for prosthesis design

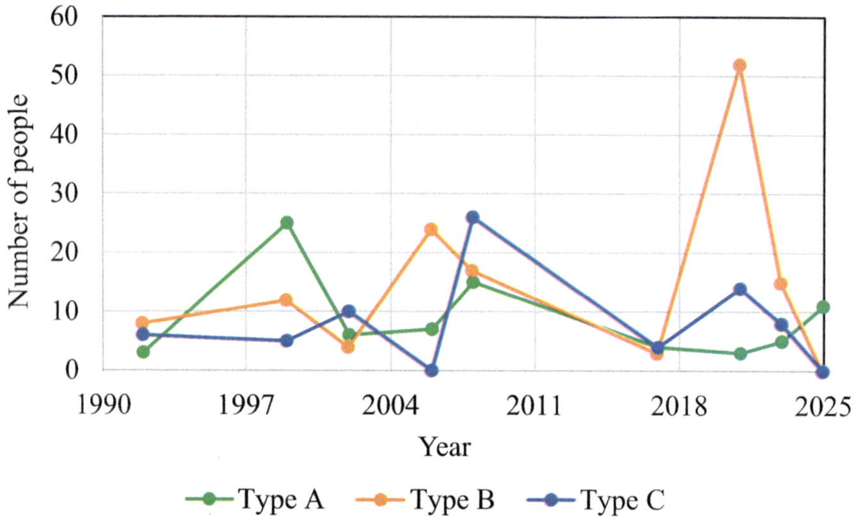

Fig. 7.6 Type A, B, and C hip injuries: literature review (Liebergall et al. 1992; Müller et al. 1999; Liebergall et al. 2002; Suzuki et al. 2006; Burd et al. 2008; Siavashi 2017; Cech et al. 2021; Yang et al. 2023; Li et al. 2025)

7.3 Results and Discussion

Based on the information collected previously, there were 284 people, 189 males (67%) and 95 females (33%), and the mean age was 36.84 years. Men are more susceptible to suffering this pathology due to the mechanism of injury. In addition, Fig. 7.6 shows the quality of each type of floating hip. The primary lesion was type B (Pelvic ring fracture associated with ipsilateral femoral fracture).

These results highlight the importance of selecting specific treatments for each type of injury. Furthermore, the treatment can differ depending on the lesion's grade, so the proposed methodology based on 3D processing and reconstruction is an alternative solution for specific treatments.

7.4 Conclusions

The hip is vital for everyday activities such as working, walking, and exercising. This study demonstrated the importance of compiling information on floating hip types to analyze the condition and establish a methodology for prosthesis development. Such research helps to create hip prosthesis prototypes due to the complexity and uniqueness of the necessary interventions, which may vary depending on the area of the injuries that occur ipsilaterally and in two different bones. These cases help to develop prosthesis models and to evaluate causes such as accidents, age, and gender.

Based on these results, techniques can be presented for developing customized prostheses. Future work will involve experimental validation and clinical trials to evaluate the feasibility and effectiveness of the proposed prosthetic framework. By addressing the biomechanical challenges associated with floating hip injuries, this research is expected to contribute to the advancement of more effective prosthetic interventions, ultimately leading to improved patient prognosis and quality of life.

Acknowledgements The authors gratefully acknowledge the grant awarded by the Instituto Politécnico Nacional, Secretaría de Ciencia, Humanidades, Tecnología e Innovación (SECIHTI), and COFFA for supporting this research.

References

Barceló M, Torres OH, Mascaró J, Casademont J (2021) Hip fracture and mortality: study of specific causes of death and risk factors. Arch Osteoporos 16:15. https://doi.org/10.1007/s11657-020-00873-7

Blankenbaker DG, De Smet AA (2010) Hip injuries in athletes. Radiol Clin North Am 48(6):1155–1178. https://doi.org/10.1016/j.rcl.2010.07.003

Burd TA, Hughes MS, Anglen JO (2008) The floating hip: complications and outcomes. J Trauma 64(2):442–448. https://doi.org/10.1097/TA.0b013e31815eba69

Cech A, Rieussec C, Kerschbaumer G, Seurat O, Corbet C, Vibert B, Tronc C, Ruatti S, Bouzat P, Tonetti J, Boudissa M (2021) Complications and outcomes in 69 consecutive patients with floating hip. Orthop Traumatol Surg Res 107(6):102998. https://doi.org/10.1016/j.otsr.2021.102998

Ferguson RJ, Palmer AJ, Taylor A, Porter ML, Malchau H, Glyn-Jones S (2018) Hip replacement. Lancet 392(10158):1662–1671. https://doi.org/10.1016/S0140-6736(18)31777-X

Giordano V, Miura KF, Calegari IT, Pires RE, Freitas A, Altamirano-Cruz MA, Taype D, Giannoudis PV (2023) Simultaneous ipsilateral floating hip and knee: the double floating extremity—a systematic review and proposal of a treatment algorithm. Eur J Trauma Emerg Surg 49(5):2057–2069. https://doi.org/10.1007/s00068-023-02277-x

Glazebrook M, Daniels T, Younger A, Foote CJ, Penner M, Wing K, Lau J, Leighton R, Dunbar M (2008) Comparison of health-related quality of life between patients with end-stage ankle and hip arthrosis. J Bone Joint Surg Am 90(3):499–505. https://doi.org/10.2106/JBJS.F.01299

Li L, Li L, Zhou D, Zhao Q, Li C (2025) Characteristics and treatment strategies of the hip fracture triad. Front Surg 12:1510344. https://doi.org/10.3389/fsurg.2025.1510344

Liebergall M, Lowe J, Whitelaw GP, Wetzler MJ, Segal D (1992) The floating hip. Ipsilateral pelvic and femoral fractures. J Bone Joint Surg Br 74(1):93–100. https://doi.org/10.1302/0301-620X.74B1.1732275

Liebergall M, Mosheiff R, Safran O, Peyser A, Segal D (2002) The floating hip injury: patterns of injury. Injury 33(8):717–722. https://doi.org/10.1016/S0020-1383(01)00204-2

Müller EJ, Siebenrock K, Ekkernkamp A, Ganz R, Muhr G (1999) Ipsilateral fractures of the pelvis and the femur—floating hip? A retrospective analysis of 42 cases. Arch Orthop Trauma Surg 119(3–4):179–182. https://doi.org/10.1007/s004020050385

Neumann DA (2010) Kinesiology of the hip: a focus on muscular actions. J Orthop Sports Phys Ther 40(2):82–94. https://doi.org/10.2519/jospt.2010.3025

Prieto-Alhambra D, Judge A, Javaid MK, Cooper C, Diez-Perez A, Arden NK (2014) Incidence and risk factors for clinically diagnosed knee, hip and hand osteoarthritis: influences of age, gender and osteoarthritis affecting other joints. Ann Rheum Dis 73(9):1659–1664. https://doi.org/10.1136/annrheumdis-2013-203355

Saputra E, Anwar IB, Jamari J, van der Heide E (2013) Finite element analysis of artificial hip joint movement during human activities. Procedia Eng 68:102–108. https://doi.org/10.1016/j.proeng.2013.12.154

Sen RK, Jha L (2017) Floating hip. J. Clin Orthop 2(1):43–48

Siavashi B (2017) Floating hip, eleven cases and literature review. J Orthop Spine Trauma 3(1):e63868. https://doi.org/10.5812/jost.63868

Suzuki T, Shindo M, Soma K (2006) The floating hip injury: which should we fix first? Eur J Orthop Surg Traumatol 16(3):214–218. https://doi.org/10.1007/s00590-006-0081-4

Thorp LE (2014) Hip anatomy. In: Nho SJ, Bedi A, Salata MJ, Mather RC III, Kelly BT (eds) Hip arthroscopy and hip joint preservation surgery. Springer, New York, pp 3–15. https://doi.org/10.1007/978-1-4614-6965-0_113

Yang Y, Zou C, Fang Y, Shakya S (2023) Medium-term clinical results in patients with floating hip injuries. BMC Surg 23(1):40. https://doi.org/10.1186/s12893-023-01927-6

Chapter 8
Biomechanical Evaluation of Upper Limb Arthroplasty in Amputees and the Effects of Phantom Limb Syndrome Through a Prosthetic Device Compliant with NOM-241-SSA1-2021

Karen Pamela Vázquez-Thierry, Juan Alfonso Beltrán-Fernández, Alejandro Tonatiu Velázquez Sánchez, Erik Omar Alvarado-Alcántara, Verónica Guzmán-Mercado, Gabriel Josue Reyes-Morales, and Alejandro González-Rebattú

Abstract This study focuses on establishing the design and engineering parameters of a myoelectric prosthetic device for upper limb amputations, developed in compliance with Mexican health regulation NOM-241-SSA1-2021, which outlines good manufacturing practices for medical devices. The prosthesis was designed based on the anthropometric and anatomical characteristics of the case study: a female patient with complete finger amputation in the right hand. In addition, the research analyzes the biomechanical effects of prosthesis use on the residual limb's functionality, as well as the potential influence of the phantom limb syndrome on the user's adaptation process.

K. P. Vázquez-Thierry · J. A. Beltrán-Fernández (✉) · A. T. V. Sánchez ·
E. O. Alvarado-Alcántara · V. Guzmán-Mercado · G. J. Reyes-Morales · A. González-Rebattú
Escuela Superior de Ingeniería Mecánica y Eléctrica, Instituto Politécnico Nacional, Ciudad de México, México
e-mail: jbeltran@ipn.mx

K. P. Vázquez-Thierry
e-mail: kvazquezt2200@alumno.ipn.mx

A. T. V. Sánchez
e-mail: atvelazquezs@ipn.mx

E. O. Alvarado-Alcántara
e-mail: ealvaradoa1800@alumno.ipn.mx

V. Guzmán-Mercado
e-mail: vguzmanm0900@alumno.ipn.mx

G. J. Reyes-Morales
e-mail: greyes1100@alumno.ipn.mx

A. Öchsner (ed.), *Progress in Biomaterials and Biomedical Engineering*, Advanced Structured Materials 249, https://doi.org/10.1007/978-3-032-13551-3_8

Keywords Myoelectric prosthesis · Electromyographic (EMG) signals · Complete finger amputation · Upper limb prosthetics · Biomechanical analysis

8.1 Introduction

The Western world has experienced an annual increase in patients undergoing amputations, mainly due to the aging population, which leads to a higher prevalence of chronic and vascular diseases (Kaur and Guan 2018).

In the United States alone, nearly 1.7 million people live with limb amputations (Kaur and Guan 2018). Regarding national figures, the National Academy of Medicine in Mexico estimates that around 75 amputations are performed daily, amounting to more than 25,000 cases per year (de Armas Mestre et al. 2021).

According to the Amputee Coalition, nearly 80% of amputee patients worldwide experience symptoms of the phantom limb syndrome. This condition represents a significant global health concern and, unfortunately, in many cases, remains undetected and undiagnosed (Amputee Coalition).

The general objective of this study is to design and develop a customized myoelectric prosthetic device tailored to the specific needs of patients with upper limb amputations.

8.2 Methodology

The research methodology, described in Fig. 8.1, is based on the design thinking approach. It is a process that employs creative tools to support decision-making and is oriented toward solutions that address end-user needs (CRN Digital Design Thinking).

The development of the device is organized into five main phases, which culminate in the production of the initial functional prototype:

A. Empathize. Identify and understand the user's needs—in this study, the clinical case—in order to establish a connection and provide solutions that create user-centered value.
B. Define. Collect and analyze information to determine the scope of the project and propose feasible solutions.
C. Ideate. Generate ideas to address the problem, including potential approaches for prototype development.
D. Prototype. Translate ideas into sketches, illustrations, and/or models that support prototype manufacturing. At this stage, mechanical and electrical instrumentation is integrated.
E. Evaluate. Conduct product validation, where all design decisions are tested and subjected to different analyses for approval or refinement.

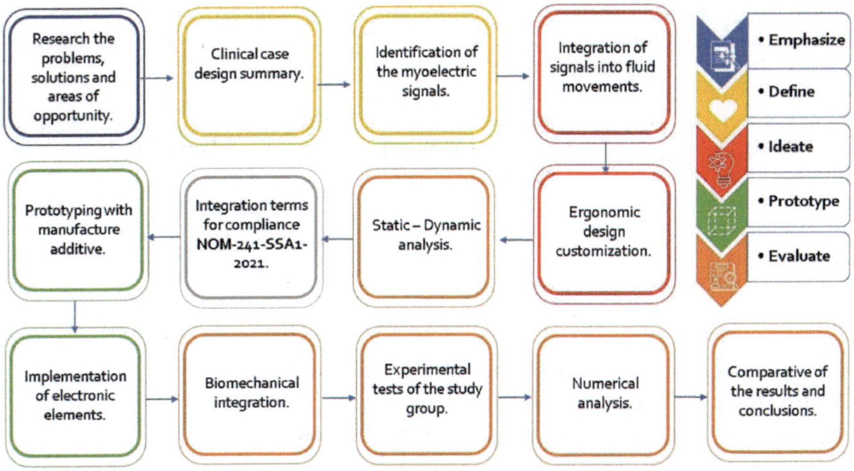

Fig. 8.1 Design and development methodology of the prosthesis

8.3 Stages of the Myoelectric Prosthesis Design

8.3.1 Design Based on Regulation NOM-241-SSA1-2021

NOM-241-SSA1-2021 establishes good manufacturing practices (GMP) for medical devices. This standard is applied to ensure a system of quality, safety, and functionality, defining the minimum requirements for the design, development, manufacturing, storage, and distribution of medical devices (Diario Oficial de la Federación Mexicana 2021) (Fig. 8.2).

Health regulations and standards are defined as a set of rules and preventive actions established by the State, "to regulate and control the sanitary conditions of human habitats, establishments, activities, products, equipment, vehicles, and individuals that may pose a risk or cause harm to the health of the general population" (Instituto de Salud del Estado de México).

This study addresses the first two stages of the regulatory process, as shown in Fig. 8.3. The processes considered during these stages are the following (Diario Oficial de la Federación Mexicana):

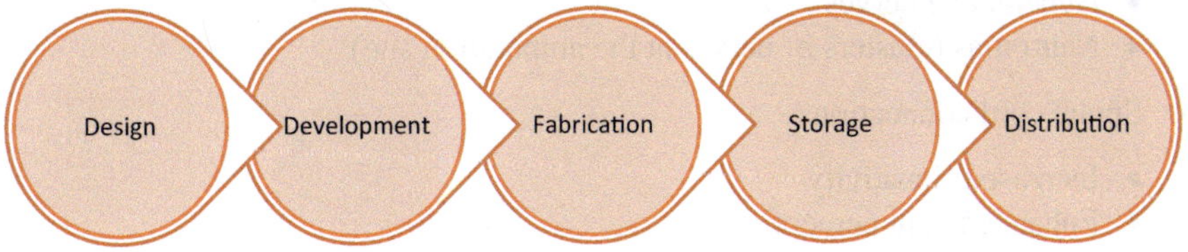

Fig. 8.2 Stages of the regulations for good practices in the design of Mexican devices

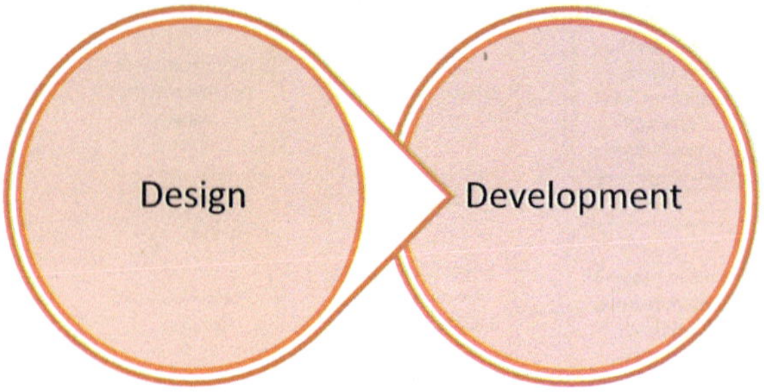

Fig. 8.3 Stages of the regulations addressed in this study

1. Document the processes of design and development.
2. Implement a change control system.
3. Establish a risk-based quality management framework.
4. Guarantee device quality.
5. Define a qualification and validation system.

8.3.2 Characterization of PLP: Neurological and Biomechanical Aspects

The phantom limb syndrome (PLP), caused by limb amputation, was first described by the French surgeon Ambroise Paré in the sixteenth century and later named by Silas Weir Mitchell in 1872. It occurs in patients who have lost a limb through accidental or surgical amputation, yet continue to experience phantom sensations from the missing limb (Angarita et al. 2013).

The main causes of PLP in amputee patients are classified into two main categories (Angarita et al. 2013):

Neurological factors

1. Cortical reorganization
   - Maladaptive cortical plasticity
   - Somatosensory reorganization leading to pain release
   - Neurons responding to adjacent stimuli
2. Spontaneous peripheral nerve activity
   - Hyperactive nerves
   - Neuromas (clusters of nerves at the amputation site)
3. Spinal cord connections
   - Increased sensitivity
   - Enhanced pain perception

Biomechanical factors

1. Loss of proprioceptive feedback
    - Absence of signals from muscles, tendons, and joints causes phantom sensations
2. Residual muscle contractions
    - Nearby muscles remain active
    - Sensation of movement
3. Difficulties in prosthesis use
    - Lack of sensory feedback may result in rejection

8.3.3 Differentiating Factors of the Prosthesis

There is a wide variety of prosthetic options. Advances in technology have transformed this into a continuously evolving field of healthcare. The customized myoelectric prosthesis proposed in this study, based on comparative analysis, demonstrates certain characteristics that distinguish it from existing solutions (Akbari 2023):

- Personalization
    - Adjustments tailored to the patient's anthropometric and anthropomorphic features (e.g., size and shape).
- Lightweight and flexible materials
    - Use of flexible polymers that mimic muscle behavior
    - Custom 3D printing for precise fit
- Improved power supply
    - Longer-lasting batteries
    - Wireless charging
    - Energy generation through movement
- Affordability
    - Open-source technologies
    - Additive manufacturing (e.g., 3D printing)
- Neural control or adaptive AI
    - Interfaces enabling natural interaction
    - Algorithms capable of learning and adapting to user routines
- Connectivity
    - Mobile application integration
    - Voice assistant compatibility

- Sensory feedback
  - Sensors to measure temperature, pressure, or textures
  - Electrical stimulation on the skin to provide tactile perception

8.3.4 Neuromuscular Basis of Myoelectric Control

The principle of myoelectric prosthesis control is based on muscle contractions producing electromyographic (EMG) signals. These imperceptible electrical signals are detectable with non-invasive sensors. Depending on the gesture performed, the prosthesis interprets the intent of movement and activates accordingly (Vicerrectorado de Investigación PUCP 2024).

Electromyographic signals are bioelectrical potentials generated during muscle contractions. They are collected through electrodes placed on the skin over the muscle. These signals are relatively small, ranging between 5 and 20 microvolts (μV) (Benavides-Álvarez et al. 2025).

There are two main types of EMG signals:

- Surface electromyography, using external electrodes
- Intramuscular (or invasive) electromyography, using needle electrodes (Benavides-Álvarez et al. 2025)

The main stages for the development of a myoelectric prosthesis are shown in Fig. 8.4 (Muñoz-Gil 2021).

A. Nervous muscle fibers. Identification of the muscle area with the highest electrical activity, representing the biopotential of the residual stump. Correct electrode placement is crucial for accurate sampling.
B. Sensors and electrodes. Surface EMG electrodes collect the user's muscle biopotentials.
C. Coding. Programming with Arduino to build a control board that translates collected signals into numerical data for interpretation.
D. Processing and visualization. Transformation of numerical data into graphical outputs and system feedback.

The development of the electrical control system is based on the biomechanical application "Design of a system for the rehabilitation of patients with symptoms caused by phantom limb syndrome in patients with total amputations" (Fig. 8.5). From signal acquisition, filtering, verification, and feedback, the process culminates in the design of a servomotor control system that enables operation of the myoelectric prosthesis.

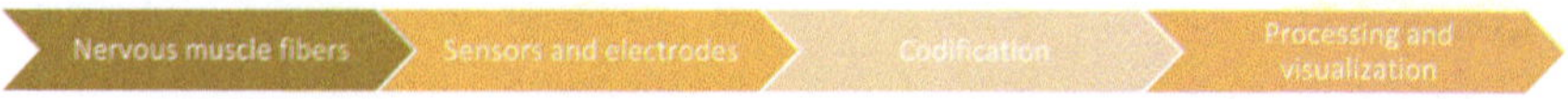

Fig. 8.4 Diagram of myoelectric signal processing, and its four main stages

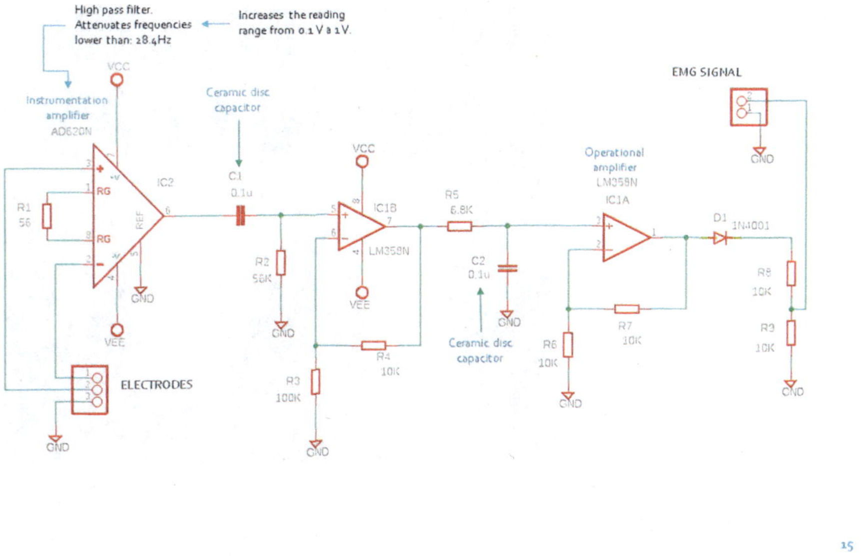

Fig. 8.5 Reference diagram of the electrical control system for an upper limb prosthesis (2024) (Vázquez-Thierry et al. 2024)

8.3.5 Personalization According to the Case Study

The need to design a customized myoelectric prosthesis enables better usability and faster adaptation. An ergonomic design tailored to the patient's specific characteristics improves pressure distribution, optimizes force transmission, and reduces discomfort. Furthermore, this approach can also lower production costs compared with conventional manufacturing processes (Aquino et al. 2018).

According to the axial tomography shown in Fig. 8.6, the case study involves a 16-year-old female patient who suffered a traumatic total amputation of four fingers on her left hand due to burns from boiling oil. The phantom limb syndrome was present, and the residual stump had been rehabilitated and was prepared for prosthetic fitting.

The process for obtaining the three-dimensional model of the patient's limb from imaging is carried out through various techniques, illustrated in Fig. 8.7:

A. Axial tomography. Obtaining the model of the region of interest from the patient's computed tomography (CT) scan.
B. Segmentation. The musculoskeletal tissues are delimited according to their density, allowing the selection of specific areas, components, or tissues to be analyzed.
C. Reconstruction and processing. The model is processed using specialized parameterization software, providing the necessary refinement and finish for subsequent manufacturing.

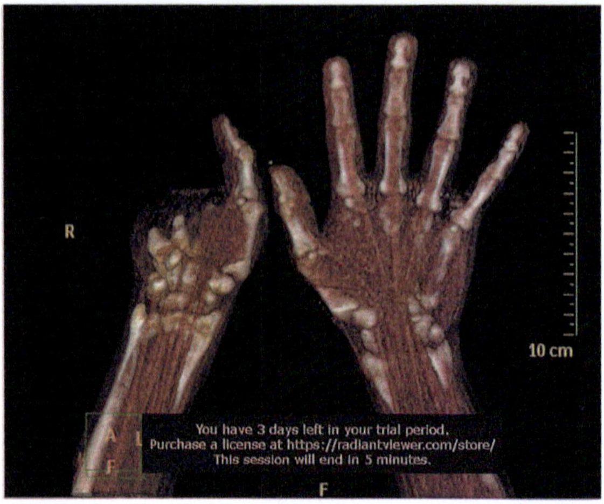

Fig. 8.6 Axial tomography of the case study

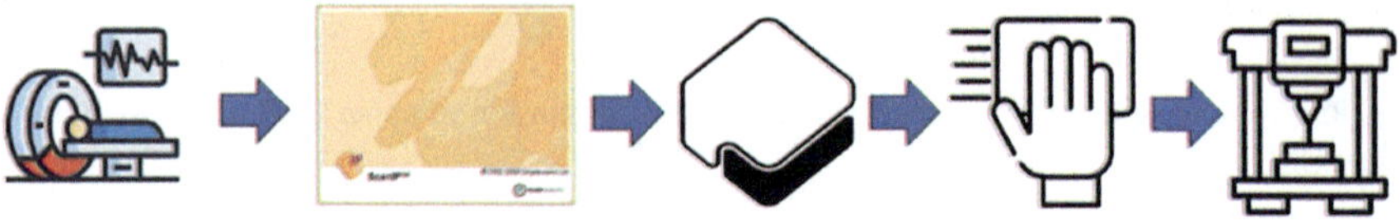

Fig. 8.7 Process of obtaining a 3D model from axial tomography

D. Experimental analysis. The digital file is subjected to validation testing through numerical simulations and experimental analyses. Components are evaluated using mechanical finite element analysis (FEA), including forces, vibration, heat transfer, and fluid flow, to assess structural integrity.
E. Additive manufacturing. Finally, the component is produced through additive manufacturing, with an appropriate selection of processes and materials.

The design of the phalanges derived from the segmentation of the case study allows for the creation of a preliminary prototype that addresses the specific needs of the patient. As illustrated in Fig. 8.8, the phalangeal components were reconstructed from the healthy hand, mirrored, and replicated in the amputated hand.

8.3.6 Preliminary Prototype

Starting from the 3D reconstruction of the phalanges in the study case, a geometric analysis was conducted to identify the articular surfaces and rotational axes (Fig. 8.9).

1. Importation of the 3D segmented models of the study case.

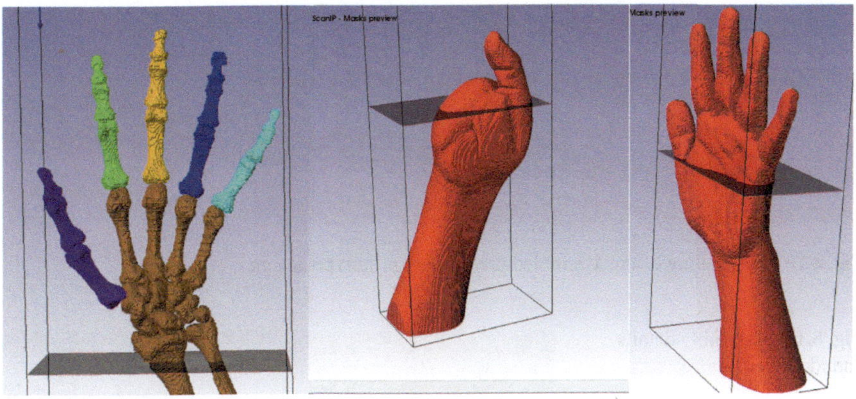

Fig. 8.8 Case study segmentation of the healthy and amputated hand

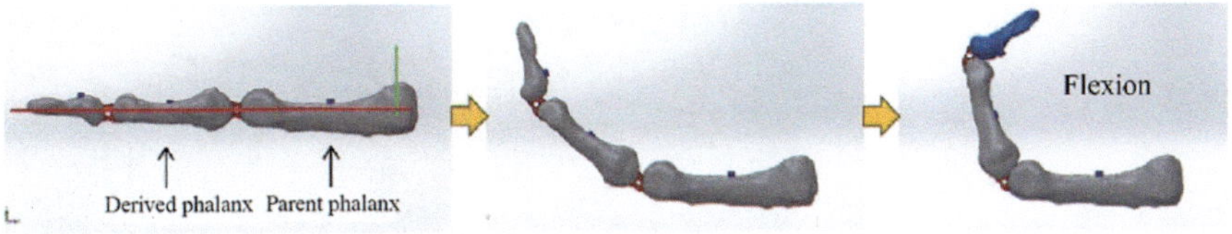

Fig. 8.9 Preliminary assembled prototype design

2. Bone alignment. Correct positioning according to anatomical landmarks based on osteology, ensuring that the axis of rotation is perpendicular to the flexion plane.
3. Establishing hierarchy. Definition of the reference phalanx as the fixed object designated as the "parent," and the mobile phalanx as the "child," which can rotate relative to its rotational axis.
4. Validation. Verification of the movements through manual sequences or animations

Finally, additive manufacturing (AM) processes were employed for fabrication. AM, for its acronym, is a manufacturing technique increasingly applied in biomedical engineering, which is based on 3D printing to create tangible, three-dimensional objects from virtual models (Zhang et al. 2024). From this principle, the preliminary prototype was produced using resin-based photopolymerization 3D printing, allowing a fine and detailed finish of the assembly (Fig. 8.10). The design incorporates a system of motion limiters that ensure physiological rotation angles, such as flexion and extension, for each finger.

The phalangeal system illustrated in Fig. 8.11 was assembled using a bolt-based connection system and each component was labeled with an identification number to ensure correct assembly.

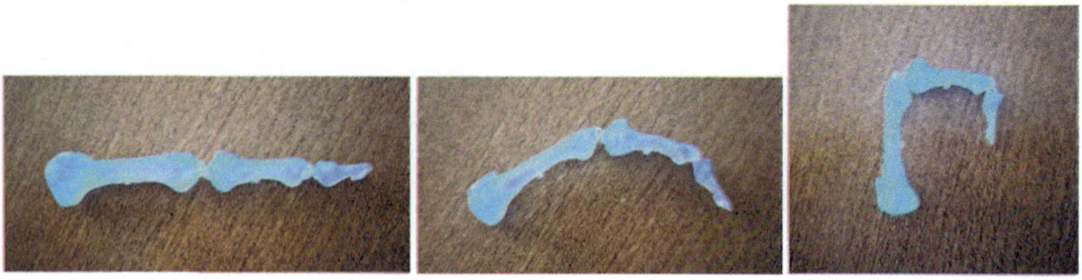

Fig. 8.10 3D printing of the assembled preliminary prototype design

Fig. 8.11 Assembly details and identifier

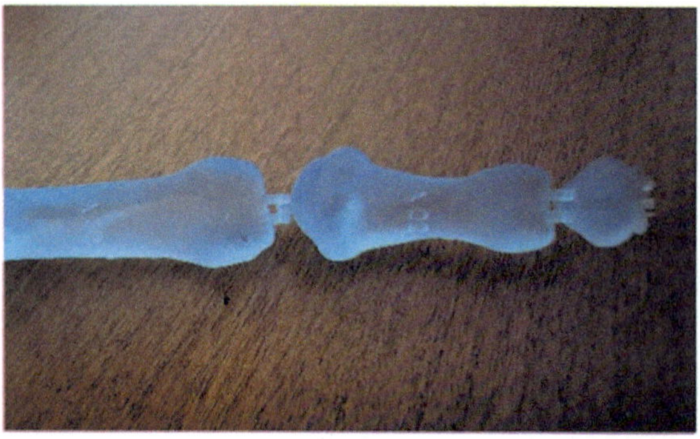

Finally, the fabrication of a base mold from the healthy hand (Fig. 8.12) enables practical experimentation with the case study and facilitates anthropometric and anthropomorphic testing for both the device design and its anchoring system. 3D printing using filament technology provides the required quality for prototype development at an affordable cost, while also eliminating the need for additional post-processing to achieve the final finish.

8.4 Conclusions

The current market for myoelectric prostheses offers mostly generic solutions, which often fail to meet the anatomical and functional requirements of patients with upper limb amputations. This study demonstrates that a personalized approach, guided by case-specific anthropometric data, can significantly improve ergonomics, adaptation, and overall patient comfort.

The integration of biomechanical analysis, axial tomography, segmentation, and additive manufacturing proved effective in developing a preliminary prototype adapted to the patient's residual limb. This workflow ensures greater precision in fitting, reduced discomfort, and a more natural distribution of forces during functional use.

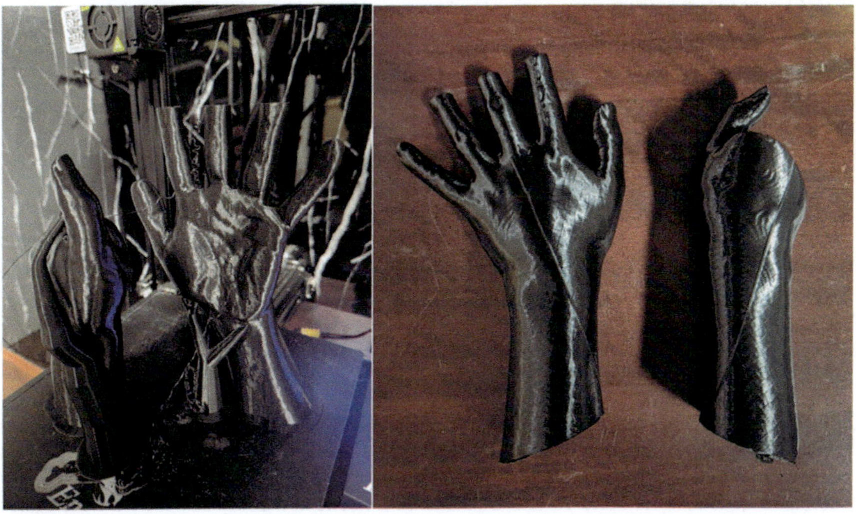

Fig. 8.12 Additive manufacturing of the healthy and amputee hand used as anatomical references for ergonomic testing and device anchoring

The case study highlights the importance of considering neurological and biomechanical aspects of phantom limb syndrome in the prosthesis design process. Addressing these factors from the early stages of development may improve adaptation and reduce rejection rates associated with lack of sensory feedback.

Additive manufacturing technologies allowed the creation of accurate, low-cost, and customizable components, enabling rapid prototyping and testing without compromising quality. This demonstrates the feasibility of incorporating accessible digital fabrication methods into clinical practice for prosthetic development.

Future work should focus on integrating advanced control strategies, such as adaptive algorithms and sensory feedback systems, to enhance usability and provide patients with a more natural interaction. Additionally, long-term clinical validation will be required to assess durability, usability, and patient satisfaction.

Acknowledges The authors would like to express their gratitude to the Instituto Politécnico Nacional (IPN) for its continuous support and contributions throughout the development of this study. Special thanks are extended to the Higher Research Scholarships Program (SECIHTI) for the financial support that made this research possible, and to COFAA for providing additional resources that facilitated the dissemination of the results.

References

Akbari M (2023) Data-driven review of additive manufacturing on supply chains: Regionalization, key research themes and future directions. Comput Ind Eng 184:109600. https://doi.org/10.1016/j.cie.2023.109600

Amputee Coalition. Controlando el dolor fantasma. https://amputee-coalition.org/resources/spanish-managing-phantom-pain/

Angarita MAM, Villa SC, Ribero OFG, García RG, Sieger FAS (2013) Fisiopatología y tratamiento del dolor de miembro fantasma. Colomb J Anesth 42(1):40–46. https://doi.org/10.1016/j.rca.2013.09.012

Aquino RP, Barile S, Grasso A, Saviano M (2018) Envisioning smart and sustainable healthcare: 3D printing technologies for personalized medication. Futures 103:35–50. https://doi.org/10.1016/j.futures.2018.03.002

Benavides-Álvarez C, Rodríguez-Martínez E, Avilés-Cruz C, Zúñiga-López A, Ferreyra-Ramírez A, Aguilar-Sánchez M (2025) Improvement in the classification of EMG signals through a convolutional neural network. Neural Comput Appl. https://doi.org/10.1007/s00521-025-11456-3

CRN Digital Design Thinking: un mundo lleno de posibilidades en la creación de nuevos productos para las empresas. https://www.crndigital.es/noticias/design-thinking-un-mundo-lleno-de-posibilidades-en-la-creacion-de-nuevos-productos-para

de Armas Mestre J, Soria Pérez R, Ibis González S, Bethencourt González M, Benavides Flores M, Rivera Somoano E (2021) Comportamiento del dolor fantasma en pacientes amputados en Cárdenas. Periodo 2015–2019. Revista Médica Electrónica 43(1):2759–2770

Diario Oficial de la Federación Mexicana. NOM-241-SSA1-2021, Buenas prácticas de fabricación para dispositivos médicos. https://dof.gob.mx/nota_detalle.php?codigo=5638793&fecha=20/12/2021 (2021)

Instituto de Salud del Estado de México. Regulación sanitaria. https://salud.edomex.gob.mx/isem/regulacion_sanitaria

Kaur A, Guan Y (2018) Phantom limb pain: a literature review. Chin J Traumatol 21(6):366–368. https://doi.org/10.1016/j.cjtee.2018.04.006

Muñoz-Gil C (2021) Electromiograma. Mapfre Salud. https://www.salud.mapfre.es/pruebas-diagnosticas/neurologicas-pruebas-diagnosticas/electromiograma/

Vázquez-Thierry KP, Beltrán-Fernández JA, Hermida-Ochoa JC, Velázquez-Sánchez AT, González MGRY, González AGRY, Moreno CA, Alvarado-Alcántara EO, Cuevas-Andrade JL (2024) Design of a system for the rehabilitation of the symptoms caused by the phantom limb syndrome for patients with full amputation. In: Advanced structured materials. Springer, pp 329–335. https://doi.org/10.1007/978-3-031-60920-6_23

Vicerrectorado de Investigación PUCP. Desarrollo de prótesis mioeléctrica [Archivo de vídeo]. YouTube. https://youtu.be/-kBmfKDQ5PQ?si=H8WSAAhQ_TQczGF_ (2024)

Zhang Y, Li J, Zou Y, Liu Y, Li L, Xu J, Li D, Rong Q, Li J, Geng Y, Lai J (2024) 3D printing technologies in water treatment: applications, challenges, and emerging trends. Chem Eng J 500:157184. https://doi.org/10.1016/j.cej.2024.157184

Chapter 9
Mechanobiological Finite Element Assessment of Dental Implant System Thread Design

Jesus Alejandro Serrato-Pedrosa, Virgilio Bocanegra-García, Ignacio Villanueva-Fierro, Absalom Zamorano-Carrillo, Erwing Irving Rendón-Ramírez, and Verónica Loera-Castañeda

Abstract Implant design optimization can maximize the performance of biological structures. Specifically, the thread pitch of implant systems is a key parameter that promotes stability, distributes loading transfer, preserves alveolar bone, and leads to complete osteointegration. Biomechanics in implantology seeks to analyze the stress and strain states within the mandibular bone and the osseointegrated implant. Numerical analyses provide accurate approximate solutions for understanding the structural behavior of components under complex clinical conditions. Hence, the primary objective of this research was to numerically analyze the biomechanical response of optimizing the thread pitch under functional loading conditions, assessing the dissipation of stress and strain fields in the jaw molar region and on the implant itself. The results of this study revealed a 25% and 22% reduction in maximum stress distribution in the gingival and cortical bone structures, respectively, under occlusal and oblique forces. Additionally, peak von Mises stress was minimized by 32% and 36% in cancellous bone. Therefore, this research contributes to understanding how

J. A. Serrato-Pedrosa (✉) · I. Villanueva-Fierro · V. Loera-Castañeda
CIIDIR-Durango, Instituto Politécnico Nacional, Durango, Mexico
e-mail: alejandroserrato@live.com.mx

I. Villanueva-Fierro
e-mail: ivillanuevaf@ipn.mx

V. Loera-Castañeda
e-mail: vloera@ipn.mx

V. Bocanegra-García
Centro de Biotecnología Genómica, Instituto Politécnico Nacional, Reynosa, Tamaulipas, Mexico
e-mail: vbocanegra@ipn.mx

A. Zamorano-Carrillo
Laboratorio de Biofísica Computacional, SEPI-ENMH Instituto Politécnico Nacional, Ciudad de México, Mexico
e-mail: azamorano@ipn.mx

E. I. Rendón-Ramírez
Vivental. Grupo Odontológico., Col. Victoria de Durango Centro, Durango, Mexico

A. Öchsner (ed.), *Progress in Biomaterials and Biomedical Engineering*, Advanced Structured Materials 249, https://doi.org/10.1007/978-3-032-13551-3_9

the optimization of thread features can lead to the advancement of more effective overall mechanical performance in implant systems, thereby enhancing osteointegration through a biomechanical criterion and preserving the well-being and quality of life in patients.

Keywords Biomechanics · Dental implants · Thread pitch · Computational biomodelling

9.1 Introduction

The most fundamental goal of dental implant surgeries is to ensure osteointegration and complete acceptance will be acquired in the patient. The long-standing success of dental implants is determined by a combination of biological and mechanical conditions, where mechanobiological behavior converges as a combination of both to have a decisive impact on promoting the osteointegration process and reducing bone loss margins based on a mechanical criterion of stress and strain patterns (Sugiura et al. 2016; Robau-Porrua et al. 2020; Alemayehu and Jeng 2021). The structural design of dental implants significantly influences initial implant stability and the capacity to resist applied forces during and after the osseointegration process (Alghamdi and Jansen 2020). A myriad of geometric conditions influences implant systems' biomechanical behavior, including thread depth, thread thickness, thread face angle, thread pitch, and thread helix angle. Among all the design parameters mentioned, thread pitch has a greater medical magnitude for operation (Pirmoradian et al. 2020; Kong et al. 2009). The thread pitch of an implant body is a crucial geometric factor that affects the contact between bone and implant and the distribution of functional and parafunctional chewing forces. Thread pitch is the distance between the centers of two threads along the same axis (Ryu et al. 2014; Desai et al. 2012). Additionally, the thread pitch significantly contributes to increasing surface contact primary stability, implant surface area and enhancing the speed of implant positioning (which is directly related to single, double, or triple lead) (Fanali et al. 2021; Kreve et al. 2024).

Dental implants exhibiting a reduced thread pitch have an increment number of threads per unit of length along the implant body, resulting in a larger implant surface area. In this regard, employing micro geometries and the augmentation in the surface area in thread design may contribute to enhanced load distribution. These micro-design parameters are directly related and contribute to improved primary implant stability. Likewise, a reduction in the pitch of V-shaped thread profiles was associated with enhanced bone-implant contact (Hsieh et al. 2023; Heimes et al. 2023). Therefore, recent studies have highlighted the importance of utilizing narrow thread pitch in evaluating primary stability and anchorage in organic tissue to consistently demonstrate that implants with thread configuration are more prone to exhibit enhanced load resistance and diminished effective stress distribution to a great extent (Ryu et al. 2014). Nonetheless, this is a design parameter governed by the thread profile. It has been explored that V-shaped provides better bone initial contact (BIC) performance and less stress on the trabecular bone than thin square shapes (Huang et al. 2023; Kim et al. 2009). Furthermore, V-shaped thread profiles are a standard in implantology practices as they are one of the most widely used and commercially available implant thread designs (Ramkumar et al. 2020; Al-Sanea et al. 2023).

Scientific published research consistently demonstrates that implant thread pitch optimization exerts a significant influence on enhancing mechanical distribution patterns in jaw and maxilla elements and the implant system itself. The finite element method (FEM) allows for the proper mathematical and numerical prediction of the structural response (Falcinelli et al. 2023; Prados-Privado et al. 2020). Thus, this research's main aim is to optimize a fundamental implant geometrical component in the thread, as it is the pitch in a commercially available implant system. Incorporating macro-geometry and reduction in thread pitch in a redesign proposal was adequate for a common V-shaped thread profile to provide insights into the biomechanical analysis effects of implant systems design parameters in assessing load distribution and primary stability.

9.2 Materials and Methods

This research employed numerical analysis through the finite element method to compare the biomechanical performance of an implant system and the thread pitch redesign version recommended for the molar region placement within a simulated environment encompassing cortical bone, cancellous bone, and gingival tissue. The analysis evaluated stress and strain distribution field patterns within the implant body, abutment, organic tissues, and implant-abutment interaction. A discretization quality analysis was conducted to validate the numerical model's accuracy and computational efficiency, necessitating a refined mesh density in critical interest regions such as implant threads and corresponding bone interfaces.

The implant system generated was based on novel clinical trends, such as the use of extremely high-quality zirconia implants in a two-piece system to avoid the risk of damaging the area surrounding the implant. The German implant manufacturer leader Albus Witar Implants (Köln D-50997, Germany) was taken as a reference to reproduce its sophisticated and versatile AWI-5008® tapered implant model for the first and second molar regions. The general dimensions for this dental implant system are 18 mm in length and a diameter of 6 mm in the upper abutment zone and 5 mm in the round apex area; also, the implant body has a 0.6 mm pitch V-shaped thread along 8 mm. The optimized thread pitch was refined to be set to 0.3 mm (which corresponds to half of the original design); changing only this geometric parameter can be beneficial to evaluate the thread pitch design factor's relevance adequately. The essential aim to adjust the pitch to how it has been described relied on assessing the impact of a macro design variation on force distribution (this selection criterion corresponds with methodologies employed in prior research of modifying thread design parameters) within cortical and trabecular bone regions under occlusal

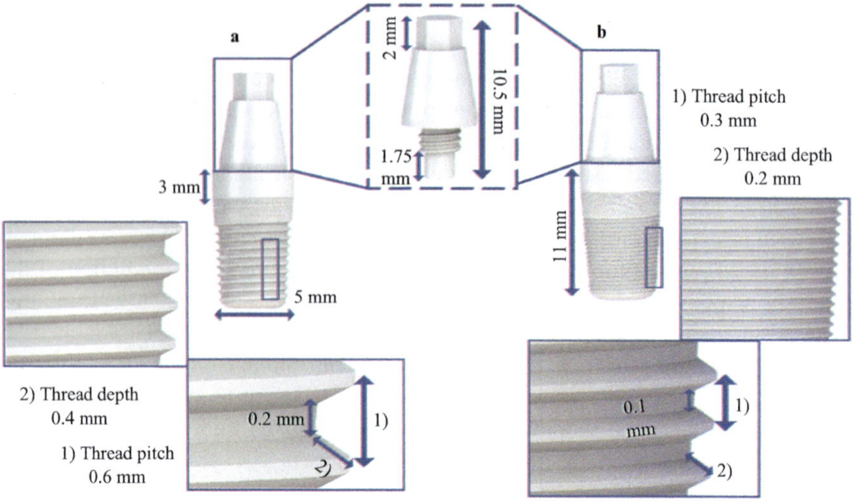

Fig. 9.1 Dental implant systems modeling. **a**. Manufacturer dental implant system. **b**. Optimized dental implant system

and oblique loading conditions (Azcarate-Velázquez et al. 2019). The creation of all implant system models was created by using the computer-aided design (CAD) software Solidworks® through reverse engineering (Fig. 9.1).

After completing the implant system geometry design, numerical simulation parameters were successfully established using the finite element analysis software (FEA) ANSYS Workbench®. This process encompassed preprocessing (assigning material properties, discretizing geometries, and applying appropriate boundary conditions and external loads) and processing and post-processing the mathematical prediction method. All materials used in the implant systems were considered isotropic, homogeneous and linearly elastic. On the contrary, bone structures were simulated with orthotropic mechanical conditions to replicate the bone's mechanical behavior better and enhance stress prediction along bone-implant interaction (Dhatrak et al. 2019). Gingival tissue was also modeled as an isotropic and linear elastic material. Furthermore, the reconstruction of biological tissues was simplified as a 3D cross-section morphology of an adult standardized mandible first/second molar region block (Tunis et al. 2017; Lenin et al. 2024). The mechanical properties of each material are properly described in Table 9.1 (Cicciù et al. 2019; Fiorillo et al. 2022; Kayabaşı et al. 2006; Alghazzawi et al. 2012; Zhang et al. 2016).

9.2.1 Loading and Boundary Conditions

Realistic clinical conditions and mechanical equilibrium were simulated by applying appropriate boundary conditions. A combination of occlusal and oblique loading

Table 9.1 Mechanical properties of the components

Component	Elastic modulus (MPa)	Shear modulus (MPa)	Poisson's ratio (ν)	Yield strength (MPa)	Density (g/cm^3)
Cortical bone Cicciù et al. 2019; Fiorillo et al. 2022)	E_{xx} 9600 E_{yy} 9600 E_{zz} 17,800	G_{xy} 3100 G_{yz} 3510 G_{xz} 3510	ν_{xy} 0.55 ν_{yz} 0.3 ν_{xz} 0.3	115	1.8
Trabecular bone (Cicciù et al. 2019; Fiorillo et al. 2022)	E_{xx} 144 E_{yy} 99 E_{zz} 344	G_{xy} 53 G_{yz} 63 G_{xz} 45	ν_{xy} 0.23 ν_{yz} 0.11 ν_{xz} 0.13	32.4	1.2
Gingival tissue (Kayabaşı et al. 2006)	19.6	7.5385	0.30	–	–
Y-TZP zirconia (Alghazzawi et al. 2012; Zhang et al. 2016)	210,000	80,769	0.3	1200	6.05

conditions was considered to replicate the main biological chewing effects in the jaw molar region from functional loading conditions. Loads were applied in the abutment component, with 100 N for occlusal (Zhang et al. 2022) and oblique directions (Lee et al. 2021; Choi and Hong 2022). Lower and lateral zones of the cross-section of the jaw molar area were restricted in all degrees of freedom for displacement ($Ux = Uy = Uz = 0$). Also, a tightening torque condition was simulated in the abutment connection with the implant body; a torque of 15 N/cm was utilized, as it is the placement tightening torque provided by the implant system manufacturer (Fig. 9.2).

Implant system and biological structures were imported into the finite element software for tetrahedral high-order three-dimensional solid elements (Solid187) and 20 nodes per element discretization generation, facilitating subsequent simulations. Consequently, an adaptive mesh refinement strategy was implemented, targeting an element size of approximately 0.1 mm in critical regions, including implant threads, abutment interfaces, and threaded biological tissue, while maintaining an element size of 0.3 mm in less critical areas. A high-quality discretization in the elements was accomplished based on ANSYS quality mesh metrics spectrums (Gok et al. 2017). The original implant system analysis was very good in the discretization quality test (average 0.26 in the skewness spectrum) with a total of 2288,453 nodes and 1484,609 elements (Fig. 9.3a). In contrast, the modified thread pitch implant design presented an extremely good mesh quality (average 0.27 in the skewness spectrum) with 2,424,972 nodes and 1,562,472 elements (Fig. 9.3b).

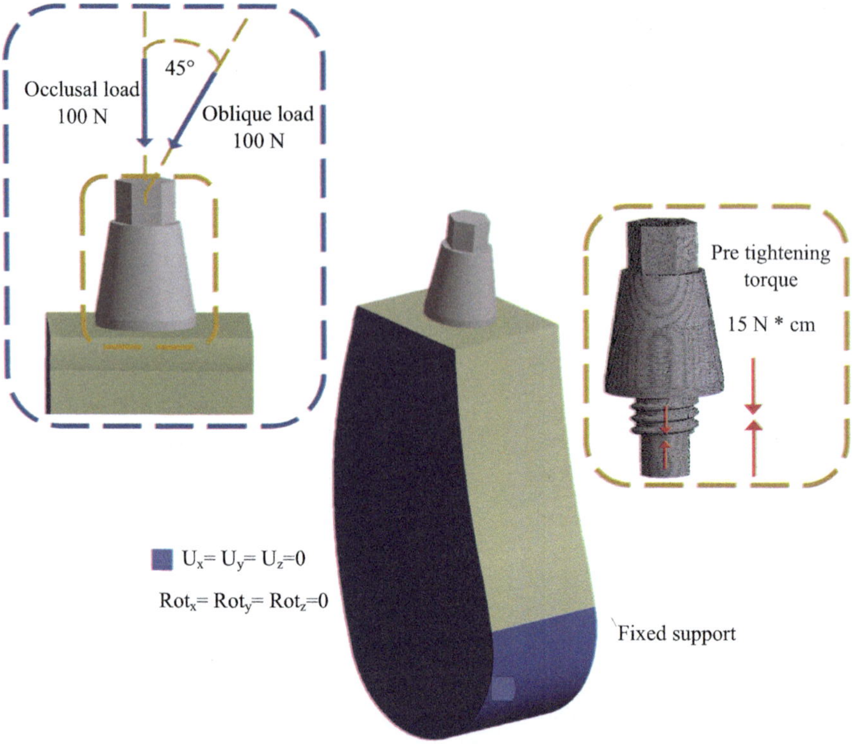

Fig. 9.2 Free body diagram of the mechanical conditions employed

9.3 Results

The principal findings of this research mainly rely on incorporating a comprehensive biomechanical predictive model, including an adequate environment of biological structures of the implant placement zone to enhance the mechanical bio-fidelity of the numerical response (utilization of appropriate properties and geometries). Hence, including the structural biological environment facilitated the comparative assessment between both implant systems, the original implant design model and the optimized thread pitch design. This integration was critical for a more comprehensive understanding of the system's mechanical behavior and response as a function of varying implant system design parameters. Figures 9.4 and 9.5 represent the comparison between the total displacement in the system for occlusal and oblique loading conditions, respectively. Figures 9.6 and 9.7 depict the data obtention for stress distribution in the gingival and cortical bone structure (occlusal and oblique loads), whereas, in Figs. 9.8 and 9.9, the occlusal force stress fields are represented within the implant systems and the effect generated in trabecular bone tissue, making a zoom-in emphasis in the mechanical behavior of the original and optimized thread configurations. Likewise, Figs. 9.10 and 9.11 represent the response of the implant system

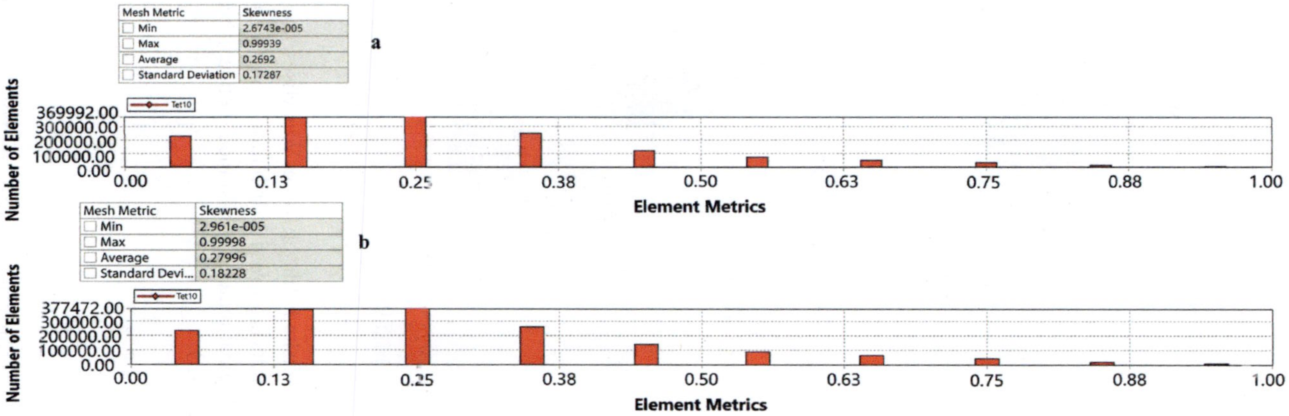

Fig. 9.3 Discretization quality test. **a**. Manufacturer dental implant system discretization process. **b**. Optimized dental implant system discretization process

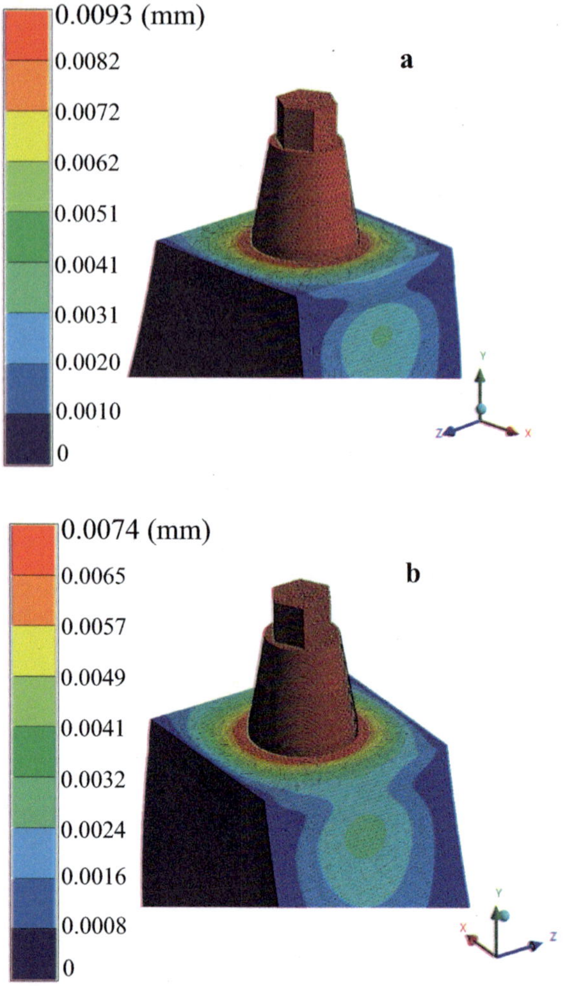

Fig. 9.4 Comparison of total displacement in the biomechanical system under occlusal loading for both implant systems. **a**. Original thread system. **b**. Optimized thread system

provided by applying the established oblique force. Von Mises stress criteria estimate total stress in a structure, considering stress distribution along planes and axes, being essential for evaluating biological material resistance; hence, it was selected for the stress analysis (Figs. 9.12, 9.13).

9.4 Discussion

The main aim of this investigation was to assess the von Mises stress fields, strain distribution, and displacement patterns in a dental implant system within its biological surrounding structures influenced by optimizing a thread design under functional

Fig. 9.5 Comparison of total displacement in the biomechanical system under oblique loading for both implant systems. a. Original thread system. b. Optimized thread system

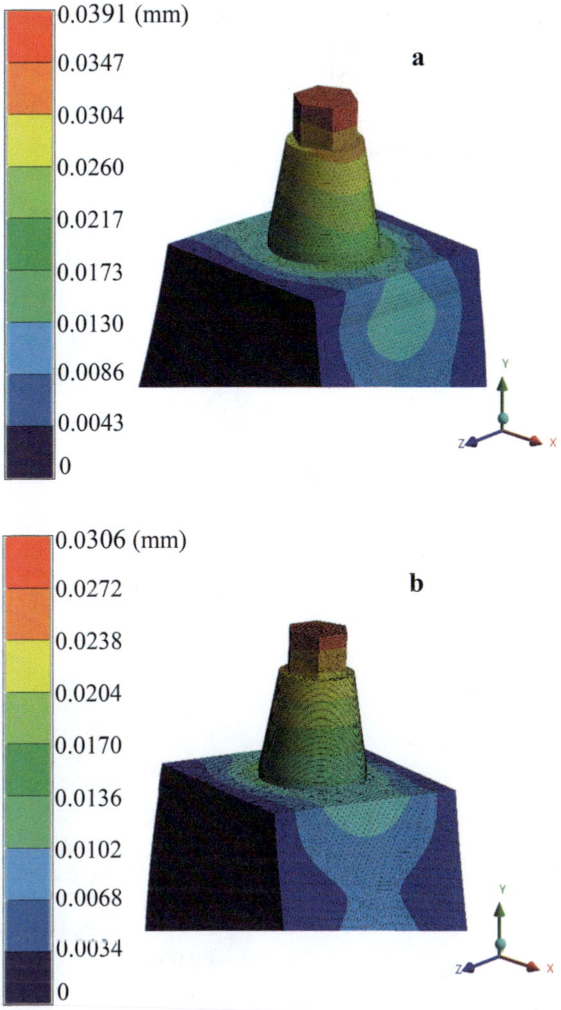

loading conditions. Implementing numerical simulation with the finite element analysis provided interesting insights to predict the biomechanical behavior of the design configuration. A direct comparison in the numerical results indicated a notable pattern in the behavior of the optimized implant system to have a stress concentrator in the body implant-abutment connection, which can be mainly attributed to the closest interaction with the application of the loading condition and the biological structures. A configuration in the abutment connection might be necessary to enhance the stress dissipation in such a zone. The optimized system has a better performance in the biomechanical effects generated in all of the biological structures under all loading conditions; the maximum stress distribution was reduced by 25% and 22% in the gingival and cortical bone structures under occlusal and oblique forces applied

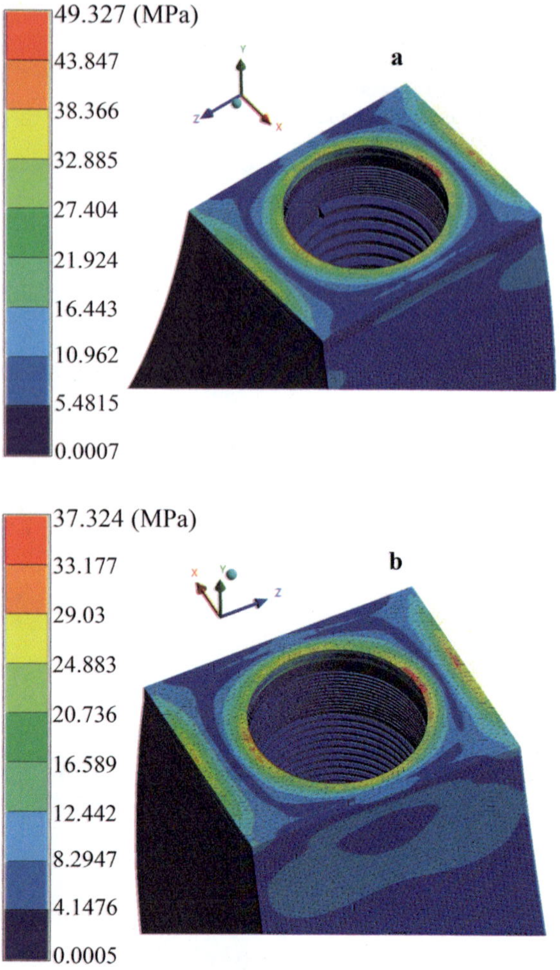

Fig. 9.6 Comparison of stress fields in gingival and cortical bone tissues under occlusal loading for both implant systems. **a**. Original thread system. **b**. Optimized thread system

respectively, this performance is similar to a previous FEM study for the cortical bone, exhibiting range stress of 5–10 MPa for a thread pitch of 0.5 (Oswal et al. 2016); in addition, it is important to point out that the increment of maximum stress of 40–50 MPa can be related to the mechanical properties of gingiva. The thread pitch optimization significantly favors the von Mises distribution, having a stress concentrator in the apex design of the implant body, suggesting that it be modified to align with the performance of the new pitch configuration. In this regard, the stress patterns in the optimized threads were more evenly dissipated along the thread length, eliminating any stress-concentrated region, having similar von Mises stress conditions in implant systems with 0.39 and 0.5 mm thread pitch design (Chang et al. 2025). Hence, this enhancement in the mechanical performance of the optimized implant system provided better mechanobiological behavior in the trabecular

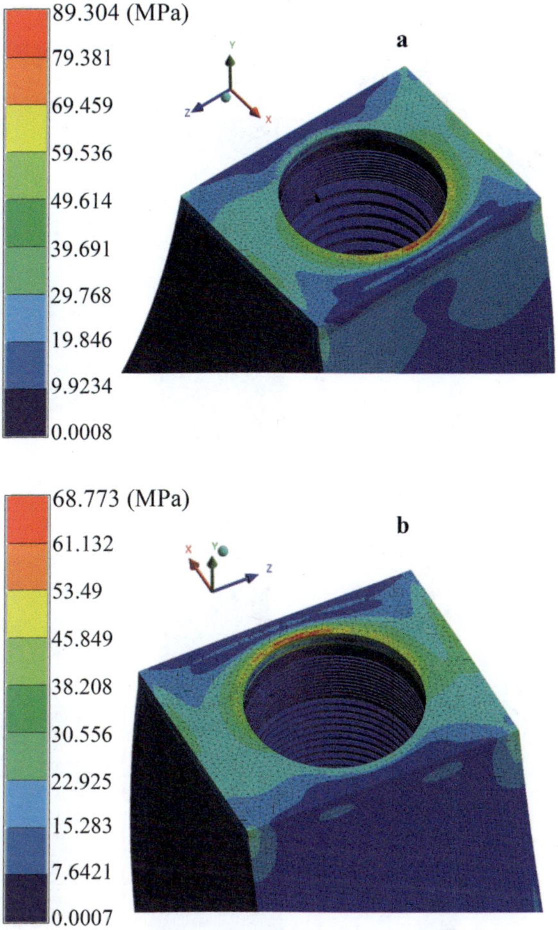

Fig. 9.7 Comparison of stress fields in gingival and cortical bone tissues under oblique loading for both implant systems. **a**. Original thread system. **b**. Optimized thread system

bone though more contact area, minimizing peak von Mises stress by 32% and 36% under the stated loads considered (oblique and occlusal). Also observed a reduction of maximum values of total equivalent strain for both loading conditions in the designed dental implant; peak values must need to be thoroughly analyzed according to the orthotropic conditions for trabecular bone (which tend to maximize the stress–strain effects), where the strain distribution behavior can be directly considered in a normal growth zone for mechanostat and principal tensile and compressive strain theories. Moreover, $\mu\varepsilon$ presented in trabecular bone in this research aligns with previous finite element findings evaluating bone resorption under occlusal loading (Epifania et al. 2023; Ausiello et al. 2021).

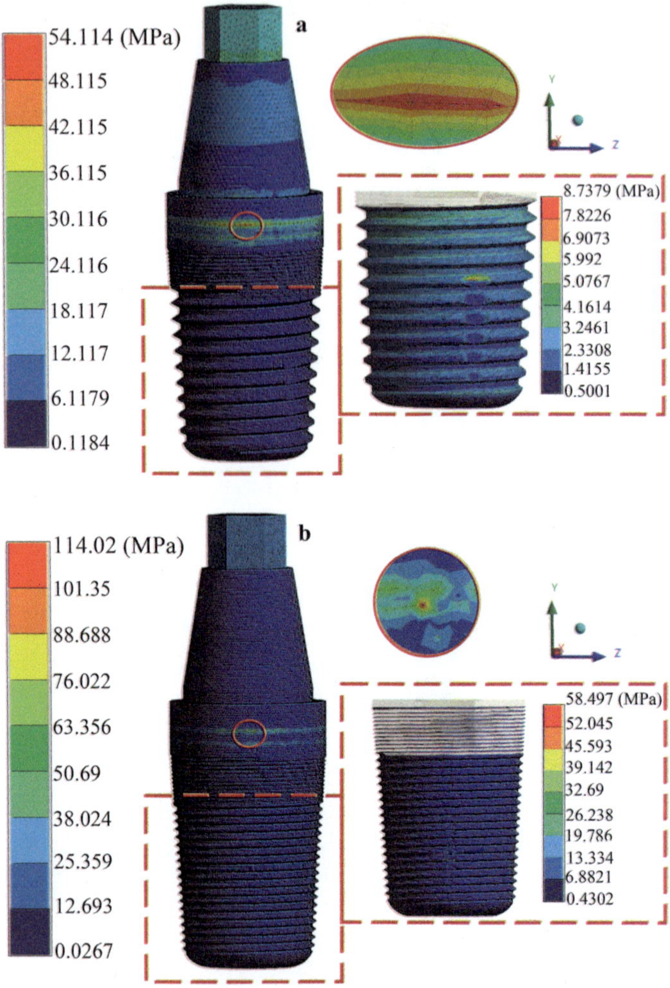

Fig. 9.8 Comparison of stress distribution in the implant systems and thread configuration under occlusal loading. **a**. Original thread system. **b**. Optimized thread system

9.5 Conclusions

The findings in this research paper indicated that the thread design is a critical parameter in the implant body geometry to maximize contact area for load transmission and thus have stress and strain field distribution. Particularly enhancing the thread pitch performance by reducing the pitch to half of the original implant system resulted in a thorough analysis of the biomechanical behavior of the implant systems evaluated and the surrounding biological structures. Numerical simulations permit having a more thorough clinical assessment, considering the mechanobiological effects generated

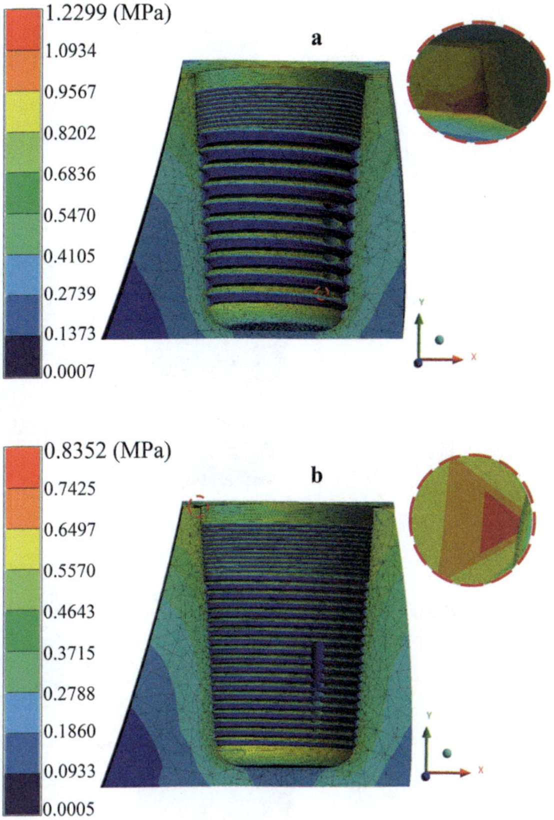

Fig. 9.9 Comparison of stress fields in trabecular bone structure under occlusal loading for both implant systems. **a**. Original thread system. **b**. Optimized thread system

in trabecular bone through to distribution stress concentrators to avoid any failure within the implant system and the strain patterns focused on the process of bone remodeling and avoidance of bone resorption, specifically in low-density trabecular bone and primary stability determination for patient-specific design criteria. Furthermore, it is relevant to acknowledge the limitations of the results found, as this paper only considered one thread profile (V-shaped) and not the effects generated by other muscles and directions in the chewing process. Nonetheless, the limitations described in the optimized thread design contribute to recent implant design parameters that utilize small thread pitch and microgeometries.

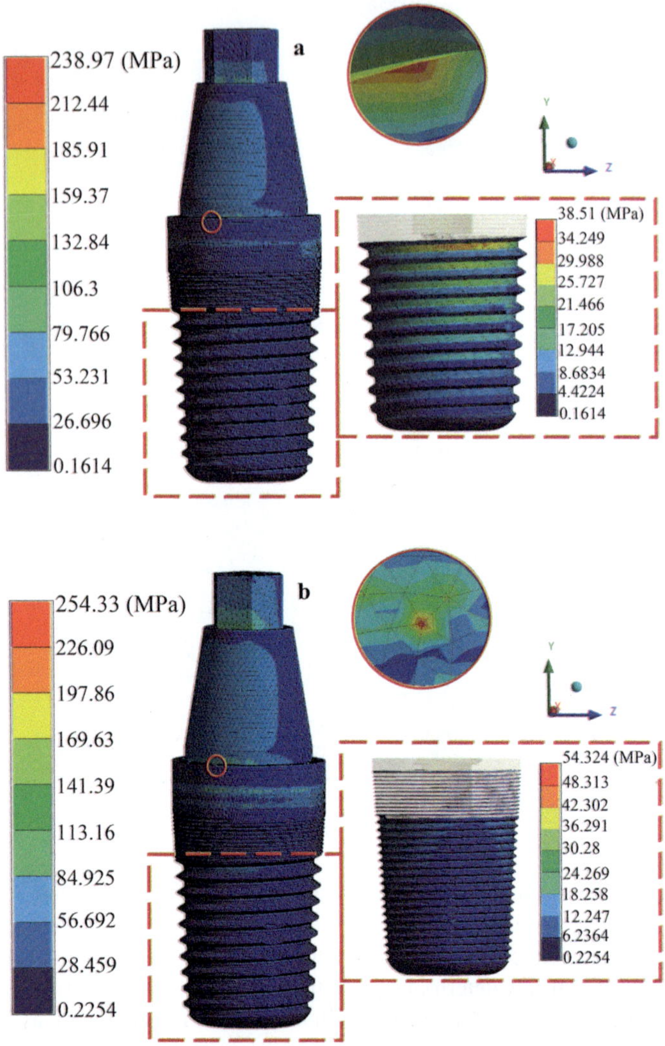

Fig. 9.10 Comparison of stress distribution in the implant systems and thread configuration under oblique loading. **a**. Original thread system. **b**. Optimized thread system

Fig. 9.11 Comparison of stress fields in trabecular bone structure under oblique loading for both implant systems. **a**. Original thread system. **b**. Optimized thread system

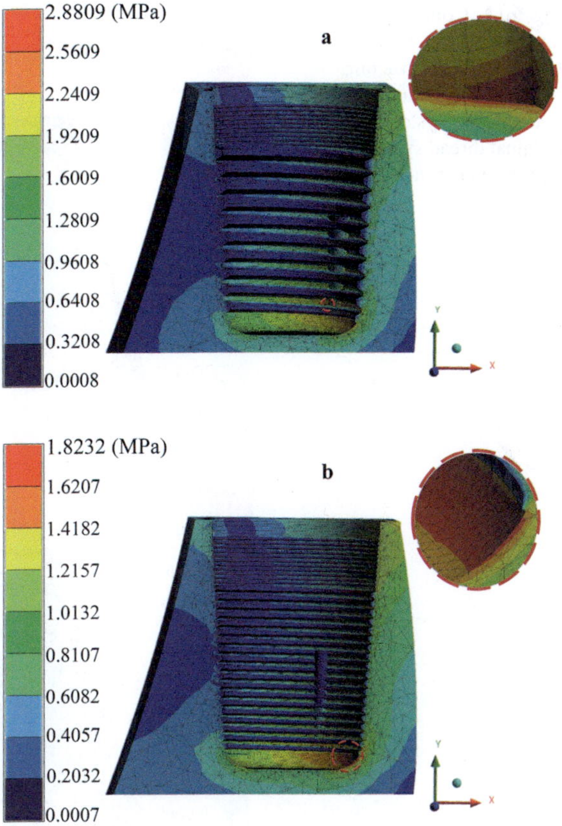

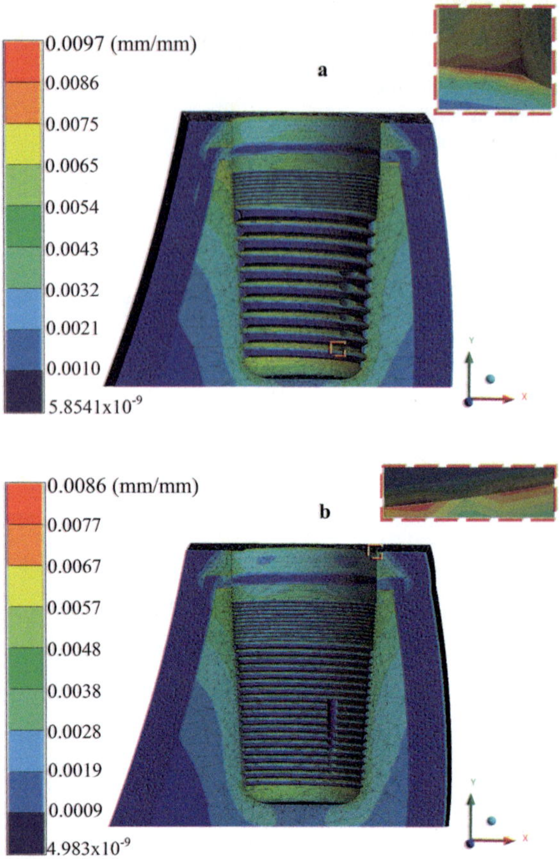

Fig. 9.12 Comparison of total equivalent strain in trabecular bone structure under occlusal loading for both implant systems. **a**. Original thread system. **b**. Optimized thread system

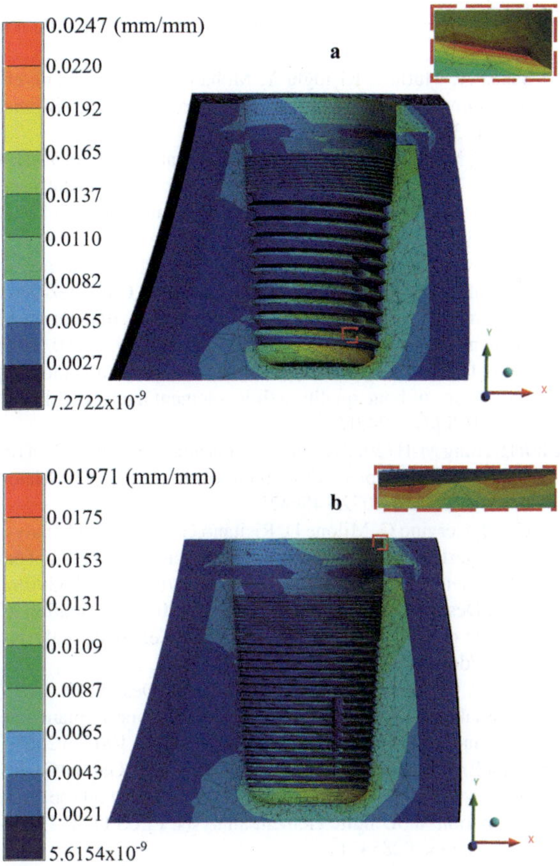

Fig. 9.13 Comparison of total equivalent strain in trabecular bone structure under oblique loading for both implant systems. **a**. Original thread system. **b**. Optimized thread system

Acknowledgements The authors kindly acknowledge the grant awarded by the Instituto Politécnico Nacional, the Comisión de Operación y Fomento de Actividades Académicas del IPN (COFAA) and the Secretaría de Ciencia, Humanidades, Tecnología e Innovación (SECIHTI) for the given support for the for the development of this research.

References

Alemayehu D-B, Jeng Y-R (2021) Three-dimensional finite element investigation into effects of implant thread design and loading rate on stress distribution in dental implants and anisotropic bone. Materials 14(22):6974. https://doi.org/10.3390/ma14226974

Alghamdi HS, Jansen JA (2020) The development and future of dental implants. Dent Mater J 39(2):167–172. https://doi.org/10.4012/dmj.2019-140

Alghazzawi TF, Lemons J, Liu P-R, Essig ME, Bartolucci AA, Janowski GM (2012) Influence of low-temperature environmental exposure on the mechanical properties and structural stability of dental zirconia. J Prosthodont 21(5):363–369. https://doi.org/10.1111/j.1532-849X.2011.00838.x

Al-Sanea A, Mutlu I, Kişioğlu Y, Mohamed E (2023) The effect of V-thread and square thread dental implants on bone stresses. J Biomim Biomater Biomed Eng 60:83–96. https://doi.org/10.4028/p-3qasy2

Ausiello P, Mendes Tribst JP, Ventre M, Salvati E, di Lauro AE, Martorelli M, Lanzotti A, Watts DC (2021) The role of cortical zone level and prosthetic platform angle in dental implant mechanical response: a 3D finite element analysis. Dent Mater 37(11):1688–1697. https://doi.org/10.1016/j.dental.2021.08.022

Azcarate-Velázquez F, Castillo-Oyagüe R, Oliveros-López L-G, Torres-Lagares D, Martínez-González Á-J, Pérez-Velasco A, Lynch CD, Gutiérrez-Pérez J-L, Serrera-Figallo M-Á (2019) Influence of bone quality on the mechanical interaction between implant and bone: a finite element analysis. J Dent 88:103161. https://doi.org/10.1016/j.jdent.2019.06.008

Chang C-L, Chen J-J, Chen C-S (2025) Using optimization approach to design dental implant in three types of bone quality-a finite element analysis. J Dent Sci 20(1):126–136. https://doi.org/10.1016/j.jds.2024.09.017

Choi H, Hong M-H (2022) Finite element analysis of the effect of tightening torque on the connection stability of a two-piece Zirconia implant system. Adv Mater Sci Eng 2022(1):1456475. https://doi.org/10.1155/2022/1456475

Cicciù M, Cervino G, Milone D, Risitano G (2019) FEM analysis of dental implant-abutment interface overdenture components and parametric evaluation of equator® and locator® prosthodontics attachments. Materials 12(4):592. https://doi.org/10.3390/ma12040592

Desai S, Desai M, Katti G, Karthikeyan I (2012) Evaluation of design parameters of eight dental implant designs: a two-dimensional finite element analysis. Niger J Clin Pract 15(2):176–181. https://doi.org/10.4103/1119-3077.97308

Dhatrak P, Girme V, Shirsat U, Sumanth S, Deshmukh VJB (2019) Significance of orthotropic material models to predict stress around bone-implant interface using numerical simulation. BioNanoSci 9(3):652–659. https://doi.org/10.1007/s12668-019-00649-5

Epifania E, di Lauro AE, Ausiello P, Mancone A, Garcia-Godoy F, Mendes Tribst JP (2023) Effect of crown stiffness and prosthetic screw absence on the stress distribution in implant-supported restoration: a 3D finite element analysis. PLoS ONE 18(5):e0285421. https://doi.org/10.1371/journal.pone.0285421

Falcinelli C, Valente F, Vasta M, Traini T (2023) Finite element analysis in implant dentistry: state of the art and future directions. Dent Mater 39(6):539–556. https://doi.org/10.1016/j.dental.2023.04.002

Fanali S, Tumedei M, Pignatelli P, Petrini M, Piattelli A, Iezzi G (2021) The effect of threads geometry on insertion torque (IT) and periotest implant primary stability: a high-density polyurethane simulation for the anterior mandible. Crystals 11(3):308. https://doi.org/10.3390/cryst11030308

Fiorillo L, Milone D, D'Andrea D, Santonocito D, Risitano G, Cervino G, Cicciù M (2022) Finite element analysis of zirconia dental implant. Prosthesis 4(3):490–499. https://doi.org/10.3390/prosthesis4030040

Gok K, Inal S, Gok A, Gulbandilar E (2017) Comparison of effects of different screw materials in the triangle fixation of femoral neck fractures. J Mater Sci Mater Med 28:81. https://doi.org/10.1007/s10856-017-5890-y

Heimes D, Becker P, Pabst A, Smeets R, Kraus A, Hartmann A, Sagheb K, Kämmerer PW (2023) How does dental implant macrogeometry affect primary implant stability? A narrative review. Int J Implant Dent 9(1):20. https://doi.org/10.1186/s40729-023-00485-z

Hsieh M-C, Huang C-H, Hsu M-L (2023) Effect of cutting flute design features on primary stability of immediate implant placement and restoration: a dynamic experimental analysis. Med Biol Eng Comput 61(2):475–484. https://doi.org/10.1007/s11517-022-02722-w

Huang Y-C, Huang Y-C, Ding S-J (2023) Primary stability of implant placement and loading related to dental implant materials and designs: a literature review. J Dent Sci 18(4):1467–1476. https://doi.org/10.1016/j.jds.2023.06.010

Kayabaşı O, Yüzbasıoğlu E, Erzincanlı F (2006) Static, dynamic and fatigue behaviors of dental implant using finite element method. Adv Eng Softw 37(10):649–658. https://doi.org/10.1016/j.advengsoft.2006.02.004

Kim J-M, Kim S-J, Han I, Shin S-W, Ryu J-J (2009) A comparison of the implant stability among various implant systems: clinical study. J Adv Prosthodont 1(1):31–36. https://doi.org/10.4047/jap.2009.1.1.31

Kong L, Zhao Y, Hu K, Li D, Zhou H, Wu Z, Liu B (2009) Selection of the implant thread pitch for optimal biomechanical properties: a three-dimensional finite element analysis. Adv Eng Softw 40(7):474–478. https://doi.org/10.1016/j.advengsoft.2008.08.003

Kreve S, Ferreira I, da Costa Valente ML, Dos Reis AC (2024) Relationship between dental implant macro-design and osseointegration: a systematic review. Oral Maxillofac Surg 28(1):1–14. https://doi.org/10.1007/s10006-022-01116-4

Lee H, Jo M, Noh G (2021) Biomechanical effects of dental implant diameter, connection type, and bone density on microgap formation and fatigue failure: a finite element analysis. Comput Methods Programs Biomed 200:105863. https://doi.org/10.1016/j.cmpb.2020.105863

Lenin V, Das S, Ganapathy S, Sahoo PP (2024) Sex estimation from mandibular morphometry using discriminant analysis–CT scan based retrospective study. Foren Imag 38:200603. https://doi.org/10.1016/j.fri.2024.200603

Oswal MM, Amasi UN, Oswal MS, Bhagat AS (2016) Influence of three different implant thread designs on stress distribution: a three-dimensional finite element analysis. J Indian Prosthodont Soc 16(4):359–365. https://doi.org/10.4103/0972-4052.191283

Pirmoradian M, Naeeni HA, Firouzbakht M, Toghraie D, Darabi R (2020) Finite element analysis and experimental evaluation on stress distribution and sensitivity of dental implants to assess optimum length and thread pitch. Comput Methods Programs Biomed 187:105258. https://doi.org/10.1016/j.cmpb.2019.105258

Prados-Privado M, Martínez-Martínez C, Gehrke SA, Prados-Frutos JC (2020) Influence of bone definition and finite element parameters in bone and dental implants stress: a literature review. Biology 9(8):224. https://doi.org/10.3390/biology9080224

Ramkumar K, Sripriya S, Meenakshi A, Sabarigirinathan C, Thulasingam C (2020) Comparison of primary stability in craniofacial implant with V-shape and buttress thread design in goat skull using resonance frequency analysis. Indian J Dent Res 31(3):403–407. https://doi.org/10.4103/ijdr.IJDR_447_17

Robau-Porrua A, Pérez-Rodríguez Y, Soris-Rodríguez LM, Pérez-Acosta O, González JE (2020) The effect of diameter, length and elastic modulus of a dental implant on stress and strain levels in peri-implant bone: a 3D finite element analysis. Biomed Mater Eng 30(5–6):541–558. https://doi.org/10.3233/BME-191073

Ryu H-S, Namgung C, Lee J-H, Lim Y-J (2014) The influence of thread geometry on implant osseointegration under immediate loading: a literature review. J Adv Prosthodont 6(6):547. https://doi.org/10.4047/jap.2014.6.6.547

Sugiura T, Yamamoto K, Horita S, Murakami K, Tsutsumi S, Kirita T (2016) The effects of bone density and crestal cortical bone thickness on micromotion and peri-implant bone strain distribution in an immediately loaded implant: a nonlinear finite element analysis. J Periodontal Implant Sci 46(3):152–165. https://doi.org/10.5051/jpis.2016.46.3.152

Tunis TS, Sarig R, Cohen H, Medlej B, Peled N, May H (2017) Sex estimation using computed tomography of the mandible. Int J Legal Med 131(6):1691–1700. https://doi.org/10.1007/s00414-017-1554-1

Zhang F, Inokoshi M, Batuk M, Hadermann J, Naert I, Van Meerbeek B, Vleugels J (2016) Strength, toughness and aging stability of highly-translucent Y-TZP ceramics for dental restorations. Dent Mater 32(12):e327–e337. https://doi.org/10.1016/j.dental.2016.09.025

Zhang W-t, Cheng K-j, Liu Y-f, Wang R, Chen Y-f, Ding Y-d, Yang F, Wang L-h (2022) Effect of the prosthetic index on stress distribution in Morse taper connection implant system and peri-implant bone: a 3D finite element analysis. BMC Oral Health 22(1):431. https://doi.org/10.1186/s12903-022-02465-y

Chapter 10
Flow in Elastic Pipes: An Experimental Study

Valeriano Salomón Álvarez Salazar, Carlos Alejandro Vargas, Franklin W. Peña Polo, Ignacio Carvajal Mariscal, Leonardo Di. G. Sigalotti, and Jaime Klapp

Abstract This article investigates the deformation behavior of elastic tubes subjected to hydrostatic pressure resulting from a constant internal fluid flow. The steady flow generates pulsatile motion within the tube, mimicking conditions commonly observed in both biological and industrial systems. Preliminary experimental findings are compared with a theoretical model that accounts for both longitudinal and transverse wave propagation. Throughout the experiments, high-resolution images were captured at various deformation stages and analyzed using advanced image processing techniques. The aim is to deepen our understanding of the mechanical response of elastic materials under dynamic loading and to validate the theoretical model through rigorous experimental observation. These insights may contribute to the improved design of fluid transport systems in biomedical and industrial applications.

Keywords Fluid–structure interaction · Elastic deformation · Pulsatile flow · Wave propagation

V. S. Á. Salazar (✉)
Departamento de Energía, Universidad Autónoma Metropolitana-Azcapotzalco, 02128 México City, México
e-mail: vsas@azc.uam.mx

C. A. Vargas · F. W. P. Polo · L. Di. G. Sigalotti
Departamento de Ciencias Básicas, Universidad Autónoma Metropolitana-Azcapotzalco, 02128 México City, México
e-mail: cvargas@azc.uam.mx

L. Di. G. Sigalotti
e-mail: ldgsd@azc.uam.mx

I. C. Mariscal
Instituto Politécnico Nacional, ESIME UPALM, México City, México
e-mail: icarvajal@ipn.mx

J. Klapp
Departamento de Física, Instituto Nacional de Investigaciones Nucleares, La Marquesa, Ocoyoacac, 52750 Estado de México, México
e-mail: jaime.klapp@inin.gob.mx

A. Öchsner (ed.), *Progress in Biomaterials and Biomedical Engineering*, Advanced Structured Materials 249, https://doi.org/10.1007/978-3-032-13551-3_10

10.1 Introduction

This study investigates the behavior of elastic pipes subjected to hydrostatic pressure under a constant internal water flow (Shukurov et al. 1997). Elastic tubes, capable of undergoing deformation in response to external forces and subsequently returning to their original shape, have long been a subject of interest in fluid–structure interaction research. The analysis of pressure wave propagation in viscous fluids within elastic conduits can be traced back to Witzig's foundational work in 1914 (E3S Web Conference 2023). Earlier still, Poiseuille pioneered the quantitative study of blood flow by modeling fluid transport through rigid cylindrical tubes, laying the groundwork for modern hemodynamics (Womersley 1957).

The interaction between a fluid and an elastic tube is highly relevant in both engineering and biological contexts. Understanding this phenomenon can contribute significantly to the development of more efficient and safer medical technologies and treatments (Rodkiewicz 1983). Recent advancements in the field, particularly in bio-engineering, include mathematical descriptions of pulse wave velocity (PWV) in arteries. For instance, Ref. (Kuchkarovich 2021) presents three-dimensional simulations of flow pulses in straight elastic pipes to analyze the propagation of pressure waves and the resulting deformation of the tube walls.

Quantitative data were obtained on the behavior of elastic tubes when different types of forces were applied, and their responses were measured. This experimental investigation seeks to identify the key mechanical properties of elastic tubes that govern their deformation behavior and structural resistance. In doing so, it also provides insight into how elastic materials respond to internal pressure fluctuations, which is crucial in the design and modeling of soft-walled fluid transport systems. The analysis of the collected data allows for drawing conclusions about the deformation capacity, stiffness, and fatigue resistance of elastic pipes, and reveals potential avenues for optimizing their performance in real-world applications.

The corresponding mathematical approach is represented by the phenomenon of fluid–structure interaction (FSI), which involves the coupling of two media with distinct physical characteristics namely, the incompressible fluid and the deformable solid boundary. These coupled problems are of great interest in mathematical physics due to their strong connection with hemodynamic models (Sarraf et al. 2022; Desjardins et al. 2001; Gilbert and Mikelic 2000), as well as with classical and modern studies on viscous flows in compliant vessels (Grandmont and Maday 2000; Canic and Mikelic 2003; Canic et al. 2006). Furthermore, these mathematical frameworks are also applicable to industrial systems transporting viscous fluids through thin-walled tubes or flexible conduits (Mikelic et al. 2007).

A crucial aspect of this work lies in bridging theory and experiment. While numerical and analytical models are indispensable tools for prediction and simulation, they often rely on simplifying assumptions. Experimental validation, especially through direct visual observation and image processing, provides an essential check on the accuracy and applicability of these models under real physical conditions. In this context, high-resolution imaging and data acquisition techniques allow the dynamic deformation of the tube walls to be recorded and analyzed.

Furthermore, this work aims not only to explore the behavior of elastic tubes under internal pressure but also to propose a methodology for validating theoretical predictions through carefully designed laboratory experiments. The results are expected to benefit researchers and engineers working in fields as diverse as biomedical engineering, soft robotics, energy systems, and materials science.

This work is organized as follows: Sect. 10.2 presents the physical model of the elastic pipe, including the theoretical background and governing equations. Section 10.3 details the experimental setup and measurement techniques employed. Section 10.4 discusses the main results, highlighting key observations and comparisons with the theoretical model. Finally, Sect. 10.5 summarizes the conclusions and outlines perspectives for future work.

10.2 Physical Model

The physical system analyzed in this study consists of an elastic cylindrical pipe with undeformed inner radius, wall thickness, and length (r, h, L). This is particularly relevant in long and slender tubes, where wall elasticity significantly influences flow behavior, as illustrated in Fig. 10.1. A steady, incompressible fluid flows through the pipe from the inlet to the outlet, inducing deformation in the compliant walls. The fluid domain is denoted by Ω_{f}, and the surrounding elastic structure by Ω_{s}. The coordinate system (x, y), defines the axial and radial directions, assuming axisymmetric behavior.

The pipe material is modeled as an isotropic, linearly elastic solid characterized by Young's modulus E, Poisson's ratio ν, and density ρ_{s}. The fluid is Newtonian and incompressible, with density ρ_{f} and dynamic viscosity μ.

Although the imposed flow is steady, the interaction between the fluid and the deformable wall leads to complex pressure and deformation fields, especially in long, thin-walled tubes. The elasticity of the wall allows for dynamic deformation and wave propagation along the axial direction, even in the absence of externally imposed oscillations.

The problem of fluid–structure interaction (FSI) is formulated by coupling the Navier–Stokes equations for the fluid inside Ω_{f} with the linear elasticity equations for the structure in Ω_{s}. At the interface between these two domains, continuity of

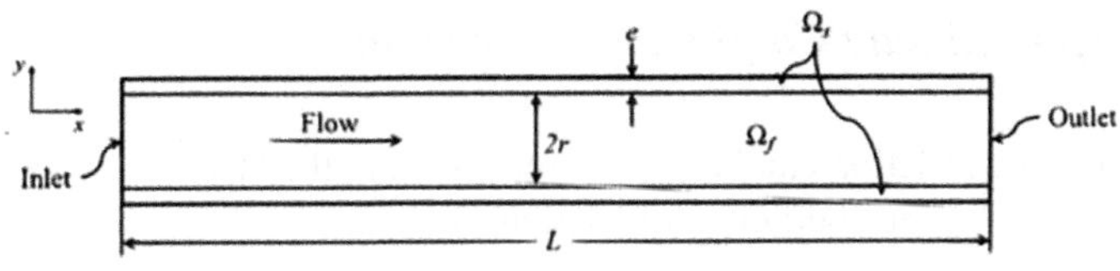

Fig. 10.1 Schematic of the flow test loop used for the experiments

velocity and stress is imposed. These coupled equations enable the modeling of deformation, pressure wave propagation, and dynamic feedback mechanisms within the system.

This configuration is representative of many biological and industrial systems, such as arteries or flexible pipelines, where soft walls play a critical role in the transport and regulation of internal flows. The schematic shown in Fig. 10.1 serves as the conceptual basis for both the experimental analysis and the theoretical modeling presented in this section.

10.2.1 Insights into Pulsatile Flow Phenomena

Pulsatile flow describes a fluid motion characterized by time-dependent variations in velocity and/or pressure, typically occurring in a periodic or cyclic pattern. In contrast to steady flow, where flow conditions remain constant over time, pulsatile flow reflects dynamic behavior influenced by rhythmic driving forces. This type of flow is prevalent in biomedical contexts—most notably in arterial blood circulation—as well as in various industrial processes involving unsteady fluid transport.

Important aspects of pulsatile flows are their time-dependent behavior, that is, the velocity at any point within the pipe varies with time, typically following a sinusoidal or other periodic profile, and their inertial effects, namely the oscillatory nature of pulsatile flow introduces significant inertial and acceleration forces that are absent in steady-state conditions.

The relationship between inertial and viscous forces in a pulsatile flow is described by the *Womersley* number (α), which is a dimensionless parameter defined as:

$$\alpha = \mathrm{Ro}\sqrt{\omega\rho/\mu} \tag{10.1}$$

where Ro is the pipe radius, ω is the angular frequency of the pulsation, ρ is the fluid density, and μ is the dynamic viscosity. Depending on the value of α, the velocity profile can range from parabolic (similar to steady laminar flow) to more complex shapes, including flow reversal near the pipe wall at high α values, while frictional losses vary depending on the pulsatile regime, making the analysis more complex than for steady flow.

10.2.2 Approximate Coefficient of Friction

For pulsating flow, friction can be approximated using the Womersley model. This simplified model for the coefficient of friction R_f is:

$$R_\mathrm{f} = 8\pi\mu/A_0 \tag{10.2}$$

where $A_o = \pi(D/2)^2$ is the cross-sectional area. This is then an approximation to the linear viscous resistance. The thickness of the elastic tube is important for the rigidity of the tube, and is given by the relation:

$$k = \mathrm{Eh}/R_0 \tag{10.3}$$

where E is the modulus of elasticity of the tube.

10.2.3 Wave Velocity in Pulsating Flow

The wave velocity c in pulsating flow in an elastic tube is related to the propagation of pressure waves generated by pulsating pumping. In this case, the wave velocity depends on both the fluid properties and the elasticity of the tube wall.

We can define the wave velocity c as the speed at which a pressure or flow disturbance propagates along the tube. In a rigid (non-deformable) tube, the speed would basically be that of sound in the fluid. But in an elastic tube, the walls expand and contract, reducing the effective velocity and coupling it to the mechanics of the wall.

For a thin tube, the most used model is the Moens–Korteweg equation:

$$c = \sqrt{\mathrm{Eh}/2}\rho\mathrm{Ro} \tag{10.4}$$

This equation assumes a thin, homogeneous tube with a linear-elastic behavior (Akaike 1969).

10.3 Experimental Setup

The experimental setup was developed to investigate fluid behavior in elastic pipes under controlled laboratory conditions. The system is housed within the Department of Energy and the Complex Systems Laboratory at the Metropolitan Autonomous University. It consists of several key components integrated to maintain a constant, measurable fluid flow throughout the apparatus, enabling precise observation and analysis of flow dynamics.

As illustrated in Fig. 10.2, the central element of the setup is a transparent acrylic container measuring 42 cm × 10 cm × 120 cm. This container enables direct visualization of the fluid during experiments, which is essential for accurate monitoring and analysis of flow behavior. Acrylic was chosen for its combination of mechanical strength and excellent optical clarity, allowing for unobstructed observation throughout the testing process.

The elastic tubes used in the experiment, depicted in Fig. 10.3, measure 30 cm in length with an average internal diameter of 8 mm. Prior to each trial, the tubes

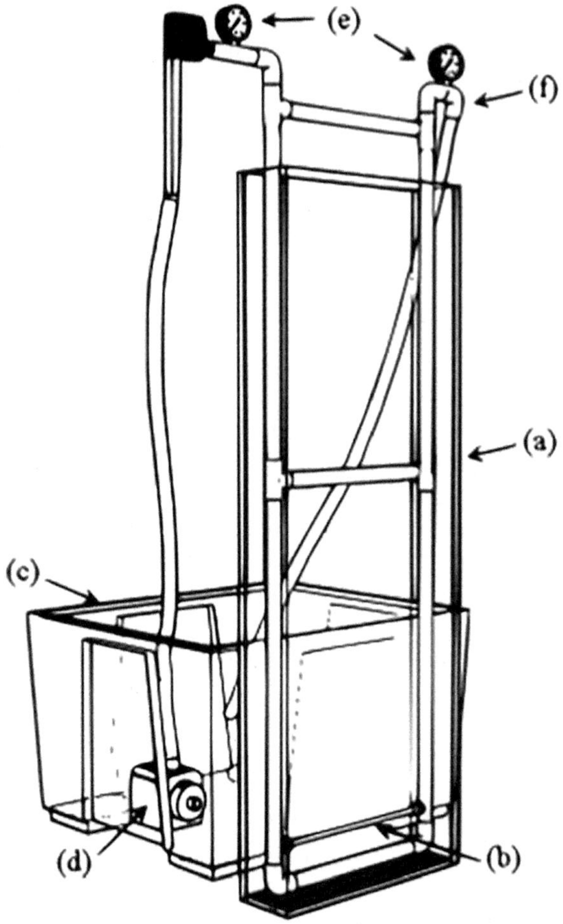

Fig. 10.2 Schematic diagram of the experimental setup. **a** Acrylic container, **b** elastic tubing, **c** water reservoir, **d** submersible pump, **e** pressure gauges, and **f** PVC piping

are thoroughly cleaned and inspected to ensure they are free from obstructions, a critical step for ensuring the accuracy and consistency of the experimental results. Their elastic properties enable them to accommodate fluctuations in fluid pressure and volume without risk of rupture. To maintain proper alignment and structural support throughout the experiments, the tubes are securely mounted at both ends using precision-engineered fixtures.

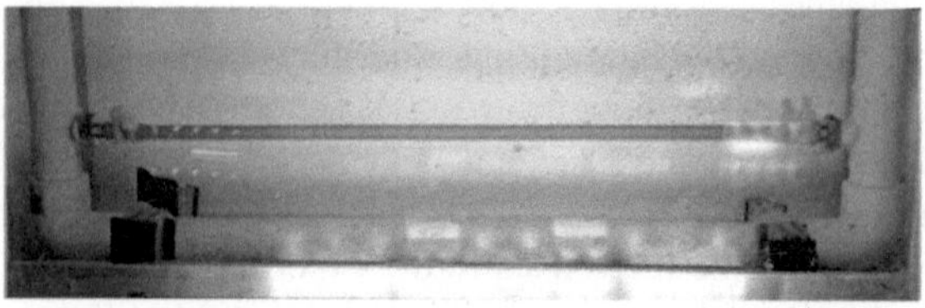

Fig. 10.3 Details of the flexible pipe immersed in water during flow evolution

The system includes a 150-L water storage tank open to the atmosphere, which serves as the primary source of double-distilled water. This reservoir ensures a constant and stable supply of fluid throughout the experiments. A submersible pump with a capacity of 1140 L per hour and a maximum piezometric head of 3.5 m is used to circulate the fluid through the system. The pump is located inside the reservoir to improve efficiency and reduce the risk of overheating.

Pressure gauges and the flowmeter are critical components of the experimental apparatus, serving to monitor and regulate fluid conditions throughout the system. These instruments are strategically positioned at key points to capture real-time measurements of pressure and flow rate during various stages of the experiment. Ensuring the accuracy of these devices through rigorous calibration is fundamental for obtaining precise and reliable data, which underpins the validity of the experimental analysis. Together, these measurement tools facilitate effective control over the fluid dynamics, enabling detailed investigation of the interactions between flow and elastic tube deformation.

PVC piping interconnects all components, ensuring a sealed and efficient flow loop. The straight pipes located upstream and downstream of the elastic tube are made of 1DN Schedule 40 PVC (25 mm). This material was selected for its durability, corrosion resistance, and ease of installation.

The volumetric flow rate is controlled using globe-type valves and measured by a flowmeter. The globe valve, connected to the inlet of the flowmeter, allows precise control of the water flow rate within a range of 3 to 20 L per minute to the elastic pipe. This ensures accurate adjustment of fluid flow throughout the experiment.

The experimental setup has been meticulously designed to study fluid behavior under controlled conditions. Each component has a specific function that contributes to the integrity of the system and the accuracy of the data collected. The use of materials such as acrylic and PVC, along with carefully calibrated measuring devices, ensures the reliability of the experimental results.

10.3.1 Data Acquisition and Image Analysis

The experiments were recorded using a Dantec Dynamics PHANTOM high-speed camera operating at 1000 frames per second (FPS), with a resolution of 512 $\times$ 200 pixels and an exposure time of 30 μs. For image analysis, we used the open-source software Fiji (Fiji Is Just ImageJ) and VirtualDub. These tools enabled accurate frame-by-frame tracking of the tube deformation.

10.3.2 Strength and Rigidity of the Material

In a tensile test, a specimen with a specific geometry is subjected to an axial force, typically until fracture (Akaike 1969). This test provides comprehensive information,

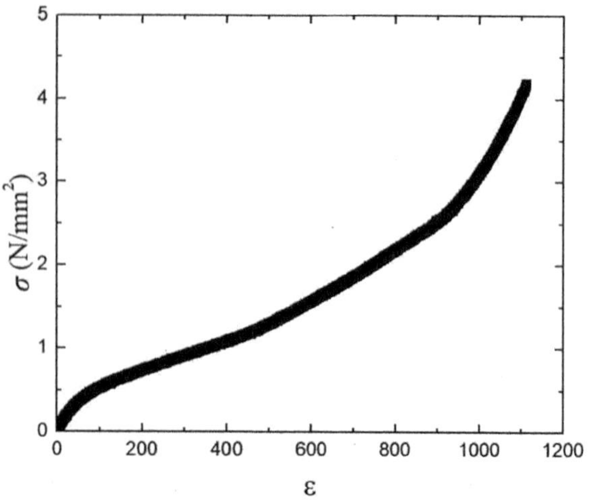

Fig. 10.4 Stress–strain diagram obtained from standard tension test

as it allows both the elastic and plastic responses of the material to be quantified through its mechanical properties such as, the elastic (Young's) modulus, the ultimate tensile strength, and the ductility (i.e., the percentage of elongation at break) (Akaike 1969; Timoshenko and Gere 1985). There are several approaches to conducting a tensile test, including those under fatigue conditions. However, the most common method involves displacement control, where the jaws move apart at a constant rate. This method was used in the present work.

The tests were carried out on a SHIMADZU universal tensile testing machine with a capacity of 10 TON, at a speed of 100 ± 50 mm/min. ISO 527-1 and ISO 527-2 describe methods for determining the tensile properties of thermoplastic materials and elastomers, respectively. ASTM D412 also describes methods for determining the tensile properties of vulcanized thermoset rubber. The results obtained from these tests are presented in Fig. 10.4. The material shows non-linear and hyper-elastic behavior (Timoshenko and Gere 1985; Shigley and Mischke 2012), and the approximate initial modulus of elasticity is:

$$E \approx 4.7 \text{ kPa} \tag{10.5}$$

The tube wall thickness is about 0.25 mm approximately.

10.4 Experimental Results

The initial test was conducted under a hydrostatic pressure of 10 cm, calculated using the relation $P_{\mathrm{H}} = \rho g h$, where$\rho$ is the fluid density,g is the acceleration due to gravity, and$h$ is the height of the fluid column. At room temperature, the corresponding pressure for a height of 10 cm was $P_{\mathrm{H10}} = 981$ Pa. Subsequent tests were performed

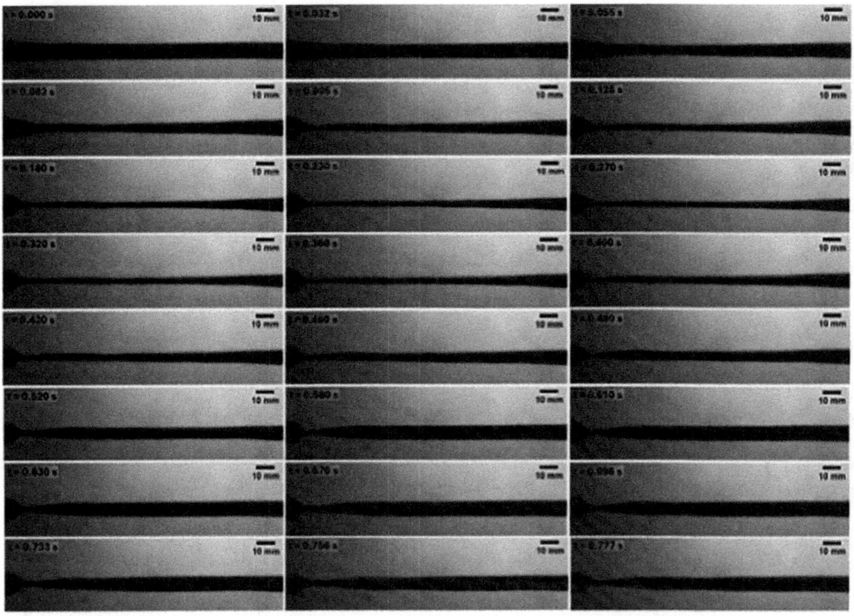

Fig. 10.5 Sequence of images obtained from the first test at a hydrostatic pressure of $P_{\mathrm{H10}} =$ 981 Pa)

at increased fluid heights: 20 cm ($P_{\mathrm{H20}} = 1.962$ kPa) and 30 cm ($P_{\mathrm{H30}} = 2.943$ kPa), allowing for the analysis of fluid–structure interactions under varying hydrostatic loads.

An increase in hydrostatic pressure was observed to induce localized necking near the tube inlet, particularly at fluid heights of $H = 20$ cm and $H = 30$ cm (see Figs. 10.6 and 10.7). Figure 10.5 shows the sequences of the first test at 10 cm of hydrostatic pressure on the elastic tube.

Frames were captured at key moments corresponding to significant changes in the deformation of the elastic tube. At $t = 400$ s, the tube reaches its minimum radius, marking the point of maximum constriction. Following this moment, the tube begins to recover toward its initial configuration. Notably, a localized necking region persists near the upstream section of the tube, although fluid flow continues through the constricted area.

The image sequence in Fig. 10.5 shows the time evolution of the behavior of a thin elastic tube through which water flows. The time progresses from $t = 0$ to$t = 0.777$ s, with snapshots captured at small time intervals. At the beginning, a localized bulge or deformation appears on the left end of the tube. This deformation travels along the tube from left to right over time. The bulge likely results from a pressure wave generated by the water flow, causing the elastic tube to expand radially in response.

The pressure wave or deformation moves steadily along the tube. The tube diameter increases locally where the wave passes, indicating internal pressurization.

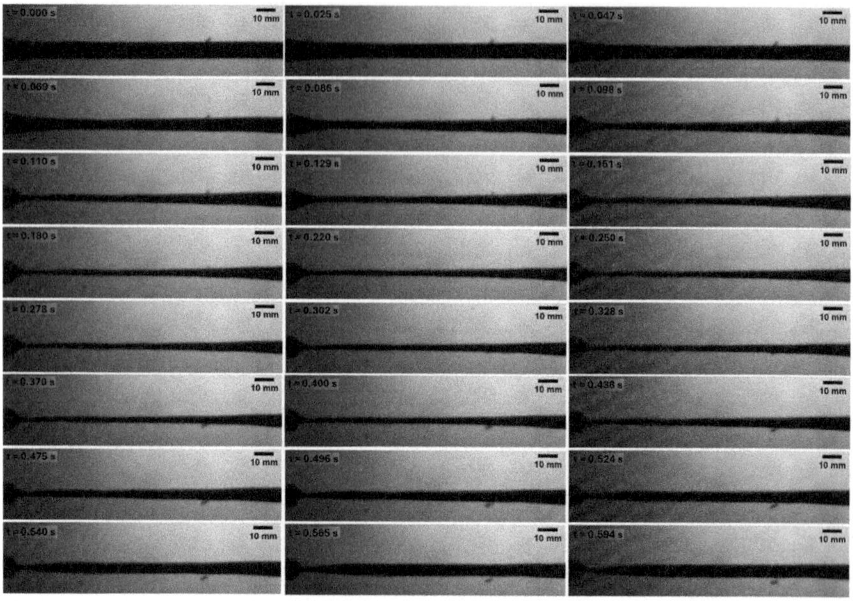

Fig. 10.6 Sequence of images obtained from the first test at a hydrostatic pressure of $P_{H20} =$ 1.962 kPa)

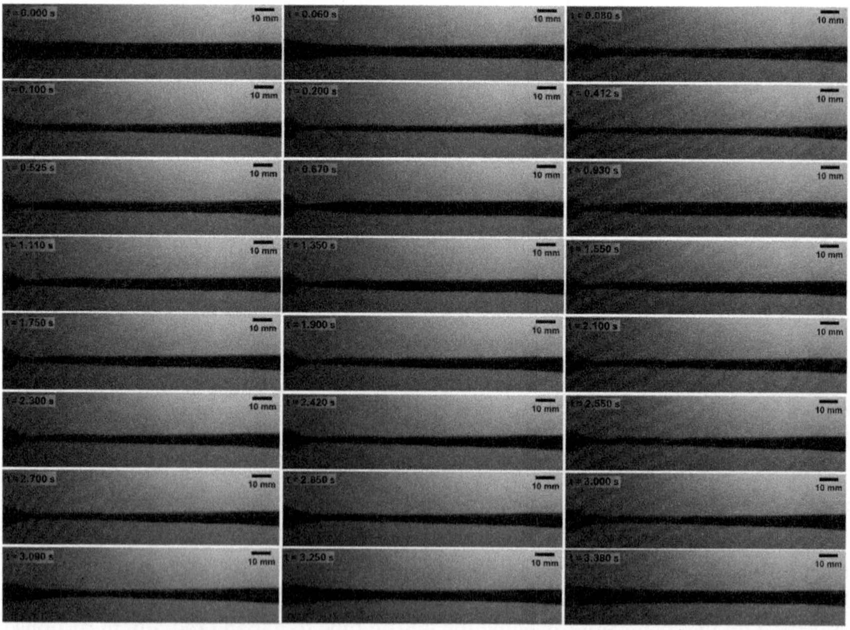

Fig. 10.7 Sequence of images obtained from the first test at a hydrostatic pressure of $P_{H30} =$ 2.943 kPa)

Therefore, the tube exhibits elastic behavior, deforming in response to internal fluid pressure without rupturing. As the wave continues to move, the section of the tube behind it gradually returns to its original diameter, indicating elastic recovery. This suggests that the tube material is reversibly elastic. In the final frames, the tube maintains a more uniform shape, possibly indicating that the pressure wave has existed in the field of view or that the flow has stabilized.

This study demonstrates that elastic pipes subjected to internal flow exhibit dynamic deformation influenced by wall stiffness, pulsation frequency, and pressure variations. The observed phase shift between pressure and flow resembles some phenomena found in biological systems, such as arteries. These findings validate the theoretical fluid–structure interaction model and provide a foundation for future investigations, including multiphase flow and non-linear wall behavior in complex geometries.

As shown in Fig. 10.6, the tube initially has a nearly uniform diameter. Around $t \approx 0.086$–0.110 s, a small, localized expansion appears near the left side of the tube. This may correspond to the onset of a pressure wave or an initial fluid impulse entering the tube. The radial deformation (bulge) progresses steadily from left to right. The deformation is more subtle and narrower compared to the first image sequence. The tube wall follows the movement of the internal pressure front, again showing elastic behavior. After the wave passes, the tube returns to a more uniform diameter, indicating elastic recovery. The deformation becomes less visible, possibly indicating damping or pressure equalization downstream.

The deformation in this sequence is less intense, more localized, and narrower than in the first sequence. This could be due to lower pressure, slower fluid velocity, increased damping, or differences in tube stiffness. The wave travels at a steady pace, suggesting that the system remains in a linear-elastic regime. This image sequence captures the propagation of a localized deformation in an elastic tube caused by internal water flow. Compared to the previous example, the deformation is less pronounced, indicating possible differences in flow conditions or material response. The tube exhibits reversible elastic deformation, with a small pressure wave traveling along its length and the material gradually returning to its initial shape.

Figure 10.7 shows the time evolution of an elastic tube under internal water flow, captured from a side view. The time progresses from $t = 0.000$ s to $t = 3.380$ s, covering a significantly longer duration than the previous two sequences.

A localized bulge or expansion forms at the left end of the tube. This deformation begins to propagate along the tube toward the right, resembling a pressure wave driven by the fluid flow. The radial expansion wave travels steadily along the tube. As the wave passes, the tube behind it maintains a uniform diameter, indicating an elastic and stable mechanical response to the internal pressure. The system enters a steady-state regime: the tube preserves a uniform shape and diameter for a prolonged period. No new bulges or dynamic deformations are observed. This suggests that the system has reached mechanical equilibrium with the flowing fluid or a quasi-steady flow condition.

Compared to the previous two sequences, this case shows a similar initial deformation, a longer wave propagation time, and a more extended stable phase, indicating a sustained and uniform internal flow. The tube demonstrates reversible elastic behavior, with no signs of collapse or permanent deformation. This behavior could be the result of the lower inlet velocity, moderate fluid pressure, higher stiffness, damping in the tube material, or a combination of these factors.

The first sequence displays a strong and fast deformation, with a pressure wave moving quickly along the tube. This suggests a relatively high flow rate or pressure pulse, resulting in a noticeable elastic response. The second sequence shows a less intense and more localized deformation, with moderate wave propagation and a smoother return to the resting state. This indicates milder internal flow conditions or slightly more damping. The third sequence covers a much longer period and demonstrates a slow, stable wave propagation, followed by a prolonged steady-state condition. The deformation is minimal, implying a low-pressure or low-velocity flow with a highly elastic and stable tube response.

By analyzing these differences qualitatively, we gain insight into how elastic conduits respond dynamically to internal flow, which is essential for applications in biomedical engineering (e.g., arteries), soft robotics, and microfluidics.

10.4.1 Data Used in the Experiment

The data used in the experiments are listed as follows:

$E = 4.7$ kPa.

$h = 0.00025$ m.

$A_0 = 5.027 \times 10^{-5}$ m^2

$\rho = 1000$ kg/m^3

$R_0 = 0.004$ m.

The velocity was calculated using the Moens–Korteweg equation with the following parameters:

$R_f = 499.6$ Pa s/m^3

$K = 293{,}750$ kg m^{-1} s^{-2} (Physically, K has dimensions of pressure).

$c = 0.113$ m/s.

10.5 Conclusions

This experimental investigation successfully characterized the fluid–structure interaction phenomena in elastic pipes subjected to pulsatile flow conditions, providing valuable insights into the complex dynamics governing deformable conduit systems. The study bridged theoretical predictions with experimental observations through high-resolution imaging and quantitative analysis, yielding several significant findings with broad implications for both biomedical and industrial applications. The main conclusions can be summarized as follows:

- Dynamic deformation and wave propagation: The elastic tubes exhibited predictable deformation patterns with wave propagation velocities ($c = 0.113$ m/s) that closely aligned with theoretical predictions from the Moens–Korteweg equation. Localized necking phenomena were observed at higher hydrostatic pressures ($P_{H20} = 1.962$ kPa and $P_{H30} = 2.943$ kPa), which demonstrate the capacity of the material to accommodate significant pressure variations while maintaining structural integrity and complete elastic recovery.
- Theoretical model validation: The experimental results strongly validated the fluid–structure interaction model and the utility of the Womersley number approach in characterizing the balance between inertial and viscous forces. The observed phase relationships between pressure waves and wall deformation confirmed the coupling mechanisms predicted by theory, particularly regarding material properties ($E \approx 4.7$ kPa) and geometric parameters.
- Material performance: The comprehensive mechanical characterization revealed non-linear, hyper-elastic behavior with excellent fatigue resistance. The material demonstrated complete elastic recovery across all tested pressure ranges without structural failure or permanent deformation, indicating strong potential for applications requiring repeated loading cycles and long-term operational reliability.
- demonstrated complete
- Applications and impact: The findings have direct relevance to cardiovascular biomechanics, providing benchmarks for arterial stiffness assessment and pulse wave analysis. For industrial applications, the characterized relationship between material properties and dynamic response enables optimized design of flexible pipelines, particularly for pulsating pump systems and variable flow conditions.
- Methodological contributions: The integration of high-speed imaging (1000 FPS) with advanced image processing proved highly effective for capturing transient deformation phenomena. This methodology provides a robust framework for future investigations involving complex geometries, multiphase flows, and non-linear material behaviors.
- Future perspectives: This work establishes a foundation for extending investigations to three-dimensional deformation analysis, bifurcated geometries relevant to vascular networks, and active flow control strategies. The experimental approach can be readily adapted to study temperature effects, material aging, and various fluid properties, contributing to the development of more efficient fluid transport systems and advancing the fundamental understanding of soft matter mechanics in engineering applications.

References

Akaike H (1969) Fitting autoregressive models for prediction. Ann Inst Stat Math 21:243–247

Canic S, Mikelic A (2003) Effective equations modeling the flow of a viscous incompressible fluid through a long elastic tube arising in the study of blood flow through small arteries. SIAM J Appl Dyn Syst 2:431–463

Canic S, Tambaca J, Guidoboni G, Mikelic A, Hartley CJ, Rosenstrauch D (2006) Modeling viscoelastic behavior of arterial walls and their interaction with pulsatile blood flow. SIAM J Appl Math 67:164–193

Desjardins B, Esteban MJ, Grandmont C, Le Talec P (2001) Weak solutions for a fluid-structure interaction model. Rev Mat Comput 14:523–538

CONMECHYDRO-2022. E3S Web Conference, vol 365, pp 03026 (2023). https://doi.org/10.1051/e3sconf/202336503026

Gilbert RP, Mikelic A (2000) Homogenizing the acoustic properties of the seabed: Part I. Nonlinear Anal Theory Methods Appl 40:185–212

Grandmont C, Maday Y (2000) Existence for an unsteady fluid-structure interaction problem. Math. Model. Numer. Anal. 34:609–636

Kuchkarovich SZ (2021) Method for determining hydraulic resistance during fluid flow in pipes. Int J Innov Eng Res Technol (IJIERT) 8(12):80–84

Mikelic A, Guidoboni G, Canic S (2007) Fluid-structure interaction in a pre-stressed tube with thick elastic walls. I. The stationary Stokes problem. Netw Heterog Media 2:397–423

Rodkiewicz CM (1983) Arteries and arterial blood flow, 3rd edn. Springer, Wien

Sarraf S, López E, D'Elía J, Craiem D (2022) Analysis of flow pulse propagation in elastic pipes for the estimation of arterial stiffness. Asoc Arg Mecán Comput 39:901–910

Shigley JE, Mischke CR (2012) Mechanical engineering design, 9th edn. McGraw-Hill, New York, pp 30–36

Shukurov ZK, Yuldoshev BSh, Begjanov A (1997) Investigation of hydraulic resistance of pulsating flows of viscous fluid in elastic pipe. In: Procceedings Annual Conference Powering Canada's Future, vol 2, pp 1–20. Canada Nuclear Soc, Toronto

Timoshenko SP, Gere JM (1985) Theory of elastic stability, vol 1. McGraw-Hill, New York, pp 1–99

Womersley JR (1957) Oscillatory flow in arteries: The constrained elastic tube as a model of arterial flow and pulse transmission. Phys Med Biol 2:178–187

Chapter 11
CAE Analysis of an Adaptive AirBike System for CrossFit Wheelchair Athletes

A. Laiseca-de la Cruz, C. Landeros-Centeno, M. Cabrera-Herrera, R. Suárez-Toscano, and I. Soto-Ayala

Abstract This study presents a computer aid engineering analysis of an adaptive system designed to enable CrossFit wheelchair users to train with an AirBike. The design process was based on a user needs assessment, considering key aspects such as equipment accessibility, device ergonomics, exercise intensity, and necessary modifications to ensure a safe and inclusive experience. The evaluation established the user profile, identifying physical factors such as upper-body mobility and strength, as well as the scope required to meet users' motivational needs. This analysis defined the key functional requirements for the system. To meet these requirements, the development process adhered to the quality function deployment methodology to prioritize technical specifications. A three-dimensional model was created in SolidWorks, integrating a rail and stop mechanism for wheelchair accessibility, along with adjustable handles. Stress analyses were conducted to assess system performance under an applied force of 1372 N, representing the expected loading conditions. The results showed that the maximum stress (230.6 MPa) remained within safe limits, as it did not exceed the material's yield strength. Finally, a full-scale prototype was manufactured, ensuring compliance with safety, comfort, and efficiency criteria for adaptive CrossFit athletes.

Keywords CAE · Adaptive design · User centered engineering · Wheelchair users · Adaptive Crossfit

A. Laiseca-de la Cruz · C. Landeros-Centeno · M. Cabrera-Herrera (✉) · R. Suárez-Toscano · I. Soto-Ayala
Universidad Iberoamericana Puebla, Unidad Territorial Atlixcáyotl, Centro Comercial Puebla, San Andrés Cholula, Puebla, México
e-mail: michelle.cabrera.herrera1@gmail.com

R. Suárez-Toscano
e-mail: 716206@iberopuebla.mx

I. Soto-Ayala
e-mail: isaura.soto@iberopuebla.mx

I. Soto-Ayala
Instituto Politécnico Nacional—Escuela Superior de Ingeniería Mecánica y Eléctrica—Sección de Estudios de Posgrado e Investigación Edificio 5, 2Do Piso, Unidad Profesional Adolfo López Mateos "Zacatenco" Col. Lindavista, Ciudad de México, México

A. Öchsner (ed.), *Progress in Biomaterials and Biomedical Engineering*, Advanced Structured Materials 249, https://doi.org/10.1007/978-3-032-13551-3_11

11.1 Introduction

CrossFit is a discipline that combines high-intensity functional exercises and has gained popularity around the world for its physical and mental health benefits. However, despite its inclusive approach, many people with disabilities, especially wheelchair users, face significant barriers to participating fully in these activities. In this context, there is a need to develop adapted sports equipment that allows these users to enjoy the benefits of CrossFit without limitations (Díaz 2024).

Exercise is essential for people in wheelchairs, as it not only improves physical health but also contributes to emotional well-being and prevents the complications associated with immobility (World Health Organization: Physical Activity 2024). Regular training helps strengthen upper-body muscles, improve circulation, maintain flexibility, and prevent problems such as muscle atrophy, obesity, and pressure ulcers. In addition, exercise has a positive impact on cardiovascular and lung health, reducing the risk of chronic diseases and increasing quality of life.

Currently, the market for adapted exercise equipment offers limited options, especially for high-intensity sports such as CrossFit. There are some devices designed for users with reduced mobility, such as handbikes (hand bicycles) and arm ergometers, but most of this equipments are oriented toward lower intensity aerobic activities or general endurance training (Batec Mobility: The Handbike: Mobility and Autonomy in Your Hands 2024). On the other hand, traditional AirBikes are widely used in gyms because of their ability to work both the upper and lower train, but they do not have features adapted for wheelchair users, as can be seen in Fig. 11.1.

Some adapted solutions include custom modifications made by specific users or gyms, but these options are often expensive, inaccessible, and in many cases do not meet ergonomic standards and adequate safety requirements. Therefore, there is a clear gap in the market for specialized design that allows people in wheelchairs to access functional, intensive, and safe training equipment aligned with the demands of CrossFit.

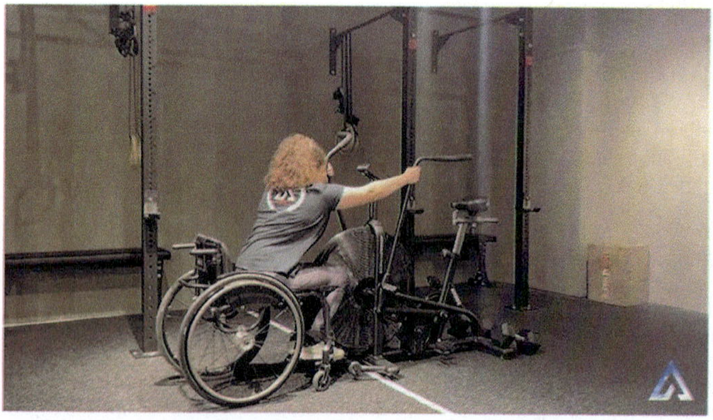

Fig. 11.1 Non-ergonomic adaptation of Crossfit for wheelchair users

This project aims to design an AirBike specifically adapted for people who use wheelchairs and want to practice CrossFit.

The proposed design will address key mechanical and ergonomic aspects, such as ease of access, safe wheelchair integration, the ability to adjust arm resistance, and a robust structure that supports the demands of intense training.

The expected result is an innovative solution that combines functionality, accessibility, and efficiency, in line with universal design principles. This project represents an important step toward the democratization of sport, demonstrating that accessibility and sports performance can coexist without compromising quality or user experience.

11.2 Methodology

11.2.1 Interview

An interview was conducted with CrossFit athletes adapted in the Kraken gym, located in Calzada Zavaleta in Puebla, in order to deepen the needs, challenges, and limitations faced by practicing this type of training. During the conversation, aspects related to the accessibility of the available equipment, the ergonomics of the devices used, the intensity of the exercises, and the modifications needed to ensure a safe, effective, and inclusive experience were explored. These inputs served as a basis for identifying areas of improvement and guiding the design of specific solutions that respond to the demands of this user group.

11.2.2 User Profile

Subsequently, a user profile was created from the information gathered in the interviews. This profile was built considering the physical characteristics, specific needs, and goals of adapted CrossFit athletes. Aspects evaluated included factors such as the level of mobility and strength in the upper train, the adaptations needed to integrate the wheelchair into the exercises, and related performance expectations with the training.

In addition, emotional and motivational aspects were taken into account, such as the search for inclusion, autonomy, and personal improvement that these athletes pursue through physical activity. This process led to the development of a comprehensive understanding of the user, facilitating the design of adapted equipment that not only meets technical and functional requirements but also promotes accessibility, comfort, and safety during use.

11.2.3 Design Proposal

Based on the needs collected during interviews and user profile analysis, a preliminary design proposal for an adapted AirBike was developed that meets the specific demands of adapted CrossFit athletes. This outline integrates innovative solutions focused on accessibility, functionality, and security, ensuring that users can perform high-intensity workouts effectively and comfortably.

11.2.4 Quality Function Deployment

An analysis of the design proposal was developed using the quality function deployment (QFD) matrix, which is a tool for deploying the quality function of a product and ranking design needs. This determines the technical specifications and requirements of the customer, qualifying them according to the priority of compliance.

11.2.5 SolidWorks Design

Once the initial concept had been defined, detailed design was developed using SolidWorks CAD software. At this stage, three-dimensional models of each component were created, ensuring that they were compatible with each other and optimizing the assembly of the equipment. During the process, several corrections and refinements were made, adjusting the design to improve key aspects. This made it possible to develop a complete and functional digital model, ready for the next validation and manufacturing stages.

This design included elements such as an adapter and handles for the wheelchair athlete, as well as a rail and stop that would prevent the movement of the wheelchair when the athlete is performing the exercise, with the aim of increasing user safety and efficiency.

11.2.6 Mechanical Analysis

A motion analysis of the device developed using SolidWorks software was performed. In this, aspects such as tension, deformation, and displacement of the device were evaluated by applying a force on components such as the end of the rail and in the connectors on the handles. For this, the base of the structure was taken into account as a fixed element and the materials corresponding to each component were added.

Rail Stop

To calculate the force applied on the stop, the maximum weight supported by the wheelchair used as model was considered, which is 140 kg, so the calculation would be as follows:

$$\text{Applied force} = \text{ma} = (140\,\text{kg}) * 9.8\frac{\text{kg}}{\text{m}^2} = 1372\,\text{N}$$

Handle Connectors

On the other hand, the force applied to the connectors of the handles was calculated using the equation of drag force or aerodynamic resistance (University of Iowa: Drag forces 2016):

$$F = \frac{1}{2}C_d \cdot A \cdot \rho \cdot v^2$$

where F is the drag force, C_d is the coefficient of drag, A is the transverse area of the object facing the flow, ρ is the density of the fluid (air), and v is the velocity of the object with respect to the fluid.

First, a drag coefficient of 0.35 was considered, based on the drag coefficient of an amateur cyclist (Aguirre 2023). On the other hand, to calculate the transverse area of the object facing the fluid, we measured the fan blades area of an Airbike, which was 0.3 m^2. As for fluid density, the air density in Puebla was considered, which is 1200 g/m^3. Finally, the average speed of an adapted CrossFit athlete was calculated when performing this exercise at a high intensity, which gave a result of 4 m/s.

Therefore, the following strength was obtained:

$$F = \frac{1}{2}(1) \cdot \left(0.3\,\text{m}^2\right) \cdot \left(1200\frac{\text{g}}{\text{m}^2}\right) \cdot \left(4\frac{\text{m}}{\text{s}}\right)^2 = 1008\,\text{N}$$

11.2.7 Manufacture of Prototype

Finally, a life-size prototype of the device was manufactured. Wood was used to produce the wheelchair rail and bumper, while PVC tubes were used for fastening element of the bumper to the rail and the user handles. As for the adapters for the AirBike handles, these were 3D printed using PLA.

11.3 Results

11.3.1 Interview

The need to adapt an AirBike so that wheelchair-friendly CrossFit athletes can perform the necessary exercise on this machine was highlighted, since the design of existing products does not include adaptations for people with motor disabilities.

11.3.2 User Profile

At the end of the interview, the device was restricted to wheelchair users who practice CrossFit adapted for people with paraplegia who have sufficient upper limb strength.

11.3.3 Design Proposal

Figure 11.2 shows the sketch of the design obtained.

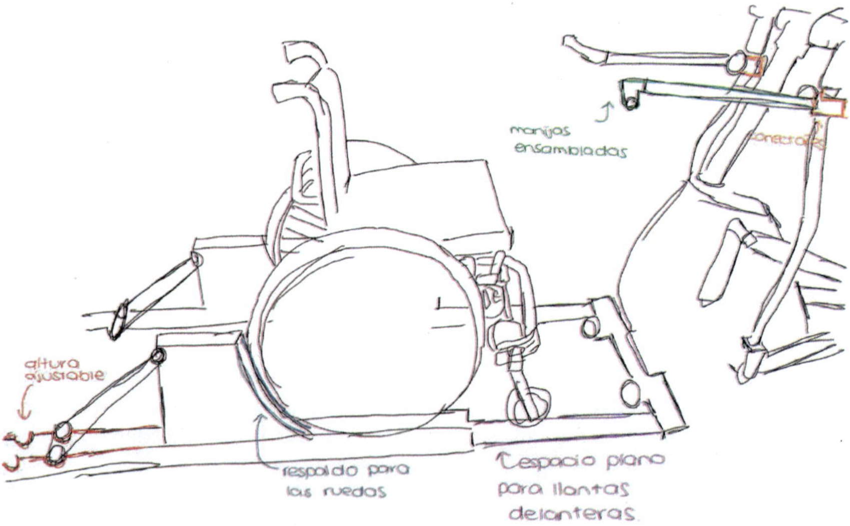

Fig. 11.2 Outline of the design with the indicated requirements

11.3.4 Quality Function Deployment

The technical and client requirements were specified to analyze their relationship and assign them a relevance score. In terms of technical requirements were defined: strong structural design, stability and safety, inclusive for wheelchair users, durability, ease of use, ergonomics, corrosion resistance, electronic safety, adjustment of resistance levels, and compliance with Mexican regulations.

On the other hand, the customer's requirements were: that the equipment can be used for users and not wheelchair users, that the handles can only be put on when used (removable), exercise safety, monitor heart rate and calories burned during training, durable and sturdy equipment for long-term use, comfortable and ergonomic handles to ensure pleasant experience, lightweight handle adaptations for easy transport and storage, easy to clean and maintain material after training, eco-friendly and recyclable material, space to secure the wheelchair and prevent it from moving during training.

After completing the matrix, aspects that obtained a higher relevance score were: inclusive for wheelchair users, stability, ease of use, durability, and strong structural design.

11.3.5 SolidWorks Design

The final design modeled in SolidWorks is shown in Figs. 11.3, 11.4, 11.5, and 11.6, showing elements such as adapters and detachable handles as well as the rail and stop for the wheelchair.

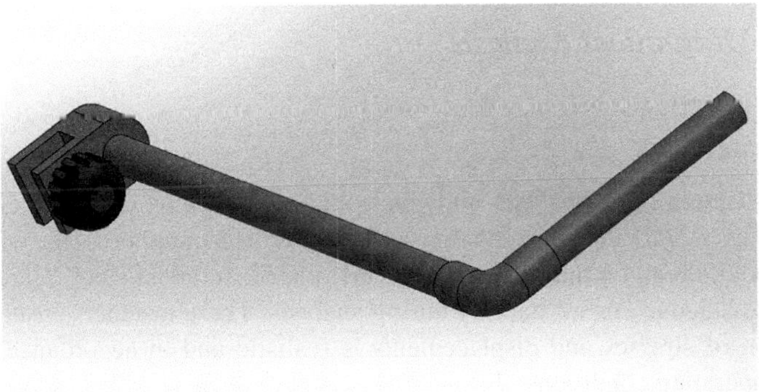

Fig. 11.3 Detachable handle with adapter

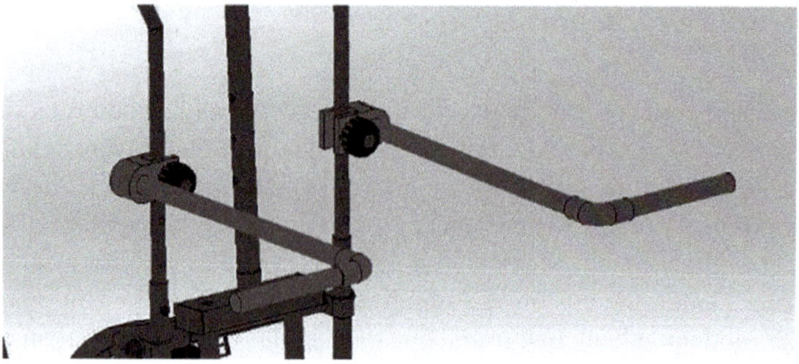

Fig. 11.4 Handles placed in the structure

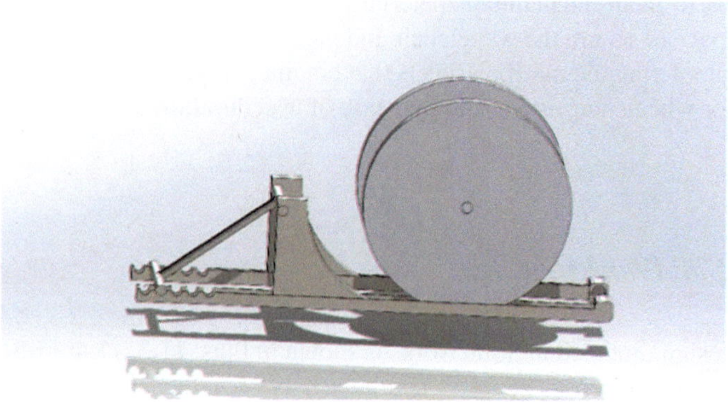

Fig. 11.5 Wheelchair rail and stop

11.3.6 Mechanical Analysis

Base Structure

In the software, a static analysis study was obtained based on the applied forces as shown in Fig. 11.7 for the assembly that was designed as the support of the wheelchair. In this model, the main material used was AISI 316L stainless steel. The assembly was double-sided to ensure stability during analysis. These fasteners ensure that the distribution of stresses and displacements is realistic and in accordance with the intended operating conditions.

The results obtained show that the maximum von Mises stress reaches $2.306 \times 105\text{N/m}^2$. The maximum displacement is 6.323×10^{-4}mm, while the single strain was determined with a maximum of 6.789×10^{-7}. These values indicate an efficient structural response under the applied load of 1372 N.

Handle Connectors

Fig. 11.6 Final device

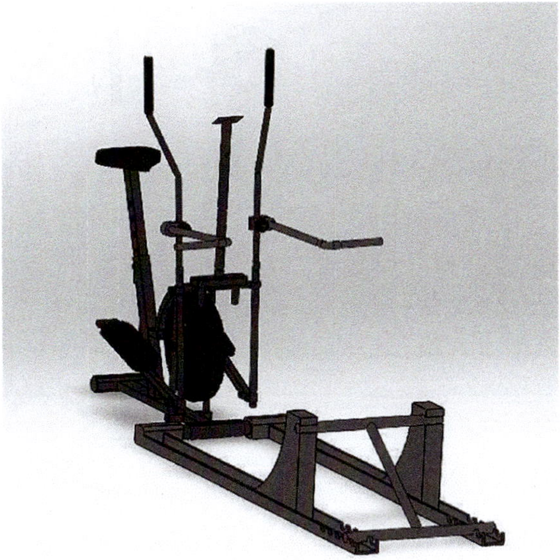

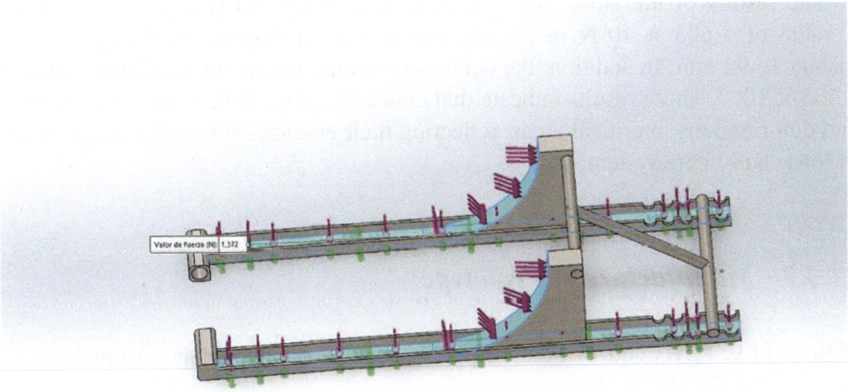

Fig. 11.7 Forces applied for the static analysis of wheelchair support

In the software, a static analysis was carried out to evaluate the behavior of the connectors under applied forces, as shown in Fig. 11.8. The main material selected for these elements was carbon steel, due to its hardness properties, low cost, and high mechanical strength. During the analysis, appropriate constraints were set on key points to ensure stability of the model and simulate realistic operating conditions.

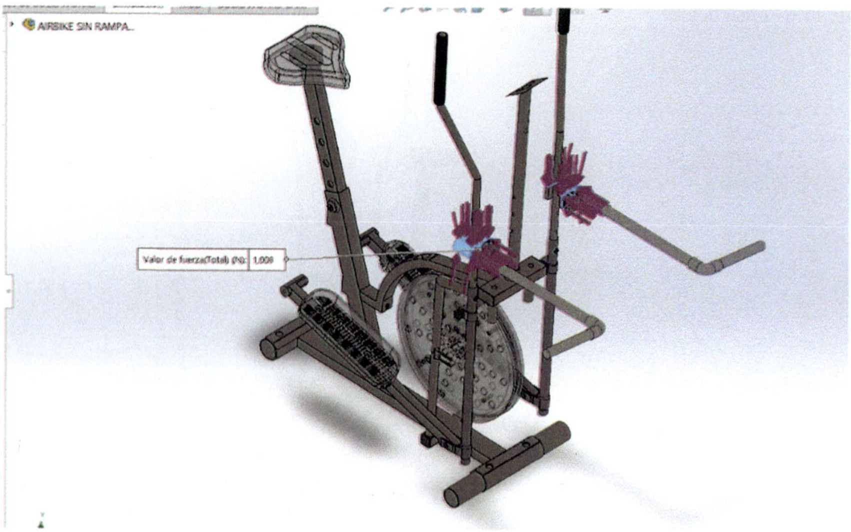

Fig. 11.8 Applied forces for the static analysis of handle connectors

The results of the study show that the von Mises' maximum stress reached a value of $1.603 \times 10^9 \mathrm{N/m}^2$, while the maximum displacement was approximately 16.92 mm. In addition, the equivalent strain presented a maximum value of 4.555×10^{-3}. These results indicate that connectors experience significant stresses and deformations in critical areas, reflecting their essential role in the transmission of loads within the system.

11.3.7 Manufacture of Prototype

Figures 11.9, 11.10, and 11.11 show pictures of the prototype manufactured.

11.4 Results Analysis

11.4.1 Rail Stop

Von Mises Stress Analysis

Figure 11.12 shows a static analysis performed in SolidWorks, where the distribution of von Mises nodal stresses is analyzed in an assembly under the application of a force of 1372 N. The color scale on the display makes it possible to identify the

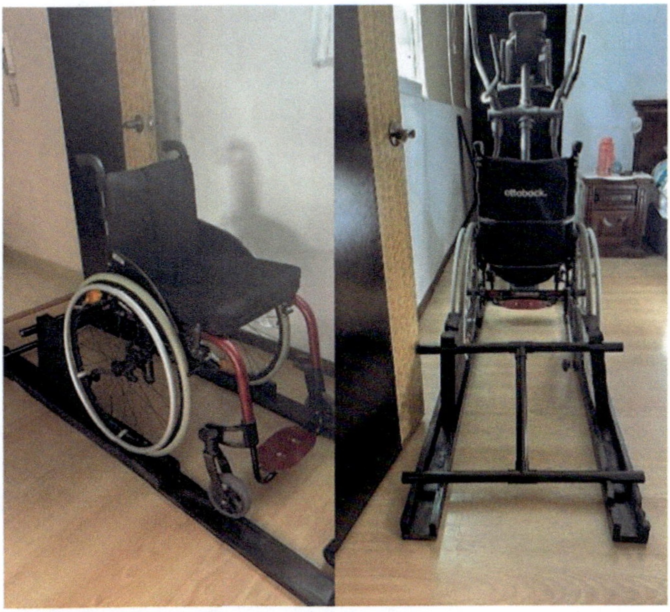

Fig. 11.9 **a** Side view of the prototype, **b** rear view of the prototype

zones of highest and lowest stress in the structure, being the dark blue indicative of low stress and the red of high stress. The maximum stress recorded in the analysis is approximately 230.6 MPa $\left(2.306 \times 10^5 \text{N/m}^2\right)$, which is observed in specific areas of the structure, mainly in the areas near the joints or curves where the force is applied.

The material used in the assembly is AISI 316L stainless steel, which has an initial yield stress of 170 MPa and a tensile strength of 485 MPa. Comparing these values with the maximum recorded stress, it is concluded that the stresses exceed the elastic limit, suggesting that the structure could be subjected to plastic deformation in the identified critical areas. However, the stresses are below the tensile limit, so a fracture is unlikely to occur under these conditions.

Analysis of Displacement

Figure 11.13 shows the displacement analysis performed in SolidWorks for the assembly under an applied force of 1372 N. The color scale in the graphical representation indicates the values of displacement in millimeters (mm), with values ranging from dark blue, representing minimum displacements, to red, which represents maximum displacements. The deformation scale in this analysis is 300.791.

The maximum displacement reported is 0.6323 mm, as seen in the red colored areas, located mainly at the ends of curved parts. These zones are more susceptible to deformation due to the application of the load and the geometrical characteristics of the assembly, which concentrate the bending at these points.

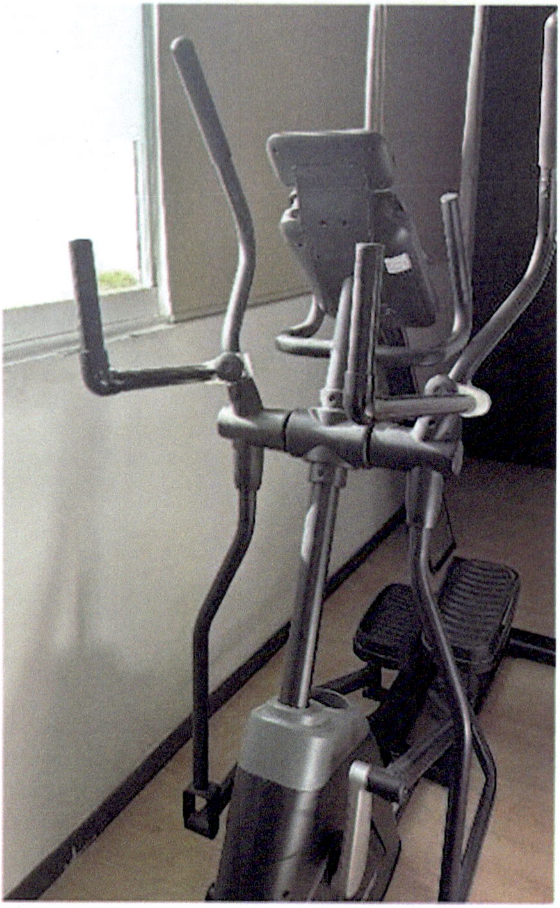

Fig. 11.10 Adapters and handles for athletes

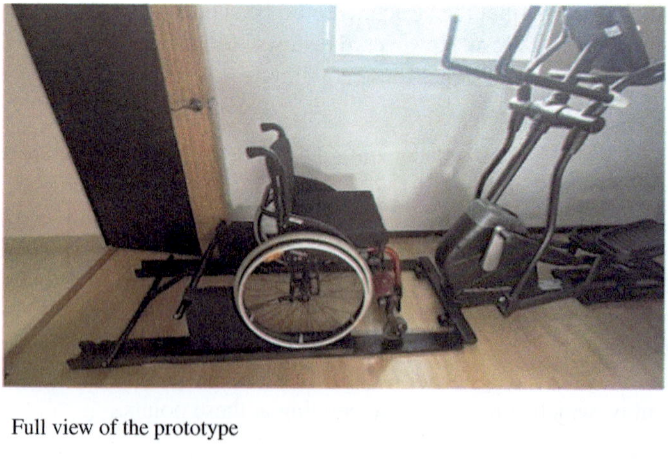

Fig. 11.11 Full view of the prototype

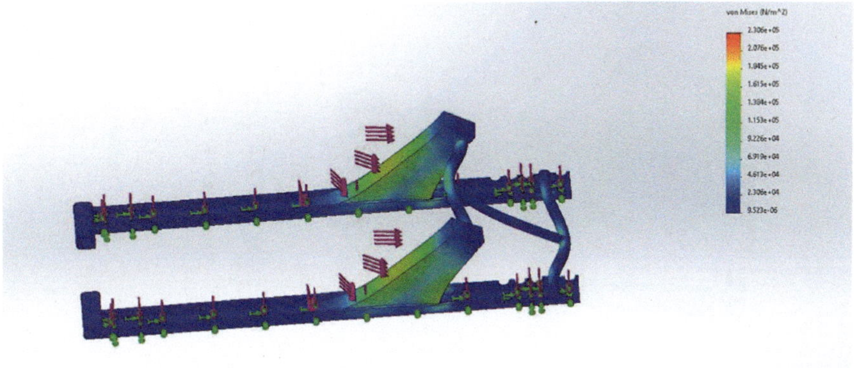

Fig. 11.12 Von Mises stress analysis

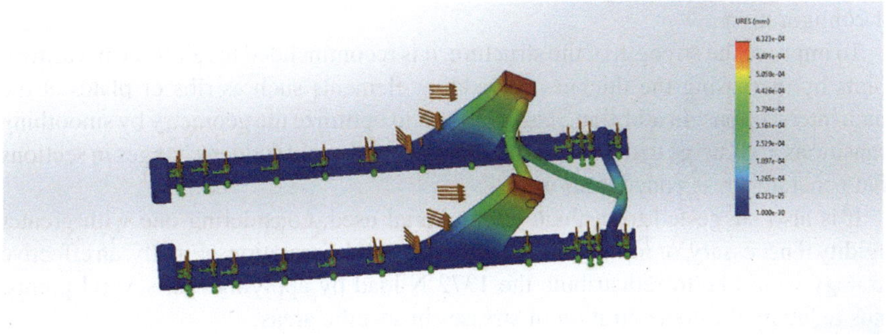

Fig. 11.13 Displacement analysis

The dark blue areas show minimal displacements, indicating that these parts of the assembly are well attached or under less stress. These results reflect a relatively rigid structure, but with some localized bending in the critical areas.

The maximum displacement of 0.6323 mm indicates good structural stability, but if greater rigidity is required, it is recommended to reinforce critical areas, modify geometry to redistribute loads or use more rigid materials. These improvements would optimize the assembly's stability and performance.

Analysis of Strains

Figure 11.14 corresponds to the analysis of strains of a structure under a force of 1372 N, represented by a color map in the SolidWorks simulation. The strain range (indicated in the color scale) shows a maximum of $6.798\ e - 07$ and a minimum close to $6.236\ e - 17$, reflecting that red areas are the most deformed.

The red areas of the analysis indicate the areas with the greatest strain, located mainly at the junctions where the diagonal bars and the central structure converge. This suggests that these zones bear the greatest load or experience the greatest strains,

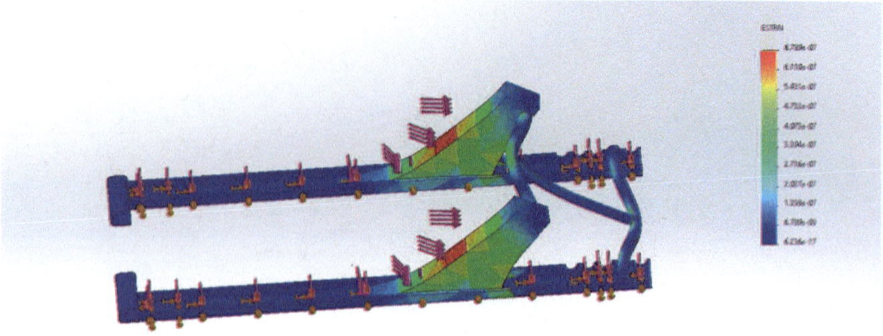

Fig. 11.14 Strain analysis

possibly due to stress concentrations caused by abrupt changes in design geometry or configuration.

To improve the strength of the structure, it is recommended to reinforce the critical joints by increasing the thickness or adding elements such as ribs or plates at the main intersections. In addition, it is important to optimize the geometry by smoothing transitions and curves to distribute forces evenly and avoid sudden changes in sections that generate stress concentrations.

It is also suggested to evaluate the material used, considering one with greater rigidity if necessary, or modify the design to reduce deformations. Finally, an effective strategy would be to redistribute the 1372 N load by applying it at several points, thus reducing the concentration of stresses in specific areas.

11.4.2 Handle Connectors

Von Misses Stress Analysis

Figure 11.15 corresponds to the von Mises stress analysis performed in SolidWorks, which shows that the critical areas of the model, represented in red and yellow, are subjected to stresses up to 1.6 GPa $\left(1.6 \times 10^9 \mathrm{N/m^2}\right)$.. These areas mainly correspond to the connectors of the handles and other structural parts close to the fasteners, which bear the highest applied load of 1008 N. On the other hand, the blue zones indicate areas with low stress, suggesting that they are not directly involved in the main charge. However, the materials considered (stainless steel and carbon steel) have much lower elastic limits, typically between 207 and 350 MPa, indicating that the calculated stresses significantly exceed their capacity, which could lead to plastic deformation or structural failure.

Analysis of Displacement

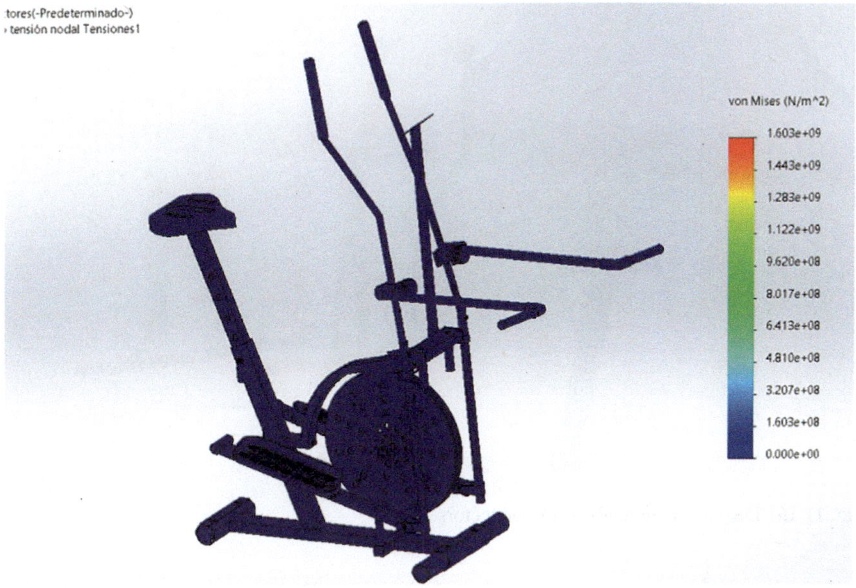

Fig. 11.15 Von Mises stress analysis of connectors

Figure 11.16 shows an analysis of displacements made in SolidWorks, in which the areas of the model that experience greater deformation under the application of a force of 1008 N are identified. According to the color scale, the areas in red show the maximum displacements, reaching approximately 16.92 mm, while the blue areas correspond to points with minimal or no displacements. The most significant displacements are observed in the upper parts of the handles, suggesting that they are subjected to bending under the applied force.

Analysis of Strains

Figure 11.17 shows an analysis of equivalent strains in SolidWorks, which evaluates the relative deformations in the model under the application of an external force of 1008 N. According to the color scale, the red areas correspond to the areas with the highest strains (maximum of approximately $4.555\,e-03$), while the blue zones indicate areas with minimal or no deformation.

In this case, the most significant strains are again concentrated on the top of the handles, especially in the areas furthest from the attachment points. This pattern suggests that the flexibility of the material and the design of the component allow for greater relative elongation in these areas under the applied load.

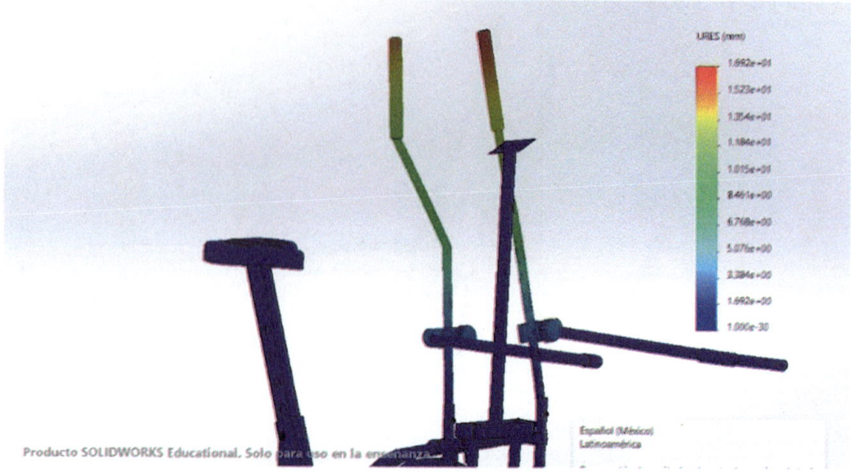

Fig. 11.16 Displacement analysis of connectors

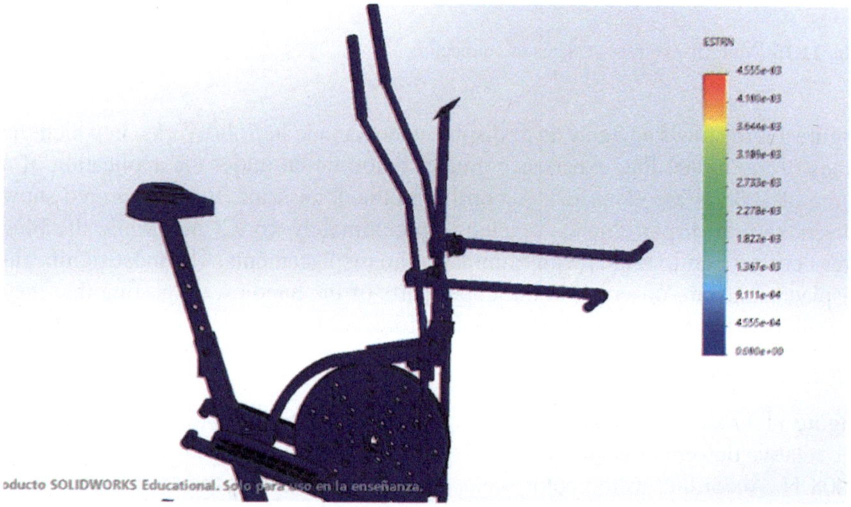

Fig. 11.17 Strain analysis

11.4.3 Analysis of Manufacturing Results

The manufactured stand whose purpose was to hold and stabilize a wheelchair together with exercise equipment.

It can be noted that the design shows clear functionality, as the support fits correctly to the wheels of the wheelchair, indicating good consideration of dimensions during the design and manufacturing process.

In addition, the integration with the elliptical ensures that it was designed correctly to facilitate simultaneous use of the equipment by people with reduced mobility.

11.5 Conclusions

This project drives sports inclusion by adapting an AirBike with handles, rails, and buffers for wheelchair users, promoting participation in adapted CrossFit competitions. It is also a key tool for physical rehabilitation, as it improves muscle strength, cardiovascular endurance and exercise safety. By ensuring stability and accessibility, the design is relevant for both sports and therapeutic use.

As a recommendation, it is suggested to evaluate the user experience to make adjustments in future versions, especially in terms of comfort and fit. It would also be useful to incorporate anti-slip rubbers in the base to improve adhesion to the floor and perform additional stress tests to ensure the durability of the support in the long term.

As regards ergonomics, it would be important to analyze whether the position of the chair in relation to the pedals of the Airbike allows a comfortable movement for the end user. The finishes should also be checked to ensure that the edges and joints do not pose a risk of injury or damage to the chair.

A proposal for future improvements of the device includes the development of an adjustable design that allows rails and handles to be adapted to different types of wheelchairs and users, optimizing ergonomics and functionality. In addition, the integration of sensors that measure the user's performance, such as applied force and pace, would allow a personalized follow-up during training.

References

Aguirre T (2023) Cycling and aerodynamics: what you need to know. https://www.sport.es/bicio/ciclismo-y-aerodinamica-lo-que-debes-saber/#:~:text=El%20coeficiente%20de%20drag%20(Cd,y%20segura%20en%20la%20bicicleta. Accessed 2 Dec 2024

Batec Mobility: The Handbike: Mobility and Autonomy in Your Hands (2024). https://batec-mobility.com/handbike/. Accessed 2 Dec 2024

Díaz M (2024) Benefits of CrossFit for Health. https://www.debate.com.mx/estiloyvida/Descubre-los-Increibles-BENEFICIOS-del-CrossFit-para-tusalud-y-bienestar-20240922-0058.html. Accessed 2 Dec 2024

University of Iowa: Drag Forces (2016). https://pressbooks.uiowa.edu/clonedbook/chapter/drag-forces/. Accessed 2 Dec 2024

World Health Organization: Physical Activity (2024). https://www.who.int/news-room/fact-sheets/detail/physical-activity. Accessed 2 Dec 2024

Chapter 12
Characterization and Numerical Simulation of Hemp-Reinforced Bio-composites Using Additive Manufacturing

Anusha Arulalan, Christopher Rockinger, and Markus Merkel

Abstract Additive manufacturing has revolutionized bio-composite applications by enabling precise material deposition and sustainable production. This study evaluates the mechanical and thermal properties of hemp-reinforced recycled polylactic acid composites fabricated using fused filament fabrication and injection molding. Tensile specimens were produced using both techniques and compared to pure recycled polylactic acid samples. Experimental tests, including thermomechanical analysis, thermogravimetric analysis, differential scanning calorimetry, and tensile testing, were conducted alongside numerical simulations to assess material performance. Results indicate that hemp-reinforced composites significantly outperform recycled polylactic acid in key mechanical properties. Results showed the elastic modulus increased by 21.15%, ultimate tensile strength improved by 33.23%, and the coefficient of thermal expansion decreased by 14.23%. These findings demonstrate that these bio-composites can serve as viable alternatives to synthetic materials in structural applications, reducing plastic consumption by 10% while maintaining superior mechanical integrity. This study paves the way for sustainable composite development in automotive, aerospace, and other high-performance industries.

Keywords Bio-composites · Additive manufacturing · Hemp · Recycled polylactic acid · Mechanical properties

12.1 Introduction

Numerous countries consented to alter it and formally promised to sign the 2015 Paris Agreement though the development has been sluggish, they do have the best of intentions. Nonetheless, a fourth industrial revolution is taking place throughout

A. Arulalan (✉) · C. Rockinger · M. Merkel
Aalen University, Aalen, Germany
e-mail: anusha.arulalan@hs-aalen.de

A. Öchsner (ed.), *Progress in Biomaterials and Biomedical Engineering*, Advanced Structured Materials 249, https://doi.org/10.1007/978-3-032-13551-3_12

the world, which could aid nations in achieving their objective. Additive manufacturing is one of the industry 4.0's technologies (Steenhuis et al. 2022). Consumer products should be flexible with replaceable parts that can be additively manufactured. The majority of the materials used in fused filament fabrication printers are not very ecologically friendly or biodegradable. In order to address this, biodegradable composites that can be printed to your specifications and utilized in replaceable parts requirements have been created. Natural fiber-reinforced composites have garnered significant attention from researchers in recent years. Bio-composites have numerous benefits, including low cost, high strength to weight ratio, biodegradable, reduced carbon footprint, and lightweight nature (Rouway et al. 2020).

Choosing hemp fiber offers a strategic balance between mechanical qualities and environmental benefits. The great strength and stiffness of hemp fibers make them perfect for structural reinforcement in bio-composites. Dimensional stability, which is essential in load-bearing applications, is provided by its moderate density and low elongation at break (Kandachar and Brouwer 2001). Polylactic acid's high tensile modulus, strong flexural strength, and compatibility with conventional manufacturing techniques make it unique among biodegradable polymers. It is an environmentally friendly substitute for plastics made from petroleum because it is biodegradable and comes from renewable resources. Polylactic acid provides the perfect mix of printability and mechanical performance for additive manufacturing, despite its heat constraints. It was chosen as the polymer matrix in this investigation because of these characteristics. Because of the literature research, biodegradability, and compatibility with additive manufacturing, polylactic acid was chosen as the matrix material in its recycled form, which was produced by turning waste polylactic acid filaments into pellets, and raw carded hemp fiber, which was obtained from Nina Heitmann Felde Fibers, was utilized as the natural reinforcement (Ranakoti et al. 2022; Wang et al. 2022).

12.2 Materials and Experimental Methods

This work builds on our previously published study (Arulalan et al. 2025) which demonstrated how to fabricate a natural fiber-reinforced composite using hemp and recycled polylactic acid and conduct preliminary tensile tests.

12.2.1 Materials

Raw carded hemp fibers were added at specified weight ratios to recycled polylactic acid, which was pelletized from waste filament. Tensile testing was carried out in accordance with ASTM D638 guidelines after the composite was produced using fused filament fabrication. To compare the created material's properties, tensile

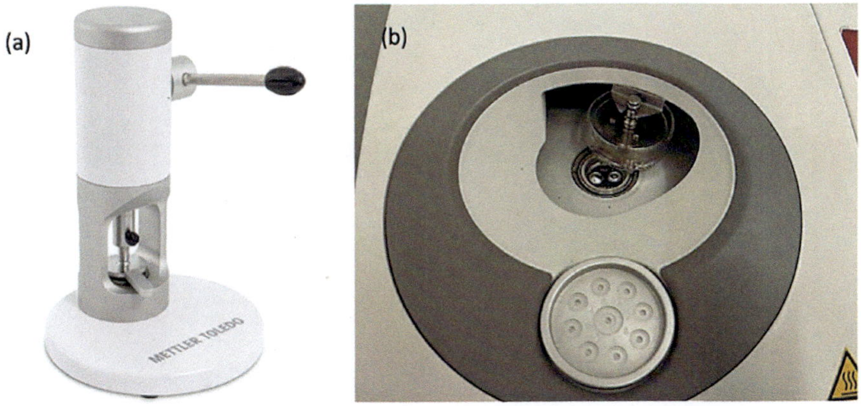

Fig. 12.1 **a** Mettler Toledo crucible sealing press, **b** samples placed in differential scanning calorimetry machine

specimens were also prepared using recycled polylactic acid. Although fundamental understanding was gained, additional thermal, microstructural and numerical analysis were required to comprehend the composite behavior under broader conditions.

12.2.2 *Differential Scanning Calorimetry*

A Mettler Toledo thermal analysis system (differential scanning calorimetry 3+) was used to assess samples' melting and crystallization behavior. Approximately 5 mg of each sample were sealed in aluminum crucibles using a Mettler Toledo crucible sealing press, Fig. 12.1a and placed in differential scanning calorimetry 3+ machine, Fig. 12.1b.

The testing procedure involved heating of the samples to 250 °C at 20 K/min, cooling to −50 °C, and a secondary heating to 250 °C. Liquid nitrogen was used for cooling. Each test lasted 51 min.

12.2.3 *Thermomechanical Analysis*

Thermomechanical analysis testing is carried out by a Mettler Toledo Thermomechanical analysis/SDTA 2+ machine, Fig. 12.2. The natural fiber-reinforced composites and recycled polylactic acid samples were precisely cut in 2324.49 μm 2278.23 μm in length, respectively.

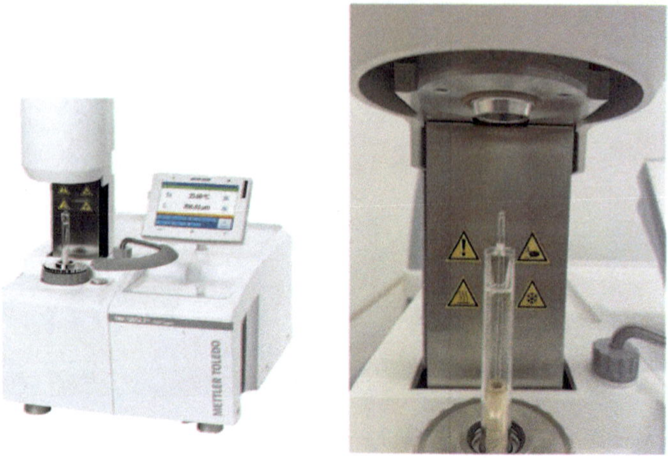

Fig. 12.2 **a** Thermomechanical analysis/SDTA 2 + machine, **b** sample placed in thermomechanical analysis machine

A temperature cycle from 30 to 150 °C, cooled to 30 °C, and reheated to 150 °C was applied at 2 K/min for heating and 20 K/min for cooling. A constant force of 0.02 N was applied. The test duration per sample was approximately 2 h and 10 min.

12.2.4 Thermogravimetric Analysis

Three natural fiber-reinforced composites and three recycled polylactic acid samples made up the total of six samples that were analyzed. The Mettler Toledo Thermogravimetric analysis/differential scanning calorimetry 3+ system was used to perform the thermogravimetric analysis, Fig. 12.3.

Sample weights ranged between 18.45 and 21.00 mg. The analysis was carried out using a nitrogen flow of 50 mL/min and heating from 20 to 800 °C. For the duration of the experiment, oxygen was used in place of nitrogen once it reached 600 °C.

12.2.5 SEM Analysis

Although the porosity in natural fiber-reinforced composites specimens was first observed using SEM in our previously published study (Arulalan et al. 2025), this work expands on the analysis by using ImageJ to calibrate fiber diameter assessments and quantitative porosity measurements, providing a deeper understanding of the impact of microstructural features on composite performance.

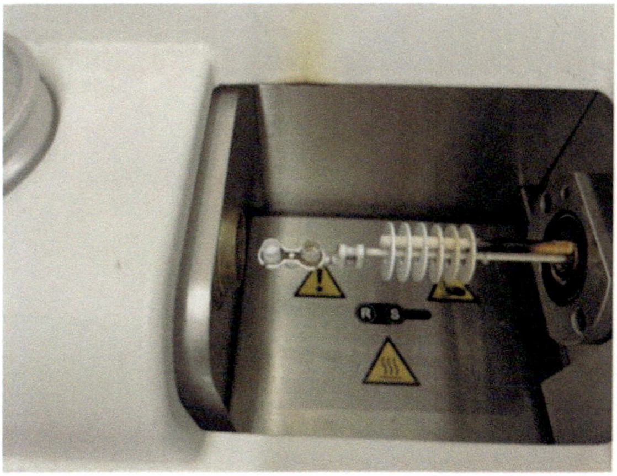

Fig. 12.3 Sample placed in thermogravimetric analysis machine

12.3 Results and Analysis

Tensile test results have been already discussed in the previous paper (Arulalan et al. 2025) and this continues with the other thermal tests.

12.3.1 Differential Scanning Calorimetry

Various thermal behaviours during heating and cooling cycles based on differential scanning calorimetry data for natural fiber reinforced composites 1, 2, and 3 are shown in Fig. 12.4. All samples exhibit distinct endothermic peaks during heating, indicating melting or softening, and exothermic responses during cooling, showing crystallization. Differences in transition temperatures and heat flow intensity show thermal stability. Recycled polylactic acid melts at 180–183 °C and crystallizes at 88–100 °C, Fig. 12.5. These thermal transitions provide information on each material's processability and temperature response.

The crystallinity values reveal material structure differences: Natural fiber-reinforced composites 1 shows the highest crystallinity at 47.39%, suggesting enhanced mechanical properties, followed by natural fiber-reinforced composites 2 (33.93%) and natural fiber-reinforced composites 3 (33.16%). Recycled polylactic acid samples exhibit crystallinity between 32.8 and 39.74%. Overall, natural fiber-reinforced composites show higher thermal stability, with melting points reaching up to 187 °C, and smoother heat flow profiles compared to recycled polylactic acid. This suggests that natural fiber-reinforced composites are better suited for high-temperature applications, while recycled polylactic acid, with more defined thermal transitions, remains well-suited for controlled-temperature processes like 3D printing.

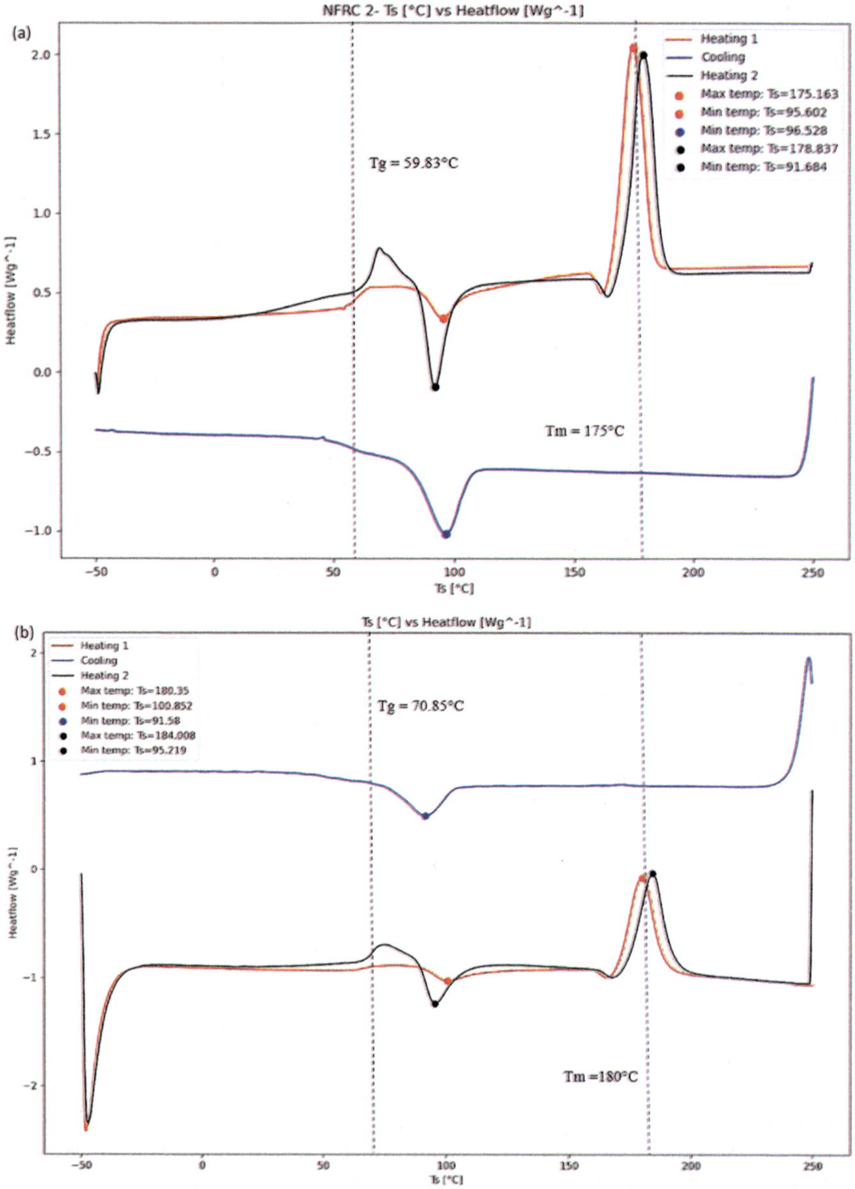

Fig. 4 **a** Differential scanning calorimetry result of natural fiber reinforced composites 1, **b** differential scanning calorimetry result of natural fiber reinforced composites 2, **c** differential scanning calorimetry result of natural fiber reinforced composites 3

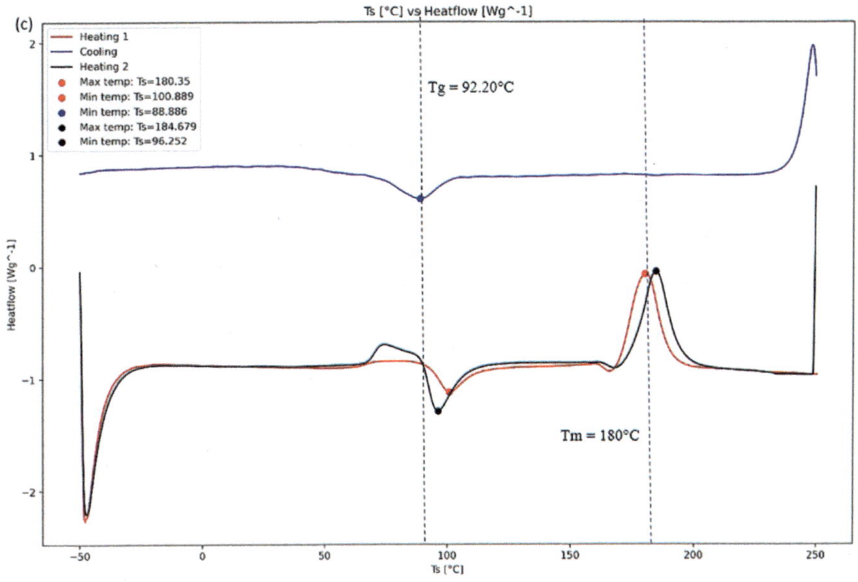

Fig. 4 (continued)

12.3.2 *Thermomechanical Analysis*

The material's rate of expansion per degree of temperature increase is indicated by the coefficient of thermal expansion, which for natural fiber-reinforced composites is 79.4 ppm/K and recycled polylactic acid is 92.57 ppm/K, Fig. 12.6a, b. When thermal load is applied, the displacement increases steadily, indicating that natural fiber-reinforced composites expand uniformly and exhibit stable and predictable thermal behavior while recycled polylactic acid may still be viable where controlled expansion is acceptable. For applications where, dimensional stability under changing temperature conditions is critical, this feature is essential.

Recycled polylactic acid has a consistent thermal expansion, but its greater coefficient of thermal expansion makes it more vulnerable to dimensional changes when heated, limiting its viability for high thermal stability applications. However, its constant response may still be valuable in situations where regulated expansion is permitted. In contrast, natural fiber-reinforced composites have a lower Coefficient of thermal expansion and higher dimensional stability, making it more suitable for high or variable-temperature situations.

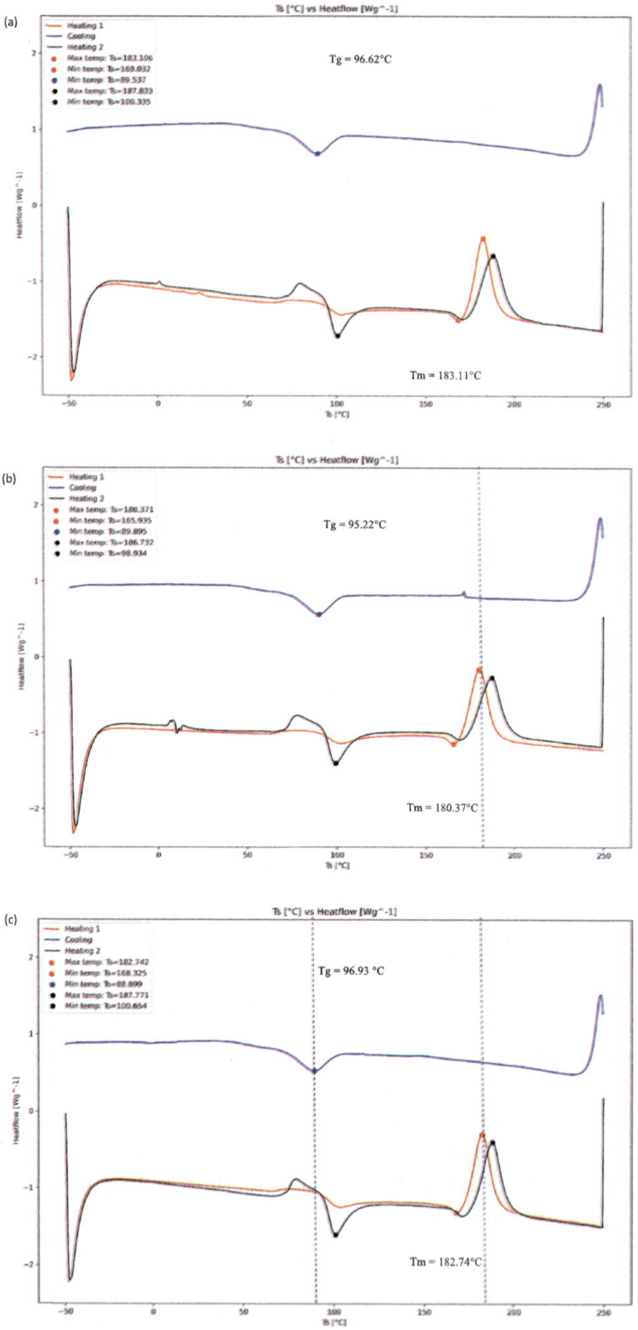

Fig. 12.5 **a** Differential scanning calorimetry result of recycled polylactic acid 1, **b** differential scanning calorimetry result of recycled polylactic acid 2, **c** differential scanning calorimetry result of recycled polylactic acid 3

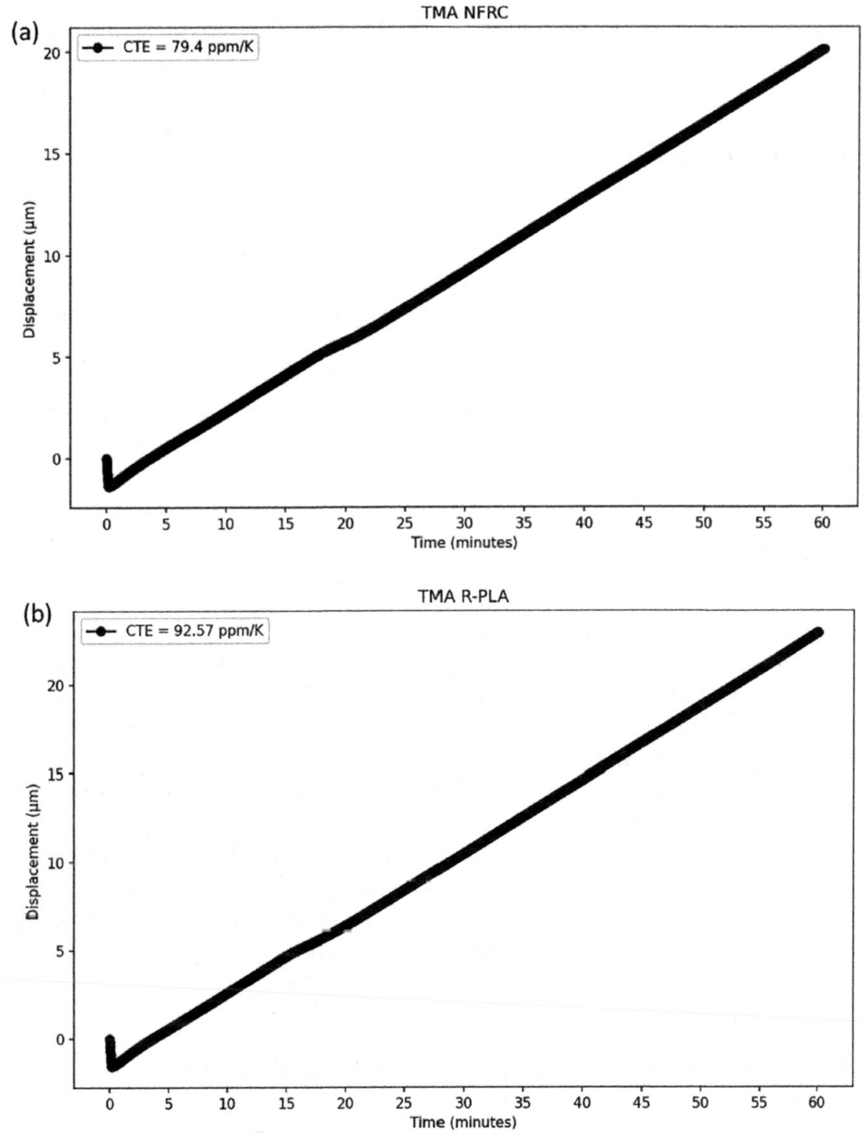

Fig. 12.6 **a** Thermomechanical analysis result of natural fiber-reinforced composites, **b** thermo-mechanical analysis result of recycled polylactic acid

12.3.3 Thermogravimetric Analysis

Thermogravimetric analysis findings for natural fiber-reinforced composites 1–3 demonstrate two stages of heat deterioration as shown Fig. 12.7. The first stage occurs between ~301–385 °C, ascribed to organic component disintegration, whereas the second stage begins over 620 °C, associated to more stable components.

These patterns show exceptional thermal stability up to 300 °C and resistance to deterioration at elevated temperatures. The natural fiber-reinforced composites ash concentrations ranged from 3.65 to 7.26%, indicating considerable inorganic residue.

Recycled polylactic acid samples similarly showed two-stage deterioration, albeit with a significantly earlier commencement (e.g., recycled polylactic acid 3 at 331.32 °C and second stage at ~616 °C), Fig. 12.8. While recycled polylactic acid is less thermally stable than natural fiber-reinforced composites, its predictable degradation may make it suitable for controlled thermal processing. The ash content was lower (2.54–4.80%), indicating fewer residual fillers.

Overall, natural fiber-reinforced composites exhibited delayed and more consistent thermal degradation, making it more suitable for high-temperature applications requiring long-term heat resistance and structural integrity.

12.3.4 SEM Analysis

A quantitative analysis of porosity in additively built natural fiber-reinforced composites specimens was conducted using ImageJ's threshold-based image segmentation. The porosity of the low-porosity sample is 0.263%, whereas the high-porosity sample has a porosity of 1.515%, Fig. 12.9. Fiber diameters were determined using calibrated ImageJ analysis from SEM images. With a mean of 19.9 μm and a standard variation of ±4.5 μm, the diameters of 17 fibers ranged from 14.0 to 28.0 μm. This distribution shows a substantial amount of fluctuation, which could be the result of irregularities in the extrusion process and random fiber orientation. These changes may have an impact on the bio-composite structure's local mechanical behavior and stress distribution. SEM analysis revealed key microstructural features, including fiber diameters (mean $\approx$ 19.9 μm) and porosity variation.

12.4 Numerical Simulation of Mechanical Behavior

Numerical simulations using ANSYS were conducted to validate experimental findings and predict material behavior under tensile and fatigue loading, building on the knowledge gathered from the manual tests.

12.4.1 Tensile Test Simulation

In accordance with DIN EN ISO 527-2:2012–06, the tensile specimen was modeled. To guarantee dependable results, a high-quality mesh was created, and color-coded

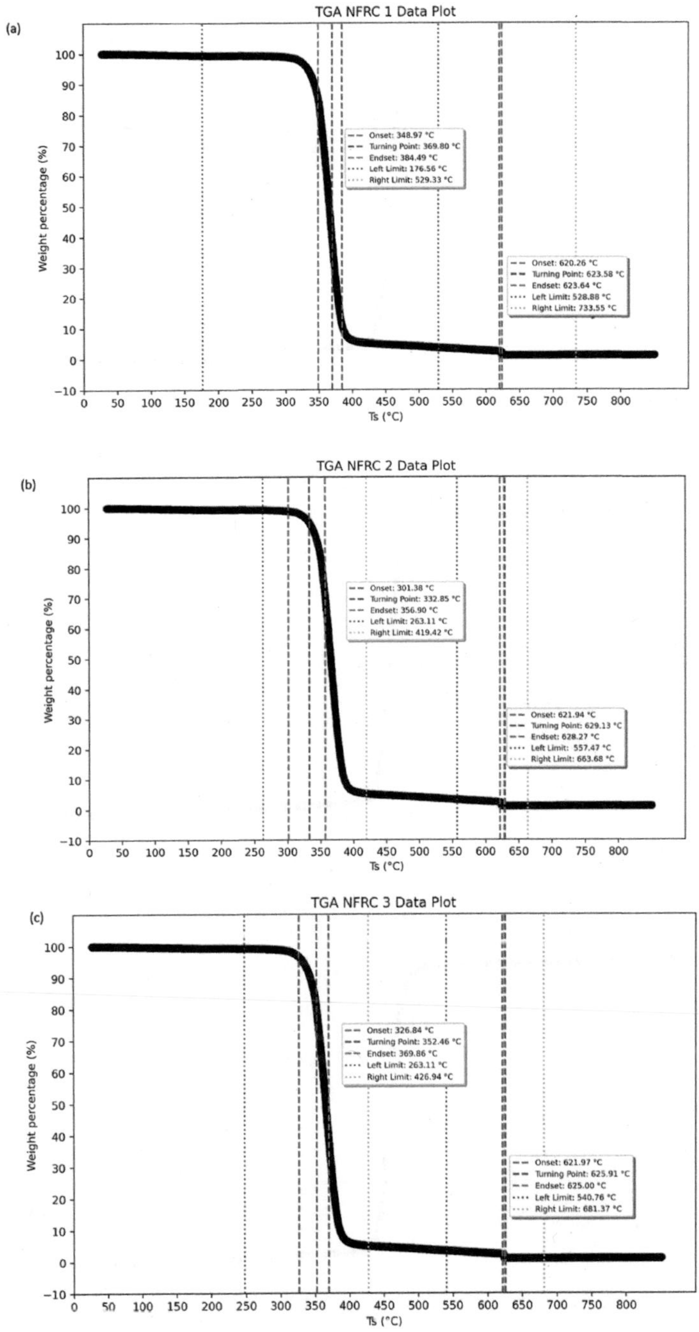

Fig. 12.7 **a** Thermogravimetric analysis result of natural fiber-reinforced composites 1, **b** thermogravimetric analysis result of natural fiber-reinforced composites 2, **c** thermogravimetric analysis result of natural fiber-reinforced composites 3

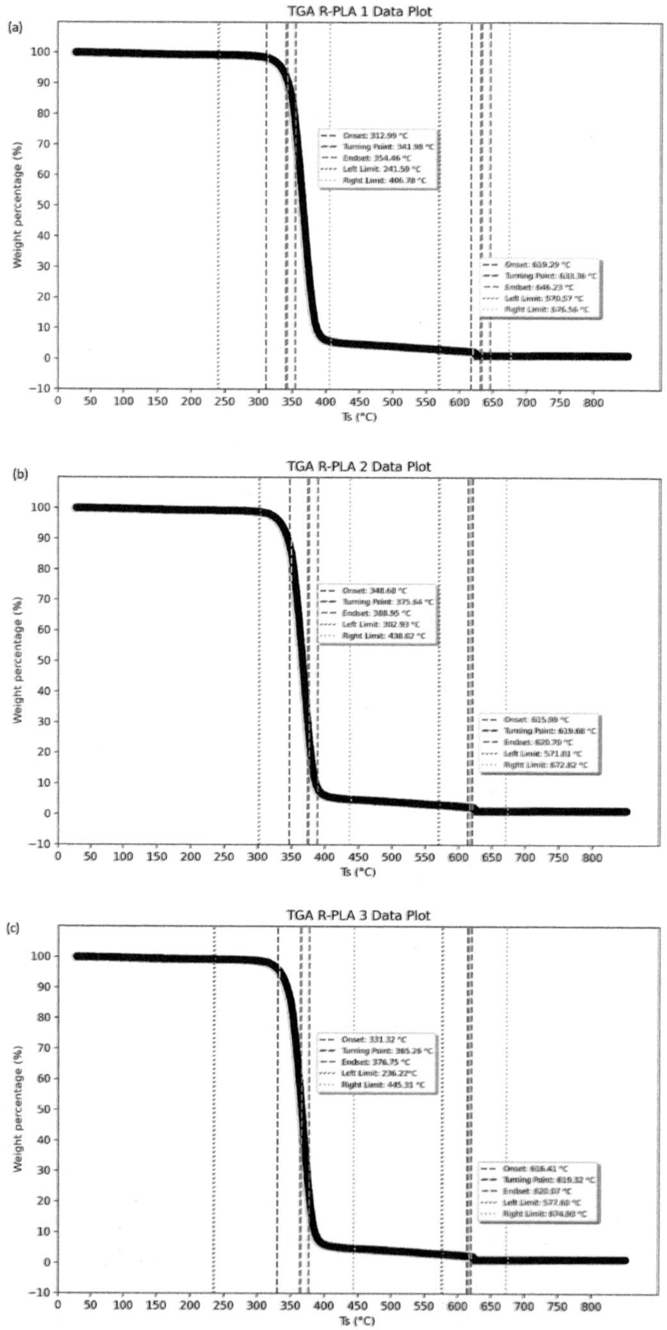

Fig. 12.8 **a** Thermogravimetric analysis result of recycled polylactic acid 1, **b** thermogravimetric analysis result of recycled polylactic acid 2, **c** thermogravimetric analysis result of recycled polylactic acid 3

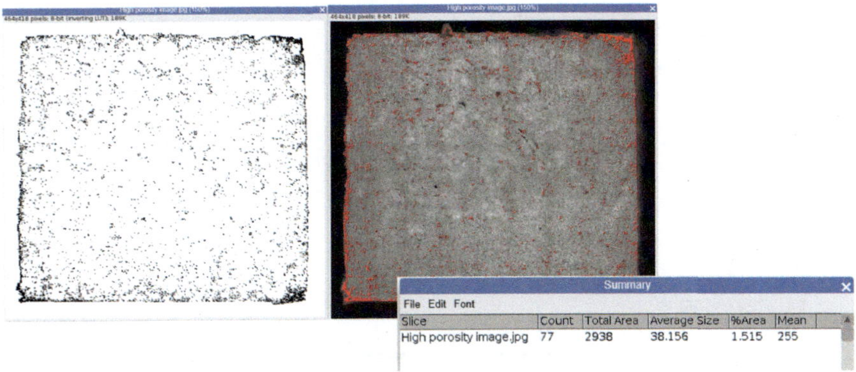

Fig. 12.9 ImageJ result of high-porosity natural fiber-reinforced composites

mapping was used to confirm mesh quality, Fig. 12.10. In order to replicate experimental circumstances, boundary conditions were applied by fixing one end of the specimen and applying a tensile force of 1106.2 N to the other end. The simulation captured deformation, stress, and strain distributions.

The maximum deformation recorded was 1.3771 mm, concentrated near the loading region. Principal stress analysis revealed a peak of 50.5 MPa at the narrowest section, consistent with expected failure locations, Fig. 12.11.

The elastic modulus was calculated using E = Stress/Strain, yielding a simulated value of 3643.36 MPa, closely matching the experimental result of 3641.18 ± 659.66 MPa. Principal strain distribution confirmed that this necking area was the most vulnerable to failure, Fig. 12.12. These findings align with the experimental behavior of the material under tensile loading. The minor variation falls within the standard deviation, validating the simulation's accuracy. This correlation

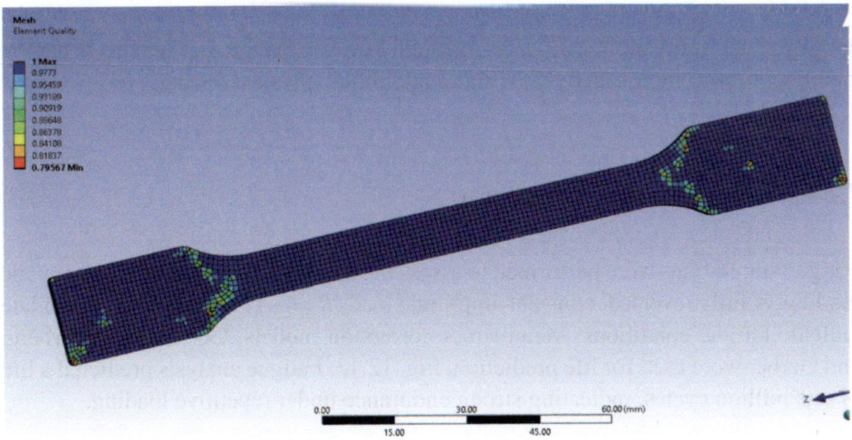

Fig. 12.10 Mesh quality of tensile specimen

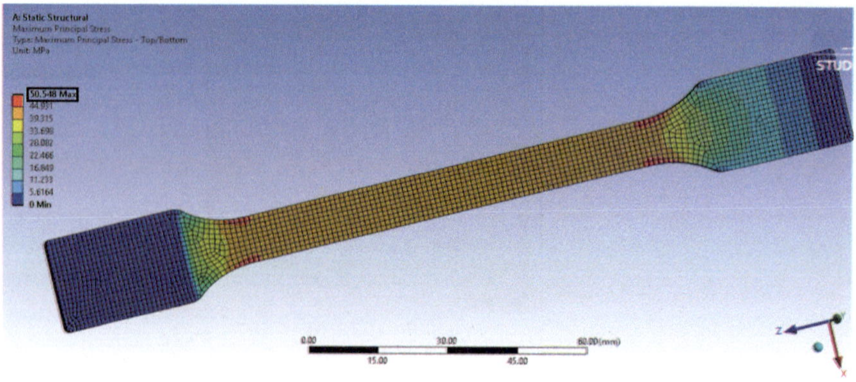

Fig. 12.11 Maximum principal stress distribution

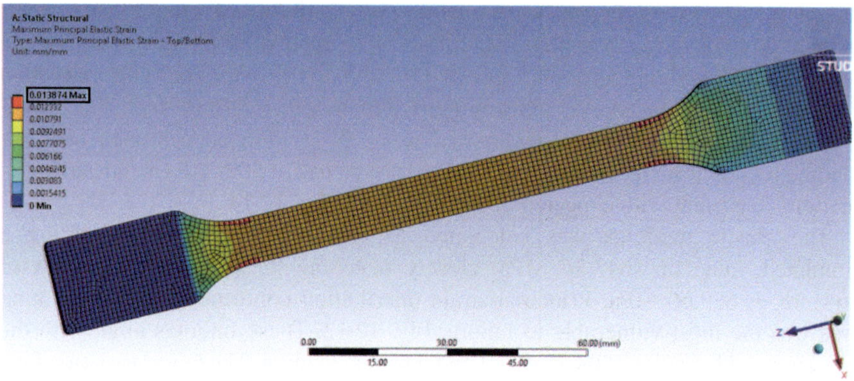

Fig. 12.12 Maximum principal strain distribution

confirms that simulation tools like ANSYS can reliably predict tensile behavior, enabling more complex analyses without additional physical testing.

12.4.2 Fatigue Test Simulation

Fatigue simulations were performed to assess the composite's durability under cyclic loading. A fully reversed, constant amplitude load ($R = -1$) was applied to simulate realistic fatigue conditions. Mean stress correction models, Goodman, Soderberg, and Gerber were used for life prediction, Fig. 12.13. Fatigue analysis predicted a life of one million cycles, indicating strong endurance under repetitive loading.

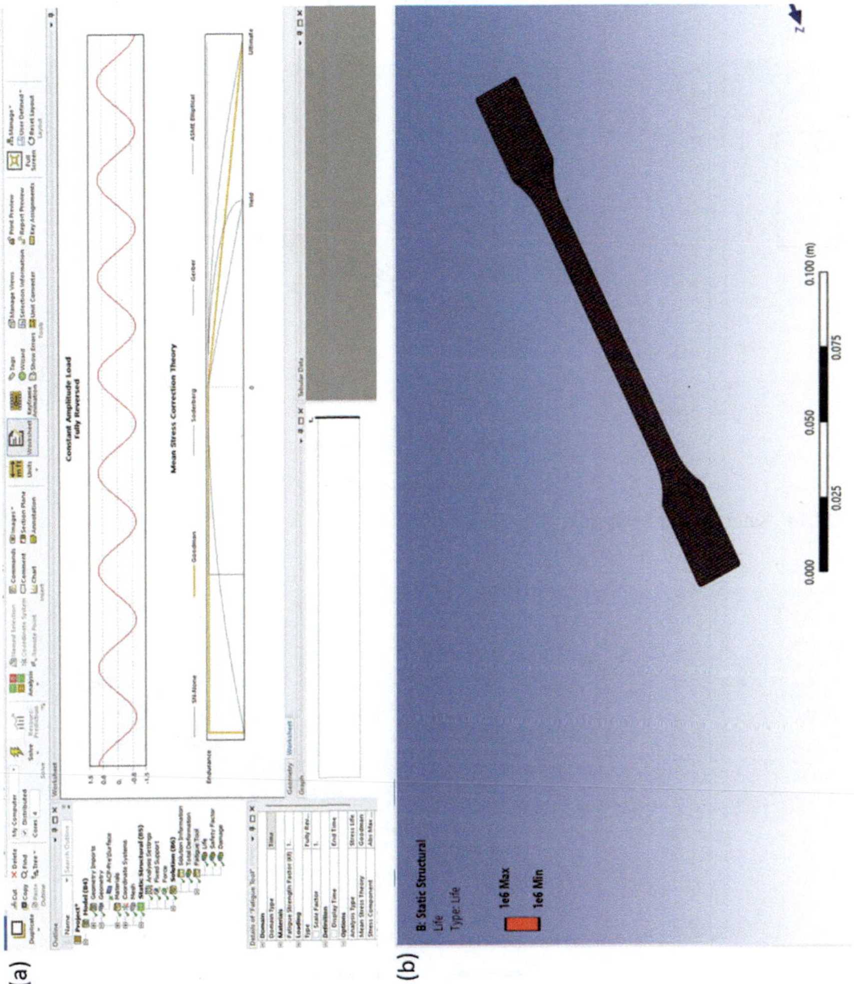

Fig. 12.13 **a** Fatigue load and mean stress correction theories, **b** fatigue life prediction results

The safety factor ranged from 2.73 to 15, with the lowest values found in regions under maximum stress, highlighting potential initiation sites for fatigue failure, Fig. 12.14.

Damage accumulation was evaluated throughout the cycle range. Notably, damage became evident after approximately 1000 cycles and continued to accumulate uniformly, Fig. 12.15. This indicates a gradual degradation pattern rather than sudden failure, suggesting the material's fatigue behavior is predictable and stable.

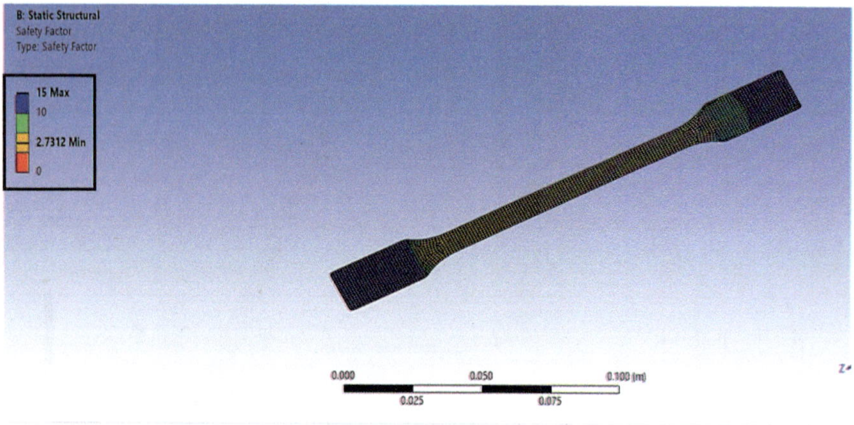

Fig. 12.14 Safety factor analysis

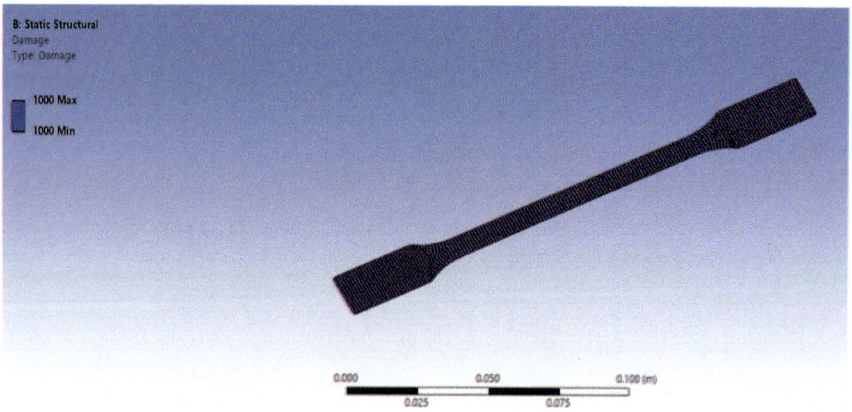

Fig. 12.15 Fatigue damage accumulation

12.5 Conclusion and Future Scope

Natural fiber-reinforced composites perform better in mechanical and thermal qualities than Recycled polylactic acid, making it a better option for industrial applications needing high strength and durability. This study compares natural fiber-reinforced composites to polylactic acid. Tensile test findings show natural fiber-reinforced composites has a substantially greater elastic modulus and tensile strength than recycled polylactic acid. Natural fiber-reinforced composites samples made using additive manufacturing and injection molding demonstrated superior yield stress and ultimate tensile strength. Injection molded natural fiber-reinforced composites showed an elastic modulus of 3641.18 MPa, higher than recycled polylactic acid's 3005.46 MPa. ANSYS fatigue tests proved natural fiber-reinforced composites is superior under cyclic loading, showing longer fatigue life, higher safety factor, and less damage accumulation than recycled polylactic acid. Thermogravimetric analysis and differential scanning calorimetry results showed natural fiber-reinforced composites have a greater melting point and crystallization temperature, a lower coefficient of thermal expansion, and degrades more gradually, withstanding temperatures up to 300 °C. Recycled polylactic acid degraded at lower temperatures, making it less suitable for high-heat applications. Environmentally, natural fiber-reinforced composites reduce dependence on petroleum-based polymers by combining recycled polylactic acid and hemp fibers. In the future, this research will examine other natural fiber combinations with recycled polylactic acid, expand natural fiber-reinforced composites production in additive manufacturing, and explore improved sustainability. Enhanced additive manufacturing processes and environmental impact assessments will support natural fiber-reinforced composites' role as a sustainable alternative to synthetic composites across automotive, aerospace, and construction industries.

References

Arulalan A, Rockinger C, Merkel M (2025) Fabrication and comparison of recycled PLA with recycled PLA/hemp composite using the FFF process. In: Altenbach H, Hitzler L, Johlitz M, Merkel M, Öchsner A (eds) Advanced structured materials, Lectures notes on advanced structured materials, vol 3. Springer, Cham, pp 103–116. https://doi.org/10.1007/978-3-031-77403-4_6

Kandachar P, Brouwer R (2001) Applications of bio-composites in industrial products. MRS Proc 702:1303. https://doi.org/10.1557/PROC-702-U4.1.1

Ranakoti L et al (2022) Critical review on polylactic acid: properties, structure, processing, biocomposites, and nanocomposites. Materials 15(12):4312. https://doi.org/10.3390/ma15124312

Rouway M et al (2020) Prediction of mechanical performance of natural fibers polypropylene composites: a comparison study. IOP Conf Ser Mater Sci Eng 948(1):012031. https://doi.org/10.1088/1757-899X/948/1/012031

H-J Steenhuis, T Ulusemre, X ang (2022) Additive manufacturing and the environment. In: International conference on additive manufacturing and the environment

Wang J, Bai J, Hua H, Tang B, Bai W, Wang X (2022) Characterization and scalable production of industrial hemp fiber filled PLA bio-composites. J Nat Fibers 19(16):13426–13437. https://doi.org/10.1080/15440478.2022.2095549

Chapter 13
Intelligent Optimization Methodology with Multiscale LBP and GLCM for the Automatic Identification of Tropical Timber Species

Xóchitl Siordia-Vásquez, Luz Yazmín Villagrán-Villegas, Luis Héctor Hernández-Gómez, Eduardo Hernández-Márquez, and José Omar Millán-Tejeda

Abstract In Veracruz, Mexico, it is challenging to visually identify endemic tropical timber species such as mahogany (*Swietenia macrophylla*), cedar (*Cedrela odorata*), parota (*Enterolobium cyclocarpum*) and rosewood (*Tabebuia rosea)* due to their highly similar textures. Reliance on visual experience alone can compromise the authenticity, quality and traceability of these species, which are critical aspects for the operation and sustainable management of small fine furniture industries and cabinet-making workshops. This study presents an automated method based on the optimized combination of multiple local binary patterns (MLBP) and grey-level co-occurrence matrices (GLCM) for efficiently identifying tropical timber species. Five key texture metrics—entropy, energy, contrast, variance and homogeneity—were extracted and their discriminatory capacity was evaluated using rigorous statistical analyses. This

X. Siordia-Vásquez (✉)
School of Electronics and Communications Engineering, Universidad Veracruzana, Poza Rica, Veracruz, Mexico
e-mail: xsiordia@uv.mx

L. Y. Villagrán-Villegas
School of Mechanical and Electrical Engineering, Universidad Veracruzana, Poza Rica, Veracruz, Mexico
e-mail: yvillagran@uv.mx

L. H. Hernández-Gómez
School of Mechanical and Electrical Engineering, Instituto Politécnico Nacional, Mexico City, Mexico
e-mail: luishector56@hotmail.com

E. Hernández-Márquez · J. O. Millán-Tejeda
Mecatronics Engineering Departament, Tecnológico Nacional de México, Campus Poza Rica, Poza Rica, Veracruz, Mexico
e-mail: eduardo.hernandez@itspozarica.edu.mx

J. O. Millán-Tejeda
e-mail: jose.millan@itspozarica.edu.mx

A. Öchsner (ed.), *Progress in Biomaterials and Biomedical Engineering*, Advanced Structured Materials 249, https://doi.org/10.1007/978-3-032-13551-3_13

highlighted significant results in the analysis of variance (ANOVA), with p-values below 0.05 for all metrics. Entropy showed the strongest results, with an F-statistic of 41.33 ($p = 0.0018$). The results indicate a statistically robust separation between species, as evidenced by comparative boxplots showing clear differences in metric distributions. This approach does not rely on supervised classifiers or large labelled databases, facilitating its application in real time and in practical environments. The findings demonstrate the method's potential for developing integrated systems for automatically identifying tropical woods in real time that are optimized to operate on hardware with limited resources.

Keywords Texture analysis · Multivariate local binary pattern · Intelligent optimization · Grey-level co-occurrence matrix (GLCM) · Gaussian maximum likelihood criterion (GMLC) · Automatic identification of timber species

13.1 Introduction

Accurate identification of tropical timber species is essential for preserving the authenticity, quality and sustainability of products in the fine furniture and high-end cabinetmaking industries. In the Veracruz region of Mexico, species such as mahogany (*Swietenia macrophylla*), cedar (*Cedrela odorata*), parota (*Enterolobium cyclocarpum*) and rosewood (*Tabebuia rosea*) have very similar textures, making them difficult to differentiate at first glance even for experts. This undermines confidence in the traceability and sustainable management of raw materials and negatively impacts the competitiveness of small industries and artisanal cabinetmaking workshops (Chila Tenorio et al. 2020; García Fernández 2018).

Traditionally, identification relied on visual and tactile experience and subjective methods that were dependent on individual knowledge. These methods were insufficient in high-demand, technically complex contexts (Velázquez Rosas et al. 2018). The development of automatic classification systems based on digital texture analysis has therefore emerged as a promising solution, offering objectivity and reproducibility. However, many existing proposals require substantial computational resources and extensive labelled databases, limiting their implementation in small industrial environments or those with limited hardware (Cano Saenz et al. 2022; Kwenda et al. 2022). In this context, it is crucial to design efficient and accurate methods that are adapted to platforms with limited resources, such as embedded devices or systems. These methods must be able to operate in real time and facilitate the automatic identification of Veracruz timber species during the manufacturing processes for fine furniture and cabinetry (Apolinario et al. 2019).This approach will strengthen product authenticity, optimize traceability, promote sustainable practices in the region and drive technological modernization in workshops with modest infrastructure. This paper therefore proposes a method based on the optimized combination of multiple local binary patterns (MLBP) and grey-level co-occurrence matrices (GLCM) that does not require supervised classifiers or large databases. This method is specially designed for implementation in hardware with limited resources. The method's feasibility and robustness are validated through statistical analyses and visualizations, demonstrating its potential for practical applications in the regional timber industry.

13.2 Materials and Methods

13.2.1 Sample Preparation

The species under study are tropical woods endemic to the Mexican state of Veracruz: mahogany (Swietenia macrophylla), cedar (Cedrela odorata), parota (Enterolobium cyclocarpum) and rosewood (Dalbergia spp.). The samples were obtained from certified local workshops and suppliers and will be accompanied by documentation guaranteeing their authenticity and origin (Merino Pérez 2019), (see Fig. 13.1). The specimens were extracted directly from solid blocks of wood, preserving their original anatomical structure and avoiding processes such as softening, impregnation and lamination. Preparation was carried out in accordance with standard wood anatomy protocols (Tian et al. 2025), cross-sections were obtained in the form of 2 × 2 cm cubes, which were then carefully sanded and cleaned to remove dust and debris in preparation for digital microscopy analysis.

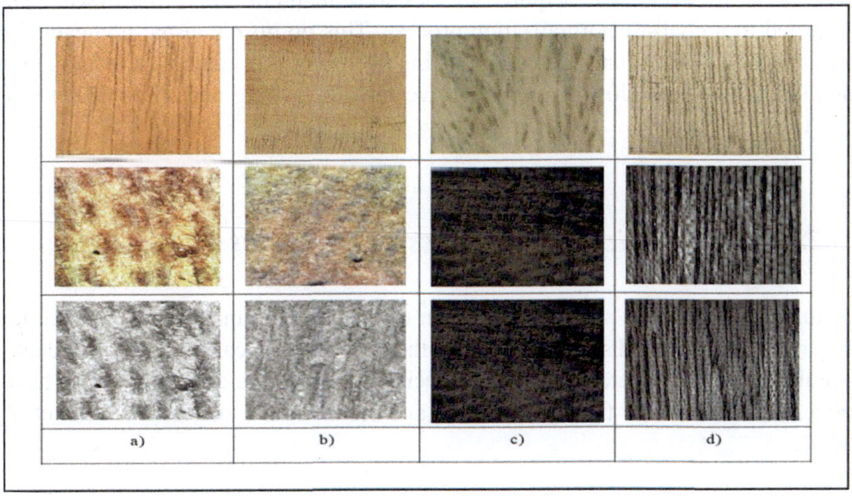

Fig. 13.1 Textural micrographs of four timber species endemics to Veracruz, México: **a** mahogany (Swietenia macrophylla), **b** cedar (Cedrela odorata), **c** parota (Cordia allaganoides), **d** purple rosewood (Tabebuia rosea)

13.2.2 Image Acquisition by Digital Microscopy

The digital images were acquired using a VEVOR LP043 digital electron microscope, which offers real-time capture and effective magnification ranging from 50 to 1000x. The microscope is equipped with a 2.0-megapixel CMOS camera to guarantee sharp, detailed images.

It also has adjustable LED lighting, enabling the user to minimize reflections, shadows and overexposure and ensure uniformity in the capture, while highlighting the natural microtextural characteristics of the samples without the need for additional treatments. The samples were placed directly on the stage of the digital microscope with an integrated camera without the need for chemical preparation or mounting on slides. Standardized procedures were implemented to minimize variability and ensure reproducibility. These procedures included fixed and oriented positioning of the samples to obtain images in consistent planes (transverse, radial and tangential), rigorous control of light intensity and white balance before each capture session, combined use of automatic and manual focus to ensure optimal clarity in the areas of interest, and capture of six images per sample to consider the intraspecific microtextural variability of each face of the analysed cube. In total, a database of 48 digital micrographs was created for analysis.

A specialized software was used to monitor and control all microscope and camera parameters, enabling the acquisition conditions to be accurately replicated for each capture. This methodology ensures the quality and uniformity of the images, which are crucial for the reliability and robustness of subsequent computational analysis (Ibrahim et al. 2017). The acquired images were then converted to greyscale and subjected to a contrast normalization process. This optimizes visual homogeneity and improves texture analysis by eliminating irrelevant chromatic information, thus facilitating the extraction of representative features (Wang and Zhao 2021) (see Fig. 13.1).

13.2.3 Characterization of the Textural Patterns

Texture, defined as the spatial distribution of pixels in an image, is imperative for discerning substantial disparities between the microanatomical structures that delineate the textural characteristics of the species examined via computer vision techniques. This facilitates the segmentation and classification stages (De Geus et al. 2021).

Multiscale Local Binary Patterns

In this context, the textural characterization of timber species is performed using the multiple local binary patterns (MLBP) operator, which is an extension of the classic local binary patterns (LBP) descriptor. MLBP characterizes the local texture of a digital image by comparing the intensity of a central pixel g with the intensity of its close neighbours P, which are located within a circular neighbourhood of radius R, Eq. (13.1). This integer value encodes a binary pattern that represents the local texture around the pixel. Mathematically, the binary comparison function S is defined by Eq. (13.2).

$$\mathrm{LBP}_{P,R}(g_c) = \sum_{p=0}^{P-1} s\left(g_p - g_c\right) \cdot 2^p, \text{ where } s(x) = \begin{cases} 1, & x \geq 0 \\ 0, & x < 0 \end{cases} \tag{13.1}$$

$$S(g(p_i), g(c)) = \begin{cases} 1, & si\ g(p_i) \geq g(c), \\ 0, & si\ g(p_i) < g(c). \end{cases} \tag{13.2}$$

In the case of multiscale LBP, several $\mathrm{LBP}_{P,R}$ operators are calculated with different P and R configurations: $(P_1, R_1), (P_2, R_2), \ldots, (P_n, R_n)$. This allows textures to be captured at various spatial scales. The multiple LBP descriptor is therefore defined as the set described in Eq. (13.3). In the case of multiscale LBP, several different P and R P configurations are calculated to allow textures to be captured at various spatial scales. The multiscale LBP descriptor is therefore defined as the set described in Eq. (13.3).

$$\mathrm{LBP}_{\mathrm{multi}} = \left\{\mathrm{LBP}_{P_1,R_1}, \mathrm{LBP}_{P_2,R_2}, \ldots, \mathrm{LBP}_{P_n,R_n}\right\} \tag{13.3}$$

In the context of this study, it has been established that, for each configuration, an LBP pattern frequency histogram will be generated. When these histograms are concatenated, they form an integrated feature vector that represents the texture at multiple scales. The resulting feature vector is shown Eq. 13.4. In this context, H_{P_i,R_i}, denotes the normalized histogram of the LBP_{P_i,R_i}., codes, calculated on the image or region of interest.

$$\boldsymbol{H} = \left[H_{P_1,R_1}, H_{P_2,R_2}, \ldots, H_{P_n,R_n}\right] \tag{13.4}$$

This procedure enables microtextural patterns to be captured at various levels of detail, thereby enhancing the robustness and discriminative power of complex analyses, such as timber species identification, which is our focus here. During this process, the space defined by the fundamental parameters of the multiscale local binary pattern (LBP) operator, the number of neighbours *(P)* and the circular neighbourhood radius *(R)* is explored.

$$P \in \{P_{\min}, P_{\min} + 1, \ldots, P_{\max}\}, R \in \{R_{\min}, R_{\min} + \Delta R, \ldots, R_{\max}\} \tag{13.3}$$

The ranges and steps of variation formed the pair *(P*, R*)* must be selected based on the resolution and scale of the anatomical features present in the analysed images. An increase is defined by Δ_R in order to find an optimal adjustment pair that allows for precise exploration of the parametric space shown in Eq. (13.5). For each pair (P, R) in Eq. (13.5), the corresponding multiple local binary pattern (MLBP) map is calculated. This is followed by the calculation of histograms and a set of five textural microdescriptors extracted from the co-occurrence matrix to characterize the species of wood under study.

Co-Occurrence Matrix and Textural Descriptors

The grey-level co-occurrence matrix (GLCM) is a statistical tool that describes how often specific combinations of grey tones appear between pixels in an image at a given distance and orientation (Comas et al. 2022). Five metrics particularly sensitive to microtextural variations are extracted from this matrix and are therefore suitable for differentiating the patterns of each timber species. Entropy quantifies randomness and complexity in pattern distribution; high values indicate greater heterogeneity and complex textures, while low values reflect uniformity and predictability (Su et al. 2025). Variance measures the overall dispersion of grey levels from the mean, indicating structural heterogeneity; high variance indicates wide textural variability, and low variance suggests uniformity (Hall-Beyer 2017). Homogeneity assesses local value similarity, with high values indicating smooth, uniform textures (Sharafudeen et al. 2021). Energy expresses the uniformity and repetitiveness of the texture pattern. Finally, contrast quantifies local variability by representing intensity jumps between neighbouring pixels and marked transitions between light and dark regions of the texture (Jackson et al. 2023).

Formally, $\{M_k\}_k^K = 1$ defines the set of descriptors that form the basis for evaluating the optimization objective function, expressed in Eq. (13.6), where each weighting coefficient ∝_k reflects the relevance of the indicated descriptor according to its ability to highlight microanatomical differences between species.

$$\mathcal{F}(P, R) = \sum_{k=1}^{K} \alpha_k M_k(P, R) \tag{13.4}$$

where $M_k(P, R)$ represents a multivariate feature vector consisting of $[M_1, M_2, \ldots, M_k]$, somewhere k is the number of statistical microdescriptors that model wood species textures. The function $\mathscr{F}(P, R)$ is then evaluated and stored, enabling the optimal pair described in Eq. (13.7) to be determined.

$$\left(P^*, R^*\right) = \arg\max_{P,R} \mathcal{F}(P, R) \tag{13.5}$$

This procedure selects the multiscale LBP operator whose configuration offers the greatest capacity for textural discrimination and reflects the microanatomical properties that are relevant for distinguishing between natural textures with very similar structures. Convergence is established either by exhaustively scanning the space or by meeting a minimum improvement criterion in $\mathscr{F}(P, R)$, thereby avoiding overfitting and ensuring the robustness of the generalization of the optimized descriptor. This method enables the automatic selection of an LBP operator configuration with multiple scales that highlights the most relevant microtextural characteristics for visually and statistically separating wood species. This approach is particularly suitable for scenarios with limitations in data labelling, as it does not require a supervised classification model. Finally, the LBP map obtained with (P^*, R^*) can be processed using the intelligent optimization method described in the next section.

13.2.4 Intelligent Optimization Methodology with Gaussian Maximum Likelihood Criterion (GMLC) Integration

If the microdescriptors $M_k(P, R) = [M_1, M_2, \ldots, M_k]$, for each species k, follow a multivariate normal distribution with parameters mean micras$_k$ and covariance covarianza$_k$ the objective function for optimization is calculated from the joint likelihood of the observations under these distributions, as expressed in Eq. (13.8).

$$\mathcal{F}(P, R) = \sum_{k=1}^{K} \alpha_k M_k^{\text{LBP}}(P, R) + \sum_{l=1}^{L} \beta_l M_l^{\text{GLCM}}(P, R) \tag{13.6}$$

where:

- $M_k^{\text{LBP}}(P, R)$ metrics are extracted from the LBP histogram (e.g. entropy and variance).
- $M_l^{\text{GLCM}}(P, R)$ metrics derived from GLCM (contrast, homogeneity, etc).
- α_k and β_l represent the weights assigned to each metric according to its relevance for microanatomical discrimination.
- K and L the total number of LBP and GLCM metrics used, respectively.

To optimize the $\mathscr{F}$ function without using supervised classifiers, the Gaussian maximum likelihood criterion (GMLC) is employed. This criterion models the multivariate statistical relationship of all combined metrics, see Eq. (9), where the joint vector of new features is formally defined for each sample i.

$$X_i(P, R) = \left[M_1^{\text{LBP}}, \ldots, M_k^{\text{LBP}}, M_1^{\text{GLCM}}, \ldots, M_l^{\text{GLCM}}\right] \tag{13.7}$$

Given the hypothesis of a multivariate normal distribution for each species y_i with parameters $\left(\boldsymbol{\mu}_{y_i}, \boldsymbol{\Sigma}_{y_i}\right)$, it is possible to define the GMLC objective function in Eq. (10).

$$\mathcal{F}_{\text{GMLC}}(P, R) = \sum_{i=1}^{N} \log\left(\mathbb{P}\left(\boldsymbol{X}_i(P, R)\boldsymbol{\mu}_{y_i}, \boldsymbol{\Sigma}_{y_i}\right)\right) \tag{13.8}$$

The objective function, $\mathscr{F}_{\text{GMLC}}(P, R)$ which incorporates the probabilistic criterion based on the generalized multivariate likelihood criterion (GMLC) model, strengthens optimization by highlighting the ability to identify texture classes of highly similar wood species in complex visual contexts. This combination provides a robust, efficient and suitable method for real-time applications (Kirbaş and Çifci 2022).

13.3 Validation and Evaluation of the Process Method

This section describes and justifies the methodology employed to validate the proposed approach. An intelligent optimization scheme was implemented to select the optimal pair (P^*, R^*) that maximizes statistical separation between species in the combined multiscale feature space extracted using local binary patterns and a grey-level co-occurrence matrix. The objective function is based on the probabilistic criterion of the generalized multivariate likelihood criterion, which strengthens the robustness of the method by highlighting its ability to resolve highly similar classes in complex visual contexts (see Fig. 13.3) in (Fahrurozi and Kosasih 2022).

To visualize the capacity of the local binary pattern descriptor to capture the textural characteristics of timber species, LBP maps were generated from images representative of natural wood textures. As can be seen Fig. 13.2, these maps encode local intensity patterns that reflect surface microstructures. This serves as a fundamental basis for constructing the combined MLBP-GLCM space and for subsequent intelligent optimization, which enhances species discrimination. During the intelligent optimization process, multiple combinations of the (P, R) parameters were evaluated to maximize the objective function, which quantifies statistical separation between species in the combined LBP-GLCM space.

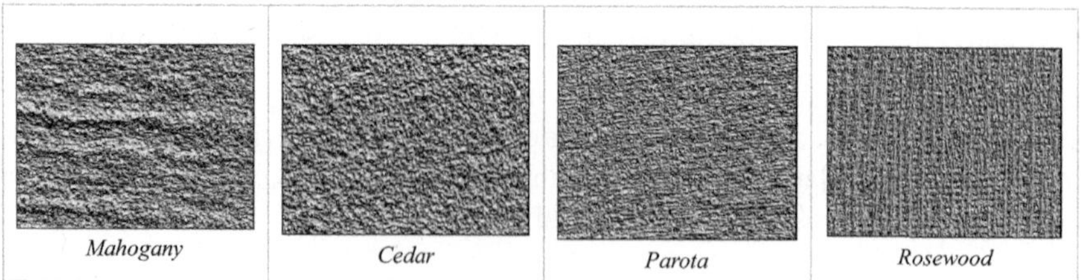

Fig. 13.2 Visual maps of local binary patterns (MLBP) extracted from samples of natural wood textures. These maps illustrate the local encoding of textures, highlighting the microstructural characteristics relevant for automatic species differentiation through joint analysis with GLCM

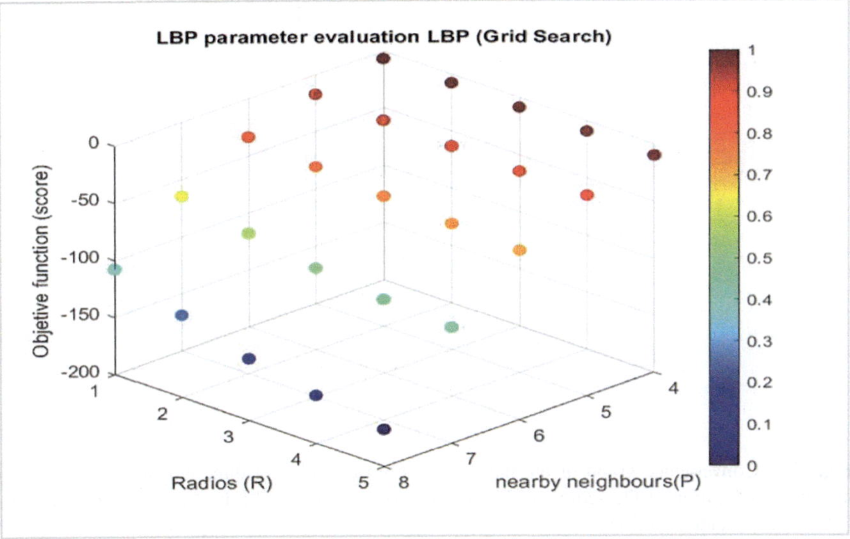

Fig. 13.3 Heat map of the objective function interpolated in the parametric space (P, R) highlighting the area where maximum statistical separation between species is achieved using the combined MLBP-GLCM descriptors

The results demonstrate a consistent improvement in scores as P and R increase, ultimately achieving an optimal value of $P^* = 8$ and $R^* = 5$ with a score of -148.13. This value represents the method's maximum discriminatory capacity, ensuring a clear and robust separation between species in the characteristic space. Figure 13.3 illustrates this performance using a heat map that shows the interpolated objective function in the parameter domain (P, R) clearly highlighting the optimal region.

Furthermore, Fig. 13.4 illustrates how the metrics were evaluated and how the optimization algorithm converged, demonstrating the stability and efficiency of the process. This adds transparency and robustness to the methodological design. The statistical validity of the method was confirmed by conducting a one-way analysis of variance (ANOVA) on the metrics extracted from the combined MLBP-GLCM space. This analysis revealed statistically significant differences ($p < 0.05$) between timber species for the primary metrics examined, particularly those derived from the GLCM descriptor.

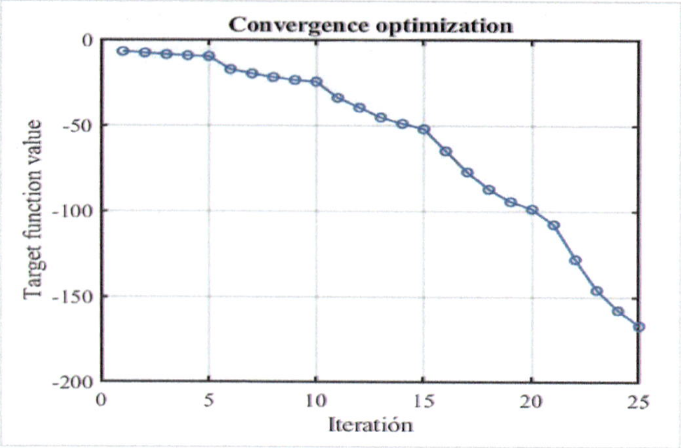

Fig. 13.4 Convergence graph of the intelligent optimization algorithm, showing the stable and downward evolution of the score, confirming the effectiveness and robustness of the method for optimal parameter selection

13.4 Discussion of Results

This section presents the findings derived from the quantitative and statistical analysis of the textural metrics obtained using local binary patterns and the grey-level co-occurrence matrix descriptors. This analysis was carried out to evaluate the discriminatory capacity of these descriptors for identifying tropical timber species. A descriptive comparison of the extracted average metrics was initially carried out to this end.

Table 13.1 shows the representative values for the LBP metric, GLCM entropy and GLCM contrast for each species. This table clearly shows differences in the means, providing initial quantitative evidence of species separation. Table 13.1 clearly shows the differences in average metrics calculated from the LBP and GLCM descriptors for the timber species studied. For instance, the entropy obtained from the GLCM descriptor varies considerably, with parota having a notably higher value (0.6304) than Cedar (0.1558), suggesting greater textural complexity in parota samples. In contrast, LBP entropy shows less variability between species, although subtle differences are still evident. Similarly, the GLCM-based contrast metric reveals that cedar also stands out with higher values (0.9249), indicating a more heterogeneous texture compared to the other species.

Other metrics, such as energy and homogeneity, also exhibit differences that complement this characterization. This suggests that the combination of MLBP and GLCM descriptors captures different aspects of the surface texture of the woods and provides a more robust description of texture.

Table 13.1 Average values of textural metrics obtained using local binary patterns and grey-level co-occurrence matrix for the timber species studied

LBP multiscale local binary pattern						GLCM co-occurrence matrix				
Especie	Entropy	Energy	Contrast	Variance	Homogeneity	Entropy	Energy	Contrast	Variance	Homogeneity
Mahogany	6.8285	0.0146	2727.8	2727.8	0.0598	0.1919	0.1943	0.5663	3.1722	1.7137
Cedar	6.7687	0.0171	2716.2	2716.2	0.0604	0.1558	0.2915	0.9249	2.2761	0.9650
Parota	6.6282	0.0197	2780.4	2780.4	0.0517	0.6304	0.0858	0.7982	4.0470	2.1181
Rosewood	6.8900	0.0156	2707.0	2707.0	0.0593	0.1716	0.2574	0.9158	2.5163	0.6860

Table 13.2 Results of the analysis of variance (ANOVA) for the textural metrics derived from the GLCM descriptor

GLCM metrics	*F*_statistical	*p*_value
Entropy	41.33	0.0018119
Energy	21.61	0.0065132
Contrast	21.17	0.0064496
Variace	22.39	0.0058107
Homogeneity	11.97	0.01819

To strengthen the statistical validity of these results, a one-way analysis of variance (ANOVA) was performed focusing exclusively on metrics derived from the GLCM descriptor: entropy, energy, contrast, variance and homogeneity. The results, summarized Table 13.2, reveal that all the metrics are statistically significant ($p < 0.05$), as indicated by high F-statistic values and p-values ranging from 0.0018 to 0.0182. Entropy showed the highest F-statistic value (41.33) and p-value (0.0018), indicating highly significant variation between species and highlighting this metric as the most powerful for capturing relevant textural differences in wood.

Energy, contrast and variance also had high F values of around 21 and 22, with p-values below 0.01, confirming that these metrics also contribute significantly to the differentiation of characteristic textures. Finally, although homogeneity had a lower F value (11.97), its p-value was still statistically significant at 0.0182, below the classic threshold of 0.05. This implies that it also contributes to discrimination, albeit to a lesser extent than the other metrics. Together, these results demonstrate that all the evaluated metrics effectively distinguish between timber species, providing robust statistical evidence in favour of constructing the combined MLBP-GLCM feature space. This differentiation is statistically robust and supports the use of the automated method for real-time applications, eliminating the need for supervised systems or extensive labelled databases. Figure 13.5 also displays the boxplots for these GLCM metrics, clearly showing the statistical dispersion and separation between species and reinforcing confidence in the inferential results. In summary, the results demonstrate that the textural features extracted using LBP and GLCM primarily constitute a robust and effective feature space for automatically differentiating tropical timber species.

This discriminatory capacity is validated both visually and statistically, confirming the applicability of the method for automatically identifying timber species without the need for labelled databases or complex supervised methods. It also maintains low computational requirements, enabling implementation in autonomous systems with real-time processing and limited hardware resources.

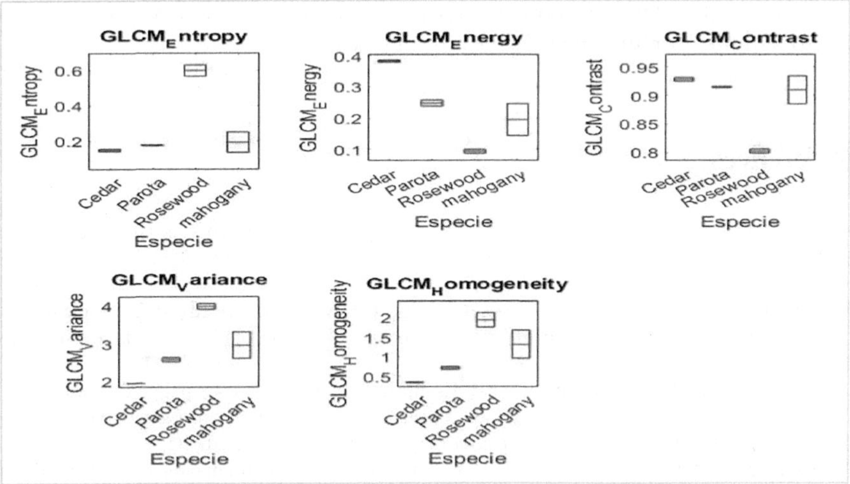

Fig. 13.5 Validation of dispersion and statistical separation between timber species

13.5 Conclusions

In conclusion, this study demonstrates the feasibility and effectiveness of an automated method that combines optimized multiscale local binary patterns and grey-level co-occurrence matrices to identify tropical timber species. Statistical validation using ANOVA and graphical analysis confirmed that the extracted metrics enable robust and clear discrimination between species, thus achieving the article's primary objective. The method's key advantages include its real-time operation, eliminating the need for supervised classifiers or extensive labelled databases, thus facilitating its application in practical environments while minimizing reliance on substantial computational and human resources. Furthermore, integrating the MLBP-GLCM feature space enhances statistical separation between species, thereby optimizing the system's accuracy and reliability. However, the method has some limitations that open up opportunities for future work. For example, the analysis focused exclusively on static metrics and did not consider variations due to environmental conditions or the physical states of the wood, aspects that could affect discrimination in more complex real-world scenarios. Likewise, the database used for feature extraction and validation can be expanded to include a greater number of species and specimens, strengthening the generalization of the method. As future work, we propose investigating the incorporation of metaheuristic techniques to complement and improve automatic feature extraction.

In summary, the developed method fully meets the set objectives, offering an efficient, robust and applicable solution for the automatic identification of tropical wood species. It strikes a favourable balance between accuracy, low computational cost and ease of implementation—characteristics that could facilitate its integration into intelligent systems for portable devices, enabling practical applications in the timber and fine furniture manufacturing industries.

References

Apolinario M, Urcia D, Huaman S (2019) Open set recognition of timber species using deep learning for embedded systems. IEEE Lat Am Trans 17(12):2005–2012. https://doi.org/10.1109/TLA.2019.9011545

Cano Saenz DA, Ordoñez Urbano CF, Gaitan Mesa HR, Vargas-Cañas R (2022) Tropical wood species recognition: a dataset of macroscopic images. Data 7(8):111. https://doi.org/10.3390/data7080111

Chila Tenorio JC, Salazar Castañeda EP, Espinoza VM (2020) Descripción organoléptica y anatómica de la madera cinco especies forestales del sector Tabiazo, Esmeraldas, Ecuador. Conciencia Digit 3(3): 164–177. https://doi.org/10.33262/concienciadigital.v3i3.1288

Comas DS, Amalfitano A, Meschino GJ, Ballarin VL (2022) Interpretación y visualización de características en texturas mediante Redes Neuronales Convolucionales. In: 2022 IEEE biennial congress of Argentina (ARGENCON). San Juan, Argentina, pp 1–8. https://doi.org/10.1109/ARGENCON55245.2022.9939876

De Geus AR, Backes AR, Gontijo AB, Albuquerque GHQ, Souza JR (2021) Amazon wood species classification: a comparison between deep learning and pre-designed features. Wood Sci Technol 55:857–872. https://doi.org/10.1007/s00226-021-01282-w

Fahrurozi A, Kosasih R (2022) Texture features and statistical features for wood types classification system. In: 2022 5th international conference of computer and informatics engineering (IC2IE), Jakarta, Indonesia, pp 186–191. https://doi.org/10.1109/IC2IE56416.2022.9970071

García Fernández E (2018) Estudio de una prueba genética de Cedrela odorata L., establecida en "La Pahua", Colipa, Veracruz. Master's thesis, Universidad Veracruzana

Hall-Beyer M (2017) GLCM texture: a tutorial. vol 3. https://www.researchgate.net/publication/316813601_GLCM_Texture_A_Tutorial. Accessed 4 Sept 2025

Ibrahim I, Khairuddin ASM, Arof H, Yusof R, Hanafi E (2017) Statistical feature extraction method for wood species recognition system. Eur J Wood Prod 76:345–356. https://doi.org/10.1007/s00107-017-1163-1

Jackson CM, Adam E, Atif I, Mahboob MA (2023) Feature extraction and classification of canopy gaps ssing GLCM—and MLBP-based rotation-invariant feature descriptors derived from WorldView-3 imagery. Geomatics 3(1):250–265. https://doi.org/10.3390/geomatics3010014

Kirbaş İ, Çifci A (2022) An effective and fast solution for classification of wood species: a deep transfer learning approach. Ecol Inform 69:101633. https://doi.org/10.1016/j.ecoinf.2022.101633

Kwenda C, Gwetu M, Dombedu JVF (2022) Machine learning methods for forest image analysis and classification: a survey of the state of the art. IEEE Access 10:45290–45316. https://doi.org/10.1109/ACCESS.2022.3170049

Merino Pérez L (ed.) (2019) Crisis ambiental en México. Ruta para el cambio. Universidad Nacional Autónoma de México, Mexico City. ISBN 978-607-30-2333-7

Sharafudeen M, Ra M, Simon P (2021) Wood texture classification using GLCM and LBP. In: National conference on smart systems and technologies pp 172–175

Su J, Zhu J, Zhu H, Zhang Y, Yang G (2025) Research on information extraction and classification of color and texture visual features of artificial board wood grain veneer based on machine visión. Measurement 256:118091. https://doi.org/10.1016/j.measurement.2025.118091

Tian Z, Zhang N, Wang J, Sha L, Liu H, Zou L (2025) Image classification of imbalanced wood microscope by integrating multi-source features. Int J Comput Intell Syst 18:184. https://doi.org/10.1007/s44196-025-00912-6

Velázquez Rosas N, Silva Rivera E, Ruiz Guerra B, Armenta Montero S, Trejo González J (2018) Traditional ecological knowledge as a tool for biocultural landscape restoration in Northern Veracruz, Mexico: a case study in El Tajín region. Eco Soc 23(3):6. https://doi.org/10.5751/ES-10294-230306

Wang C-K, Zhao P (2021) Classification of wood species using spectral and texture features of transverse section. Eur J Wood Prod 79:1283–1296. https://doi.org/10.1007/s00107-021-01728-9

Chapter 14
Development of an Artificial Intelligence System for NAFLD Detection in the Mexican Population

Verónica Guzmán-Mercado, Juan Alfonso Beltrán-Fernández, Enrique Granados-Sandoval, Alejandro Tonatiu Velázquez-Sánchez, Karen Pamela Vázquez-Thierry, and Gabriel Josué Reyes-Morales

Abstract Non-alcoholic fatty liver disease (NAFLD) has shown an increase in prevalence worldwide in recent decades, which has led to several investigations focused on its early and non-invasive detection. In countries such as Argentina, Chile, and Spain, multiple image-based diagnostic methods have been developed to improve accuracy. In contrast, Mexico still requires further technological development to address this condition with advanced computational tools. The aim of this work is to implement the use of convolutional neural networks for the classification of medical images based on patterns present in patients with hepatic steatosis. To this end, a computational model was designed and trained with clinical studies of both positive and negative NAFLD cases for the automatic detection of fatty liver.

V. Guzmán-Mercado · J. A. Beltrán-Fernández (✉) · A. T. Velázquez-Sánchez · K. P. Vázquez-Thierry · G. J. Reyes-Morales
Instituto Politécnico Nacional, Sección de Estudios de Posgrado e Investigación, Escuela Superior de Ingeniería Mecánica y Eléctrica, Unidad Zacatenco, "Unidad Profesional Adolfo López Mateos", Ciudad de México, México
e-mail: jbeltran@ipn.mx

V. Guzmán-Mercado
e-mail: vero_guzmanm94@hotmail.com

A. T. Velázquez-Sánchez
e-mail: atvelazquezs@ipn.m

K. P. Vázquez-Thierry
e-mail: kappa.thierry@gmail.com

G. J. Reyes-Morales
e-mail: greyesm1100@alumno.ipn.mx

E. Granados-Sandoval
Hospital Regional "1 de Octubre" del ISSSTE, Gustavo A. Madero, Ciudad de México, CDMX, México
e-mail: henryluz18@yahoo.com.mx

A. Öchsner (ed.), *Progress in Biomaterials and Biomedical Engineering*, Advanced Structured Materials 249, https://doi.org/10.1007/978-3-032-13551-3_14

Keywords Neural network · Steatosis · Liver · Convolutional networks · Diagnosis · Hepatic fat

14.1 Introduction

Hepatic steatosis is the accumulation or infiltration of fat in the liver. This condition can be reversible if detected in time; the main treatment consists of following a diet prescribed by a specialist, engaging in physical exercise, and avoiding the consumption of alcohol and certain medications (Barraza and Stalnikowitz 2025).

The prevalence of fatty liver disease ranges from 17 to 33%. In the early stage of this condition, patients may present with abdominal discomfort, fatigue, hepatomegaly, and hepatic hyperechogenicity. Approximately 32% of individuals with this disorder develop fibrosis, and 20% may progress to cirrhosis, with a mortality probability of 10% (Ramachandran and Kakar 2009).

Obesity is considered the primary cause of hepatic steatosis. This pathology is a chronic disease characterized by the excessive accumulation of body fat. In Mexico, it is estimated that 70% of the population is overweight (García 2004).

The diagnosis of NAFLD depends on the specialist treating the patient. In some cases, the physician may detect it through ultrasound; however, for an accurate clinical analysis, it is necessary to perform various tests, which may include clinical, biochemical, imaging, or invasive procedures (Wu and Feng 2017).

This research focuses on parallel interpretation with imaging techniques, with the aim of developing and implementing a supportive tool capable of recognizing atypical patterns in early detection cases of hepatic steatosis. The purpose is to anticipate the risks associated with disease progression in patients, who at a minimum should undergo additional radiological studies or even invasive interventions.

14.2 Development

14.2.1 Methodology

Figure 14.1 shows the methodology used in the project. The project begins with data acquisition, which is used solely for consultation purposes and does not involve access to any sensitive patient data.

After this, data preprocessing is carried out using the selected image segmentation programmes.

The model architecture was developed in order to perform training with the preprocessed data.

Finally, the results will be obtained to corroborate the efficiency of the model.

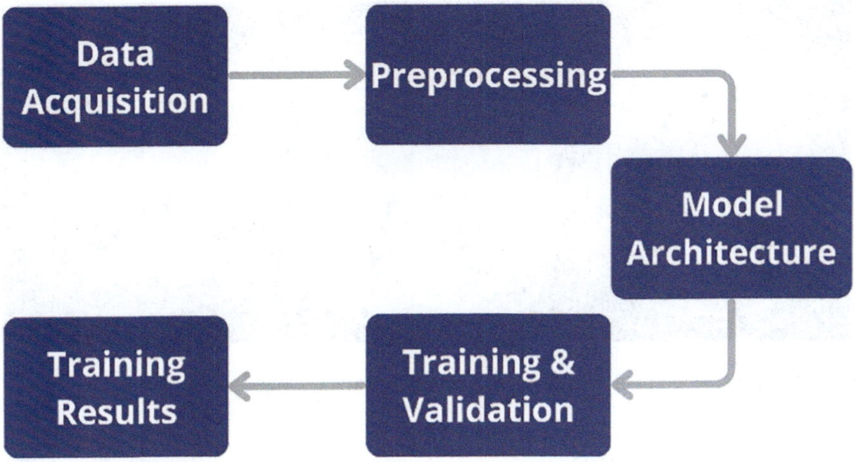

Fig. 14.1 Methodology

14.2.2 Data Processing

The present research focused on the Mexican population. To achieve greater efficiency, a smaller sample was selected with the aim of obtaining results in a timely manner. The study sample consisted of anonymized clinical studies provided by national medical institutions. This information was used for training and validating the proposed model.

The data processing included: cleaning, segmentation, resizing, format conversion, and labelling. A database of medical images from computed tomography (CT) clinical studies was used, which were processed to obtain a homogeneous and representative dataset, thus creating a suitable database for the model.

The following processes were carried out:

- **File Cleaning**

To maintain control over the cases received, a registry was created in which patient data were recorded, and in cases where they were discarded, the reason was documented.

- **Image Segmentation**

For image segmentation, the 3D Slicer® software was used. Segmentation was performed manually, since hepatic anatomy varies among patients (Fig. 14.2).

- **Resolution and Data Format Adjustment**

To establish a balance between data quality and the computational resources available for the project, image dimensions were set to 512 × 512 pixels. The format selected

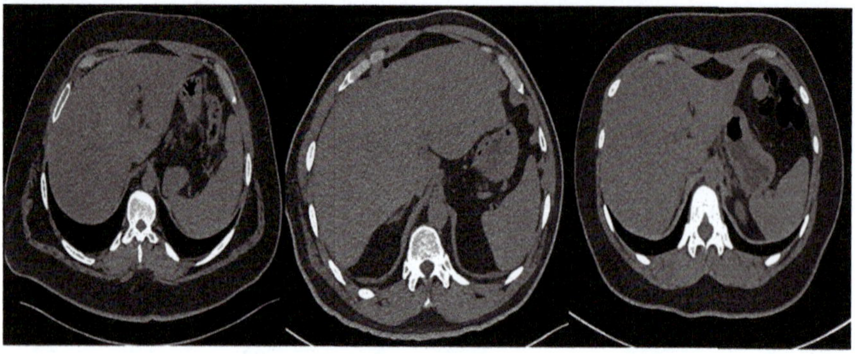

Fig. 14.2 Hepatic morphological comparison in three axial CT slices

for the images was NRRD, to ensure correct processing through the SimpleITK library in Python®.

To adjust each file, a Python® script was developed (Fig. 14.3), which defined the desired dimensions and performed the format conversion.

- **Organization and Labelling**

The files were divided into three groups:

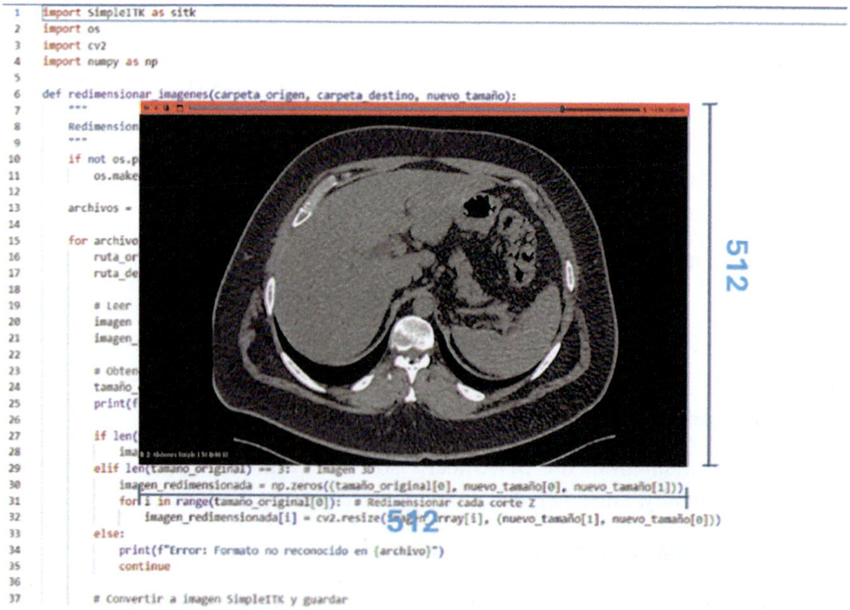

Fig. 14.3 Python® code snippet for image feature adjustment

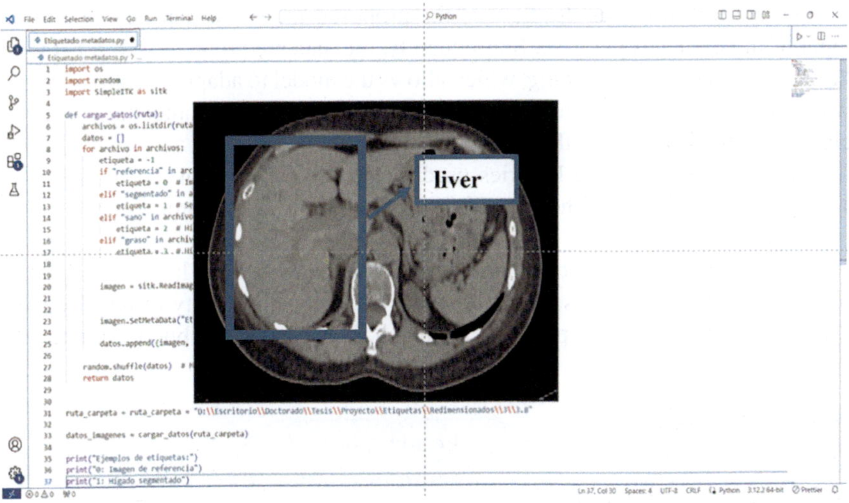

Fig. 14.4 Label generation using Python®

- Reference image.
- Segmented liver.
- Labels.

To ensure that each group of images was correctly identified by the model, a label was included within the metadata of each file. Four labels were defined:

- 0 for the reference image.
- 1 for the segmented liver.
- 2 for the healthy liver.
- 3 for the fatty liver.

As with the format conversion, this step was carried out using a Python® script (Fig. 14.4).

14.2.3 Model Development

Model Architecture

The model was based on a CNN, in which a system of three input channels was created for each acquired case. This model was trained for the classification of healthy and fatty liver, using a ResNet18-based architecture, as it provides high computational efficiency and strong performance in medical classification tasks (Wu and Feng 2017; Smrekar et al. 2008; Mount 1998).

Figure 14.5 illustrates the flow of the proposed model, which begins with the input of three images per case. Subsequently, the data are preprocessed for training through a CNN with *fine-tuning*, which allows the model to adapt to future retraining with additional cases without losing its current accuracy. The outcome consists of classifying the liver as healthy or fatty.

Table 14.1 presents the libraries used in the development of the model, along with a brief description of their functions. These tools were essential for processing, training, and evaluation.

The first version of the model consisted of basic convolutional layers, *max pooling* operations, and a final dense layer for binary classification (fatty or healthy liver). This version validated the project's approach; however, it exhibited limitations in

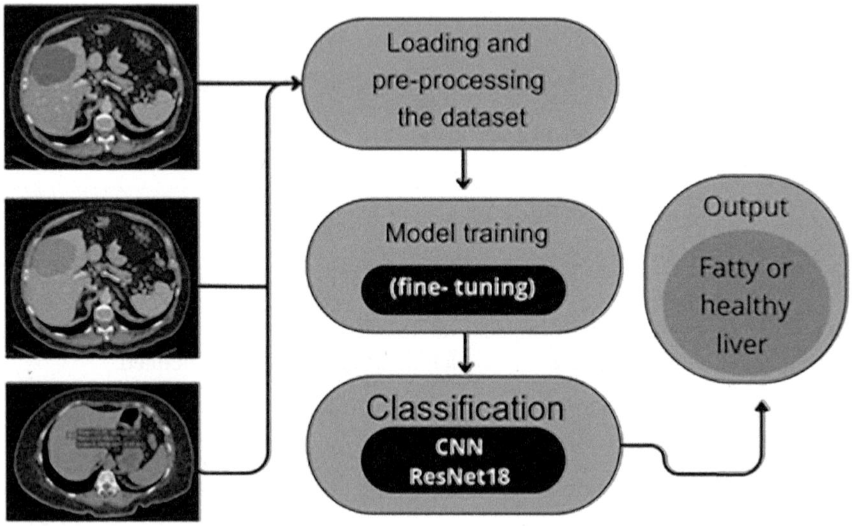

Fig. 14.5 Flowchart of the proposed classification model

Table 14.1 Libraries used in the model (Challenger-Pérez et al. 2014; Mirjalili and Raschka 2020)

Library	Function
Torch	Used for building and training the network
Torchvision	Enables handling of medical images
Numpy	Performs mathematical operations and manages numerical arrays
Os	Facilitates the interaction between the model and the operating system
SimpleITK	Allows reading, processing, and handling of images in NRRD format
Collections.Counter	Counts elements for class analysis and data distribution
Sklearn	Computes metrics such as accuracy, precision, recall, and F1-score
Time	Measures execution times to assess training performance

Table 14.2 Parameters of the new architecture (Challenger-Pérez et al. 2014; Mirjalili and Raschka 2020)

Parameter	Description
Epochs	Allow training to be performed over multiple cycles
Transformations	Apply image normalization and convert tensors to be processed by the network
Batch normalization	Normalizes the output of each layer, which stabilizes and accelerates learning
Dropout	Reduces overfitting by randomly disconnecting neurons
DataLoader	Facilitates batch data loading, which reduces memory usage and processing time during training

Table 14.3 Training parameters

Parameter	Value
Batch size	8 images per batch
Loss function	CrossEntropyLoss
Optimizer	Adam (Learning rate = 0.001)
Number of epochs	50
Data split	80% training and 20% validation
Applied transformations	Normalization and tensor conversion

identifying complex patterns and generalizing to new data. Subsequently, a modification was implemented to strengthen the architecture. Table 14.2 describes the new elements and outlines, in a simple manner, the benefits they provide.

Training

For training, 345 cases were used, representing a total of 1035 files. For each case, three views were integrated as independent channels into a single network input. This feature was implemented using a customized DataLoader. Table 14.3 presents the training parameters; training was performed in epochs, and data transformations such as normalization and tensor conversion were applied.

Adjustments, Testing, and Bias Control

Table 14.4 presents the limitations encountered during training and the solutions applied in each case.

Table 14.4 Training issues (Challenger-Pérez et al. 2014; Mirjalili and Raschka 2020)

Issue	Solution
Dimension error in layers	The input and output parameters were adjusted in layers *'nn.Linear'*
Incompatibility of tensor types	The tensors were explicitly converted to 'float32'
Unsupported loss function	The functions *'squeeze()'* and *'long()'* were used to adapt the dimensions
Duplicate tensors	*'clone().detach()'* was used to separate the copies of the tensors
Memory saturation	Batch loading was used for training
Model fine-tuning	The model was retrained using *'model.load_state_dict(...)'*
Class imbalance	The weights were adjusted based on the loss and application of *'DataAumentation (rotation and scaling)'*
Bias evaluation	The following metrics were implemented: precision, recall, and F1-score

Table 14.5 Training results

Metric	Value (%)
Accuracy	98
Precision	96
Recall	98
F1-score	97

Model Training Results

Table 14.5 presents the results obtained during training, which demonstrate that the model achieved high performance in classifying healthy and fatty liver.

The *accuracy* metric indicates the total percentage of cases in which the model made correct predictions, while precision represents its effectiveness in predicting fatty liver. On the other hand, *recall* shows that the model was able to detect nearly all actual cases of fatty liver. Finally, the *F1-score* is the combination of recall and precision, and expresses the balance of the model between diagnostic capacity and the detection of all cases in the dataset. The high percentages of these metrics indicate that the model is reliable for detecting both healthy and fatty liver.

Figure 14.6 shows the confusion matrix, which allows visualization of the correctly classified cases. The evaluation was performed with 345 clinical cases, of which 252 corresponded to healthy liver and 93 to fatty liver. From these cases, the model classified 244 as healthy and 101 as fatty, which indicates that it misclassified 8 cases, corresponding to a misclassification rate of 2.32%. However, this margin is considered acceptable in the clinical context, since the errors were false positives, which confirms that the model maintains accuracy in fatty liver classification.

Figure 14.7 shows the training curves of the model. In the left graph, it can be observed that the loss progressively decreased as the epochs advanced, indicating

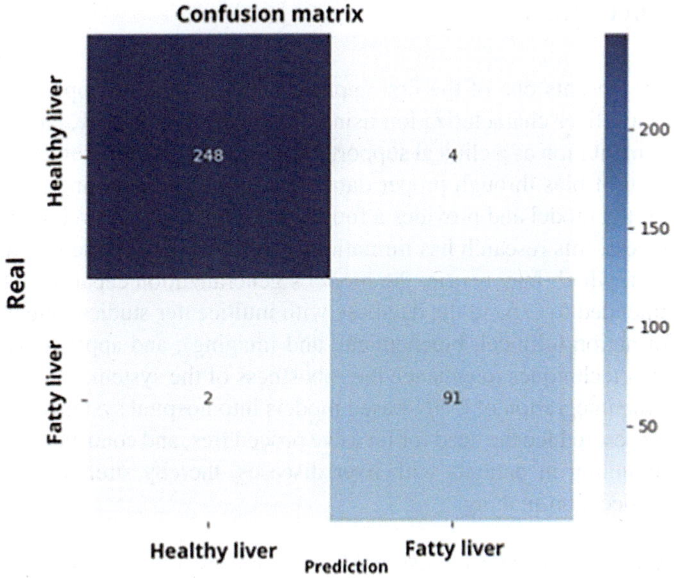

Fig. 14.6 Confusion matrix of the training obtained by Python

the proper adjustment of parameters to minimize classification errors. The right graph illustrates the evolution of accuracy, which started with moderate values and followed an upward trend until stabilizing at 95%. This metric confirms that the model increased its predictive capability.

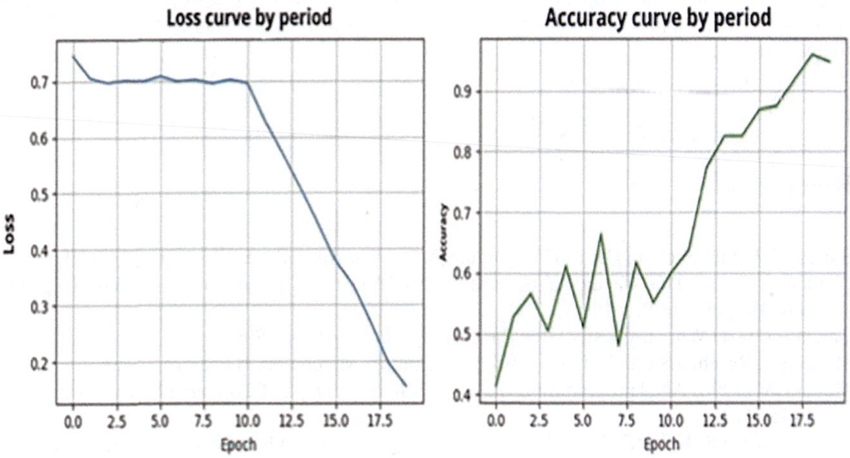

Fig. 14.7 Training curves of the model by Python

14.3 Conclusions

This study represents one of the first approaches in Mexico to apply deep 9 techniques for fatty liver characterization using computed tomography, paving the way for its implementation as a clinical support tool for early detection of this pathology. The reduction of bias through proper data preparation and labelling reinforces the reliability of the model and provides a foundation for future research in the field.

Nevertheless, this research has limitations, mainly related to the size and source of the dataset, which may restrict the model's generalization capability. Therefore, it is recommended to expand the database with multicenter studies, integrate multimodal information (clinical, biochemical, and imaging), and apply advanced *data augmentation* techniques to enhance the robustness of the system.

Finally, the integration of CNN-based models into hospital systems could enable faster diagnoses, reduce the need for invasive procedures, and contribute to improved treatment planning in patients with liver diseases, thereby strengthening clinical practice and decision-making.

Acknowledgements This research acknowledges the invaluable participation of the various institutions that made its consolidation possible.

Special thanks are extended to the Instituto Politécnico Nacional (IPN) for providing the infrastructure necessary for the development of this project.

We also acknowledge the support of the Comisión de Operación y Fomento de Actividades Académicas del IPN (COFAA), which promotes the participation of researchers in academic events of international scope.

Likewise, we thank the Secretaría de Investigación y Posgrado (SIP) for its contribution to academic training and the promotion of scientific projects.

In addition, we recognize the Secretaría de Ciencia, Humanidades, Tecnología e Innovación (SECIHTI), whose contribution has been key to the progress of this research.

Finally, we thank the Hospital Regional "1° de Octubre" for its collaboration in this research through advisory support in the interpretation of patterns and in the reading of information from clinical studies.

References

Barraza EW, Stalnikowitz DK (2025) Non-alcoholic steatosis and steatohepatitis [Article]

Challenger-Pérez I, Díaz-Ricardo Y, Becerra-García RA (2014) The Python programming language. Cienc Holguín 20(2):1–13

García E (2004) What is obesity? Rev Endocrinol Nutr 12(4):S88–S90

Mirjalili V, Raschka S (2020) Python machine learning. Marcombo, Barcelona

Mount DM (1998) ANN programming manual. Tech. Rep., Dept. of Computer Science, University of Maryland

Ramachandran R, Kakar S (2009) Histological patterns in drug-induced liver disease. J Clin Pathol 62:481–492. https://doi.org/10.1136/jcp.2008.058248

Smrekar J, Assadi M, Fast M, Kuštrin I, De S (2008) Development of artificial neural network model for a coal-fired boiler using real plant data. Energy 34:144–152. https://doi.org/10.1016/j.energy.2008.10.010

Wu Y-C, Feng J-W (2017) Development and application of artificial neural network. Wireless Pers Commun 102:1645–1656. https://doi.org/10.1007/s11277-017-5224-x

Chapter 15
Quantum Circuit Proposal to Understand the Health Status Perception Related to Mobility Factors in Urban and Rural Diabetic Persons

Vanessa Zorrilla-Muñoz, Gema Martinez-Navarrete, Nicanor Morales-Delgado, Ramon Peral-Orts, Nicolas Garcia-Aracil, Eduardo Fernandez, and Jose Maria Sabater-Navarro

Abstract More than 422 million people worldwide are affected by diabetes, with a significant proportion living in low- and middle-income countries, particularly in rural areas with limited resources. Diabetic persons often face complications such as limited joint mobility syndrome or diabetic foot, which are more prevalent among older people. Despite the recognized role of technology in managing diabetes-related factors, evidence on its potential to enhance mobility remains limited. This study

V. Zorrilla-Muñoz · G. Martinez-Navarrete (✉) · N. Garcia-Aracil · E. Fernandez · J. M. Sabater-Navarro
Bioengineering Institute, Miguel Hernández University of Elche, Elche, Spain
e-mail: gema.martinen@umh.es

V. Zorrilla-Muñoz
e-mail: vzorrilla@umh.es

N. Garcia-Aracil
e-mail: nicolas.garcia@umh.es

E. Fernandez
e-mail: e.fernandez@umh.es

J. M. Sabater-Navarro
e-mail: jsabater@umh.es

V. Zorrilla-Muñoz
University Institute on Gender Studies, University Carlos III of Madrid, Getafe, Madrid, Spain

G. Martinez-Navarrete · N. Morales-Delgado
Department of Histology and Anatomy, Miguel Hernandez University, Sant Joan d'Alacant, Spain
e-mail: nmorales@umh.es

R. Peral-Orts
Department of Applied Mechanical Engineering, Miguel Hernandez University, Elche, Spain
e-mail: ramon.peral@umh.es

N. Garcia-Aracil · J. M. Sabater-Navarro
Department of System Engineering and Automation, Miguel Hernandez University, Elx, Spain

A. Öchsner (ed.), *Progress in Biomaterials and Biomedical Engineering*, Advanced Structured Materials 249, https://doi.org/10.1007/978-3-032-13551-3_15

explores the lived experiences of older diabetic people ($N = 1822$, aged 65 years and older) with mobility challenges in urban and rural Spain, using data from the "Encuesta de Discapacidad, Autonomía personal y Situaciones de Dependencia, EDAD" (2020). Results revealed correlations between mobility challenges and health deterioration, influenced by socio-spatial factors such as urban or rural living. Urban residents reported challenges with "changing posture," "walking/moving at home," and "traveling by transport," while rural residents noted adverse technology perceptions related to difficulties in the case of "driving vehicles" and "manipulating objects." To address these complexities, a quantum circuit framework, including the quantum approximate optimization algorithm, variational quantum algorithm, and quantum support vector machine, is proposed to model multidimensional relationships among mobility, health perception, technology perception, and socio-spatial factors. This approach leverages quantum computing to uncover nonlinear patterns, offering insights for personalized technology design. These findings guide the customization of technology to address chronic condition challenges within socio-spatial constraints, with further research needed to incorporate additional sociodemographic variables and a gender perspective.

Keywords Urban/rural areas · Diabetes · Socio-spatial · Gender · Older people · Technology

15.1 Introduction

Diabetes is a chronic metabolic disorder characterized by elevated blood glucose levels, affects over 422 million people worldwide, with a disproportionate burden in low- and middle-income countries (World International Organization 2025). The global prevalence of diabetes has surged over recent decades, driven by factors such as aging populations, urbanization, and lifestyle changes (Sun et al. 2021). Annually, diabetes contributes to more than 1.7 million deaths (Global Burden of Disease Collaborative Network: Global Burden of Disease Study 2021), underscoring its status as a major public health challenge and most important disease to take attention among the global healthcare systems (World International Organization 2024). Beyond mortality, diabetes significantly impairs quality of life, particularly through complications that affect physical function and mobility. Complications in diabetes, include conditions such as diabetic neuropathies (Hicks and Selvin 2019), and diabetic foot (Hicks and Selvin 2019; Vibha et al. 2018), among others, which can severely disrupt daily activities and independence.

While technological advancements, such as wearable devices, telemedicine, and mobile health applications, have shown promise in improving diabetes management

E. Fernandez
Networking Research Centre of Bioengineering, Biomaterials and Nanomedicine (CIBER-BBN), Elx, Spain

and monitoring (Domingo-Lopez et al. 2022; Johnston et al. 2021; Ahmad et al. 2020; Beach et al. 2021; Bolanos et al. 2019), their application in addressing mobility-specific challenges remains underexplored. In particular, there is limited evidence on how technology can enhance the mobility and overall well-being of older diabetic persons, especially when viewed through the lens of their lived experiences and diverse socio-spatial contexts. Factors such as gender, urban–rural disparities, and personal health perceptions further complicate the design of effective interventions, as these elements shape how it is the personal experience and how it is managing their conditions. For instance, women and men may perceive and report health challenges differently, while rural residents often face barriers to healthcare access that urban dwellers do not (Miao et al. 2025; Hamasaki 2024).

To address these gaps, this study explores the lived experiences of adult and older diabetic persons with mobility challenges, considering both urban and rural contexts and incorporating a gender perspective. By examining personal health status perceptions, we aim to understand mobility limitations impact daily life and whether technology can serve as a transformative tool in mitigating these challenges. Central to this investigation is a novel approach: the application of quantum circuits to analyze complex, multidimensional health data. Unlike traditional computational methods, quantum circuits offer the potential to process intricate datasets, such as those capturing subjective health perceptions, mobility metrics, and socio-spatial variables. This study proposes a quantum circuit framework to model and interpret the interplay of these factors, providing insights into how technology can be tailored to improve mobility and quality of life for diabetic persons.

By integrating qualitative insights from lived experiences with cutting-edge quantum computing techniques, this research seeks to bridge the gap between technology-driven solutions and the unique needs of diabetic populations. The findings aim to inform the development of personalized, context-sensitive interventions that enhance mobility, promote independence, and improve overall well-being for those affected by diabetes.

15.2 Method

A descriptive analysis was performed using the public "EDAD 2020" database in Spain (Instituto Nacional de Estadística: INE base/Sociedad /Salud /Encuestas de discapacidades/Resultados 2025). The study included a cohort of older people diagnosed with diabetes, encompassing a total 1822 participants aged 64 years and older (699 males, accounting for 38.36% and 1123 females, constituting 61.64%). The average age was 79.84 years, with a standard error of $\pm$ 0.19 (78.64 $\pm$ 0.29 for males, and 80.57 $\pm$ 0.24 for females). The distribution of municipal sizes by sex is detailed in Table 15.1.

The results include various categories of municipal size, including provincial capitals, municipalities with more than 100,000 inhabitants, and rural areas with less than 10,000 inhabitants. The statistical method used in the study considered Pearson

Table 15.1 Distribution related to the municipally size by sex

Municipal sizes	Total ($N = 1822$)			Males ($n = 699$)			Females ($n = 1123$)		
	Freq	%	Cum	Freq	%	Cum	Freq	%	Cum
Provincial capital and municipalities with more than 100,000 inhabitants	698	38.31	38.31	264	37.77	37.77	434	38.65	38.65
From 50,000 to 100,000 inhabitants	173	9.50	47.80	71	10.16	47.93	102	9.08	47.73
From 20,000 to less than 50,000 inhabitants	234	12.84	60.65	84	12.02	59.94	150	13.36	61.09
From 10.000 to less than 20.000 inhabitants	227	12.46	73.11	95	13.59	73.53	132	11.75	72.84
Less than 10.000 inhabitants	490	26.89	100.00	185	26.47	100.00	305	27.16	100.00

correlation test with significance levels set at $p < 0.01$ and $p < 0.05$. All variables were measured using a Likert scale for mobility factors (16 in total). These factors were rated on a scale of 1 to 4 points, where 1 represented the minimum level of difficulty and 4 indicated the maximum level of difficulty. The dependent variable "How is your overall health?" was evaluated on a scale of 1 to 5 points, where 1 indicated very good health and 5 indicated very poor health. Similarly, the dependent variable "Do you think that the use of new technologies has improved aspects of your daily life?" was assessed on a scale of 1 to 4 points, with 1 signifying a substantial improvement and 4 indicating a deterioration in daily life.

Following the identification of statistically significant correlations ($p < 0.01$) between mobility difficulties, health perception, and technology perception in older adults with diabetes, a possible exploratory approach involving **quantum computing models** is proposed for future analysis. Specifically, the design of a **quantum circuit for multidimensional correlation analysis** is considered as a potential tool to represent and examine the complex interdependencies between physical, subjective, and contextual factors, such as gender and urban–rural disparities.

15.3 Results

The results presented in Table 15.2 indicated correlated variables between mobility difficulties and poor health perception in diabetes affected patients, regardless of the socio-spatial approach (rural–urban areas). Overall, the variables showed a significant correlation at $p < 0.01$, except for "drive vehicles…" and "manipulate small objects with hands and fingers when you receive personal help/assistance." Nevertheless, different mobility variables were correlated with health perception of older persons who are residing in rural and urban areas. Specifically, urban residents reported a deterioration in overall health with respect to the difficulty level to "…keep the body in the same position when you receive personal help/assistance" and "… walk/move outside your home when you receive personal help/assistance ($p < 0.01$). On the other hand, in urban areas, a significant correlation at $p < 0.01$ was observed for the variable "…changing posture when you receive personal help/ assistance."

Several differences were founded in terms of unfavorable technology perception attributed to challenges such as "change posture," "walk/move at home…" or "travel by using transports…," which exhibited correlations among persons residing in urban areas. However, these correlations were absent in rural areas. Conversely, in rural areas, variables such as "drive vehicles…" and "manipulate objects…" demonstrated associations with a decline in overall health, further exacerbated by technology utilization.

After the calculation of the Pearson correlations among the 16 Likert-scale mobility variables (independent variables) and dependent variables: health perception (D_1), technology perception (I_17), and contextual factors such as gender and urban–rural disparities, a quantum circuit-based approach is proposed to model these complex interdependencies.

Three quantum circuit approaches are proposed: the quantum approximate optimization algorithm (QAOA), the variational quantum algorithm (VQA), and the quantum support vector machine (QSVM). These circuits will encode mobility variables (e.g., changing posture, walking outside the home), health and technology perceptions, and contextual factors into quantum states, enabling efficient analysis of interactions across these dimensions as Table 15.3 shows. This approach is particularly suited to capture urban–rural differences (e.g., significant correlations in urban areas regarding difficulties for "change posture" or "driving vehicles without adaptation") and gender disparities, optimizing the design of tailored technological interventions.

Each proposed quantum circuit addresses the multidimensional analysis from a unique perspective. The QAOA will optimize the identification of complex correlations by mapping variables to a combinatorial optimization problem, ideal for exploring interactions between mobility and health perception. The VQA, with its flexibility to adjust parameters in variational quantum circuits, will model nonlinear relationships between subjective (health perception) and objective (mobility difficulties) factors, adapting to gender and urban–rural disparities. The QSVM will classify persons based on their health and technology perceptions, using a quantum feature space to enhance accuracy in identifying context-specific patterns. Quantum computing surpasses classical methods by processing large datasets more efficiently, providing deeper insights into how technology can enhance mobility and well-being in diabetic populations across diverse settings.

Table 15.2 Statistical analysis test on Likert-scale variables

	Difficulty level to…	Total (N = 1822)						Urban areas (n = 698)		Rural areas (n = 490)	
		Mean	±	S.D	α Cronbach	Pearson (D_1)	Pearson (I_17)	Pearson (D_1)	Pearson (I_17)	Pearson (D_1)	Pearson (I_17)
Mobility variables	… change posture	2.1875	±	0.2085416	0.8843	0.1356**	0.1162**	0.0827	0.1298*	0.1763*	0.1401
	…change posture when you receive personal help/assistance	2.8125	±	0.2771695	0.8839	0.1997**	0.0711	0.1404	0.1063	0.2508**	0.0042
	…keep the body in the same position	2	±	0.2041241	0.8875	0.1448**	0.0350	0.1031	0.0431	0.0821	0.0511
	…keep the body in the same position when you receive personal help/assistance	2.9375	±	0.1929756	0.8857	0.1779**	0.0047	0.1939**	0.0655	0.1156	0.0118
	… walk/move at your home	2.3125	±	0.1983001	0.8844	0.1139**	0.1145**	0.0688	0.1629**	0.0549	0.0633
	… walk/move at your home when you receive personal help/assistance	2.875	±	0.2561738	0.8830	0.2092**	0.1273**	0.1639*	0.1176	0.1777*	0.0616

(continued)

Table 15.2 (continued)

	Difficulty level to…	Total ($N = 1822$)						Urban areas ($n = 698$)		Rural areas ($n = 490$)	
		Mean	±	S.D	α Cronbach	Pearson (D_1)	Pearson (I_17)	Pearson (D_1)	Pearson (I_17)	Pearson (D_1)	Pearson (I_17)
	… walk/move outside your home	2.375	±	0.2212653	0.8864	0.1234**	0.0785*	0.0854	0.0761	0.0481	0.1014
	… walk/move outside your home when you receive personal help/assistance	3.125	±	0.2393568	0.8843	0.2114**	0.0619	0.2195**	0.0888	0.1826*	0.0567
	…travel by using transport as a passenger	2.625	±	0.125	0.8900	0.0515	0.0981**	0.0385	0.0804	-0.0762	0.1236
	…travel by using transport as a passenger when you receive personal help/assistance	3.4375	±	0.1572882	0.8868	0.1129**	0.0409	0.1540*	0.0440	0.0197	0.0732
	…drive vehicles without adaptations	2.75	±	0.1113034	0.8983	0.0713	0.0377	0.0077	-0.0437	0.1241	0.2755**

(continued)

Table 15.2 (continued)

	Difficulty level to…	Total ($N = 1822$)						Urban areas ($n = 698$)		Rural areas ($n = 490$)	
		Mean	±	S.D	α Cronbach	Pearson (D_1)	Pearson (I_17)	Pearson (D_1)	Pearson (I_17)	Pearson (D_1)	Pearson (I_17)
	…drive vehicles without adaptations when you receive personal help/assistance	3.375	±	0.2393568	0.8883	0.2094	0.2763	-0.1290	-0.2394	0.1855	0.2296
	…manipulate and move objects by using hands and arms	2.1875	±	0.1875	0.8880	0.1765**	0.1097**	0.1099	0.1036	0.1989*	0.1710*
	… manipulate and move objects by using hands and arms, when you receive personal help/assistance	2.6875	±	0.2366212	0.8869	0.1392**	0.1429**	0.1365	0.0703	0.1417	0.1955*

(continued)

Table 15.2 (continued)

	Difficulty level to…	Total ($N = 1822$)						Urban areas ($n = 698$)		Rural areas ($n = 490$)	
		Mean	±	S.D	α Cronbach	Pearson (D_1)	Pearson (I_17)	Pearson (D_1)	Pearson (I_17)	Pearson (D_1)	Pearson (I_17)
	…manipulate small objects with hands and fingers	2.375	±	0.1796938	0.8878	0.1310**	0.1169*	0.0136	0.0328	0.1206	0.2362*
	…manipulate small objects with hands and fingers when you receive personal help/ assistance	3	±	0.2415229	0.8873	0.1047	0.1801**	0.0796	0.1040	-0.0221	0.1182
	How is your overall health? (D_1)	3.8125	±	0.1875	0.9044						
	Do you think that the use of new technologies has improved aspects of your daily life? (I_17)	2.625	±	0.1547848	0.9077						

Pearson $^{**}p < 0.01$, $^{*}p < 0.05$
The total sample consisted of older persons affected by diabetes ($N = 1822$), including older people residing in urban areas ($n = 698$) and rural areas ($n = 490$)

Table 15.3 Analysis of boundaries between quantum computing circuit proposed according to the description, advantages and specific applications

Quantum circuit	Description	Advantages	Specific application
Quantum approximate optimization algorithm (QAOA)	Maps mobility, health, and technology perception variables to a combinatorial optimization problem, using superposition and entanglement to find optimal correlations	High efficiency in complex combinatorial problems; captures multidimensional interactions	Identify correlation patterns between mobility (e.g., "changing posture with assistance") and health perception in urban vs. rural areas
Variational quantum algorithm (VQA)	Uses variational circuits with optimizable parameters to model nonlinear relationships, iteratively adapting to the data	Flexible for heterogeneous data; suitable for modeling subjective perceptions	Model nonlinear interactions between technology perception (I_17) and mobility difficulties, considering gender and socio-spatial context
Quantum support vector machine (QSVM)	Projects data into a quantum feature space to classify persons based on health and technology perceptions, improving class separation	Enhances accuracy in classifying complex patterns; efficient for large datasets	Classify persons by health perception (D_1) based on mobility variables and context (urban vs. rural), identifying groups for targeted technological intervention

15.4 Conclusion

The findings revealed a significant relationship between "overall health perception" and "the use of new technologies to improve daily life" (dependent variables) in relation to mobility challenges across all diagnosed diseases. Furthermore, these results were influenced by socio-spatial factors, specifically the living environment (urban or rural areas) of the older people.

This chapter emphasizes the importance of designing technologies that prioritize enhanced usability, ergonomic considerations, minimal invasiveness, and aesthetically appeal. Additionally, it underscores the importance of incorporating socio-spatial factors (Zorrilla-Muñoz et al. 2022). However, further research is required to include additional sociodemographic variables and adopt a gender perspective (Agulló-Tomás and Zorrilla-Muñoz 2020). The integrations of emerging technologies must to prioritize enhancing the autonomy and independence of people suffering from diabetes, taking into account socio-spatial considerations. The results from this analysis offer insights into tailoring technology design based on living environments and their potential application to address complications arising from various chronic conditions. This approach considers socio-spatial limitations, aiming to achieve enhanced and more effective outcomes, which could help future researches in more comprehensive perspective with the possibility of incorporating additional sociodemographic variables and gender perspective highlights the intent to expand and enhance research in this field.

To further advance this research, a quantum circuit framework is proposed, encompassing the quantum approximate optimization algorithm (QAOA), the variational quantum algorithm (VQA), and the quantum support vector machine (QSVM). These circuits leverage quantum superposition, entanglement, and feature spaces to efficiently analyze the multidimensional relationships among mobility, health perception, technology perception, and contextual factors like gender and urban–rural disparities in the EDAD 2020 dataset ($N = 1822$). Unlike classical methods like Pearson correlation, quantum computing uncovers nonlinear patterns and context-specific insights, enabling personalized technological interventions. For instance, QAOA optimizes correlation identification, VQA models subjective–objective interactions, and QSVM classifies persons for targeted solutions. Future research should focus on implementing these circuits in practical settings, validating their efficacy, and developing technology-driven interventions to enhance mobility and well-being, ultimately improving the quality of life for older diabetic persons across urban and rural contexts.

Funding This contribution takes parts of the grant "Multimodal telerehabilitation assisted by robotic devices to maximize motor recovery" co-financed by FEDER funds, within the FEDER operational program of the Valencian Community (2014–2020) and the grant PROMETEO/2019/119 from the Generalitat Valenciana and the Bidons Egara Research Chair of the University Miguel Hernandez to Eduardo Fernandez. Moreover, this contribution has been supported by the Spanish Ministry of Science and Innovation, through the projects PID2019-108310RB-I00, TED2021-130431BI00 and PLEC2022-009424, the Luciano Navarro Tripodi Foundation Grant; the Caser Foundation Grant; and the AVI (https://innoavi.es/es/) through the project INNTA1/2024/11.

References

Agulló-Tomás MS, Zorrilla-Muñoz V (2020) Technologies and images of older women. In: Lecture notes in computer science (including subseries lecture notes in artificial intelligence and lecture notes in bioinformatics). https://doi.org/10.1007/978-3-031-05654-3_30

Ahmad A, Rasul T, Yousaf A, Zaman U (2020) Understanding factors influencing elderly diabetic patients' continuance intention to use digital health wearables: extending the technology acceptance model (TAM). J Open Innov: Technol Market Complexity 6. https://doi.org/10.3390/JOITMC6030081

Beach C, Cooper G, Weightman A, Hodson-Tole EF, Reeves ND, Casson AJ (2021) Monitoring of dynamic plantar foot temperatures in diabetes with personalised 3d-printed wearables. Sensors 21. https://doi.org/10.3390/s21051717

Bolanos L, Vicente JM, Vivas OA, Sabater-Navarro JM (2019) Electrodermal activity in relation to diabetes, autonomic neuropathy and aging: a preliminary study. Ingenieria e Investigacion 39. https://doi.org/10.15446/ing.investig.v39n3.74982

Domingo-Lopez DA, Lattanzi G, Schreiber HJL, Wallace EJ, Wylie R, O'Sullivan J, Dolan EB, Duffy GP (2022) Medical devices, smart drug delivery, wearables and technology for the treatment of diabetes mellitus. Adv Drug Delivery Rev 185:114280. https://doi.org/10.1016/j.addr.2022.114280

Global Burden of Disease Collaborative Network: Global Burden of Disease Study (2021) Results. Institute for Health Metrics and Evaluation. https://vizhub.healthdata.org/gbd-results/

Hamasaki H (2024) Patient experience in older adults with diabetes: a narrative review on interventions to improve patient experience and research gaps. Healthcare 12. https://doi.org/10.3390/healthcare12242530

Hicks CW, Selvin E (2019) Epidemiology of peripheral neuropathy and lower extremity disease in diabetes. Curr DiabRep 19(10):86. https://doi.org/10.1007/s11892-019-1212-8

Instituto Nacional de Estadística: INE base / Sociedad /Salud /Encuestas de discapacidades / Resultados (2025). https://www.ine.es/dyngs/INEbase/es/operacion.htm?c=Estadistica_C&cid=1254736176782&menu=resultados&idp=1254735573175#_tabs-1254736195764

Johnston L, Wang G, Hu K, Qian C, Liu G (2021) Advances in biosensors for continuous glucose monitoring towards wearables. Front Bioeng Biotechnol 9:733810. https://doi.org/10.3389/fbioe.2021.733810

Miao Y, Li X, Shen Z, Zhu D, Bai J, Zhang J, Ren R, Guo D, Tarimo CS, Cui J, Zhen M, Zhang J, Song Y (2025) Exploring influencing factors of healthy lifestyles in rural area among older adults with diabetes based on socioecological model. Sci Rep 15:2829. https://doi.org/10.1038/s41598-025-85163-3

Sun H, Saeedi P, Karuranga S, Pinkepank M, Ogurtsova K, Duncan BB, Stein C, Basit A, Chan JCN, Mbanya JC, Pavkov ME, Ramachandaran A, Wild SH, James S, Herman WH, Zhang P, Bommer C, Kuo S, Boyko EJ, Magliano DJ (2022) IDF diabetes Atlas: global, regional and country-level diabetes prevalence estimates for 2021 and projections for 2045. Diabetes Res Clin Pract 183. https://doi.org/10.1016/j.diabres.2021.109119

Vibha SP, Kulkarni MM, Kirthinath Ballala AB, Kamath A, Maiya GA (2018) Community based study to assess the prevalence of diabetic foot syndrome and associated risk factors among people with diabetes mellitus. BMC Endocr Disord 18. https://doi.org/10.1186/s12902-018-0270-2

World International Organization (2024) Urgent action needed as global diabetes cases increase four-fold over past decades. https://www.who.int/news/item/13-11-2024-urgent-action-needed-as-global-diabetes-cases-increase-four-fold-over-past-decades. Accessed 20 July 2025

World International Organization: Diabetes (2025). https://www.who.int/health-topics/diabetes#tab=tab_1. Accessed 28 July 2025

Zorrilla-Muñoz V, Agulló-Tomás MS, Rodríguez-Blázquez C, Ayala A, Fernandez-Mayoralas G, Forjaz MJ (2022) Ageing perception as a key predictor of self-rated health by rural older people—a study with gender and inclusive perspectives. Land (Basel) 11. https://doi.org/10.3390/land11030323

Chapter 16
Implementing Text-to-Speech (TTS)-Based Generated Voice in the Pyttsx3 Synthesizer as Support for People with Speech Impairments

Marcial Margarito Sánchez-Sánchez, Alejandra Armenta-Molina, Luis Héctor Hernández-Gómez, and Rita Trinidad Rodríguez Márquez

Abstract This paper reports on the processing of generated voice for users with speech impairments, such as diglossia, harelip, and laryngectomy. The generated voice enables users to interact with the voice assistant through communication between the control interface and the voice assistant, eliminating the need for a human voice. For this purpose, speed and sound pressure level are considered. The voice is processed using a text-to-speech system in the Pyttsx3 synthesizer. It is compatible with Windows, macOS, and Linux systems. It also allows switching between male and female voices, as well as among different languages. The control system was programmed in Python. Voice assistants with noise reduction and far-field speech recognition systems can capture remote commands in noisy environments. Therefore, the limits for determining the adequate performance distance are evaluated with a 40 dB noise background, and two critical factors were identified: playback speed and sound pressure level (SPL). The system loses effectiveness if the speed is outside the range between 90 and 200 words per minute (wpm), or if the sound pressure level

M. M. Sánchez-Sánchez · R. T. Rodríguez Márquez
Departamento de Ingeniería en Comunicaciones y Electrónica, Escuela Superior de Ingeniería Mecánica y Eléctrica Unidad Zacatenco, Instituto Politécnico Nacional, Edificio 5, PB, Av. Luis Enrique Erro S/N, Unidad Profesional Adolfo López Mateos, Gustavo A. Madero, Mexico City, Mexico
e-mail: mmsanchezs@ipn.mx

R. T. Rodríguez Márquez
e-mail: rtrodriguezm@ipn.mx

A. Armenta-Molina (✉) · L. H. Hernández-Gómez (✉)
Sección de Estudios de Posgrado e Investigación, Escuela Superior de Ingeniería Mecánica y Eléctrica Unidad Zacatenco, Instituto Politécnico Nacional, Edificio 5, 2do Piso, Av. Luis Enrique Erro S/N, Unidad Profesional Adolfo López Mateos, Gustavo A. Madero, Mexico City, Mexico
e-mail: aarmentamo@ipn.mx

L. H. Hernández-Gómez
e-mail: lhhernandez@ipn.mx

A. Öchsner (ed.), *Progress in Biomaterials and Biomedical Engineering*, Advanced Structured Materials 249, https://doi.org/10.1007/978-3-032-13551-3_16

is below 50 dB. 100% recognition was achieved by the assistant under the following conditions: SPL $\geq$ 50 dB and 170 wpm.

Keywords Text-to-speech · Pyttsx3 · Synthesized speech · Speech impairment

16.1 Introduction

The motivation for this work arises from an urgent need: to reduce the communication barriers faced by people with speech disabilities. Although advances have been made in artificial intelligence and accessibility, many solutions still face problems of cost, complexity, and adaptability, highlighting the need for innovative alternatives.

This problem is significant in Mexico. According to the National Institute of Statistics and Geography in 2020, 13.6 million people live with some disabilities, and two million have difficulty speaking or communicating. These figures reveal the magnitude of the challenge to be addressed (Cuéntame de México 2025).

Advances in speech synthesis and recognition have enabled the development of tools that improve interaction between users and devices. Recent works by Zheng et al. (2024) and Leung et al. (2024) demonstrate that fine-tuning automatic speech recognition (ASR) systems with dysarthric or Parkinsonian speech, including synthetic data augmentation, can reduce word error rates by over 30% compared to general models. However, individuals with speech impairments still face barriers due to the reliance on specific voice patterns. Automatic speech recognition has been primarily developed for standard voices, which can cause people with speech disorders, such as blocks, repetitions, or unusual pronunciations, as seen in dysarthria or stuttering, to encounter systematic errors and difficulties in using the system (Lea et al. 2023; MacDonald et al. 2024; Mujtaba et al. 2024; Wilson and John 2000).

Augmentative and alternative communication (AAC) systems (Beukelman and Mirenda 2020), like Tobii Dynavox or Proloquo2Go, use symbols. They make the expression easy, while personalized synthetic voices and neural speech prostheses offer more individualized solutions (Moses et al. 2021). Educators support literacy in AAC users, and the Convention on the Rights of Persons with Disabilities CRPD upholds communication rights for people with disabilities (United Nations 2006).

Unlike pictogram-based systems that require visual interpretation, TTS allows real-time verbal communication using written input. They give greater flexibility, accessibility, and integration into everyday devices like phones and laptops. On the other hand, brain-computer interfaces (BCIs) technologies (Brumberg et al. 2018) are still experimental and costly. TTS tools, such as the Python-based pyttsx3, are widely available, customizable, and practical for daily use. They are accessible and effective options for communication support.

16.2 Statement of the Problem

The objective was to determine the viability of the Pyttsx3 synthesizer as a solution for individuals with speech disabilities, such as diglossia, harelip, and laryngectomy (Fig. 16.1). Its effectiveness in interacting with voice assistants and in environments with varying noise levels has been determined.

The developed system consists of a text-to-speech module based on Pyttsx3. A synthesized voice command is generated. It is sent to a virtual assistant (voice assistant).

The implementation was carried out in a home automation environment. The setup was tested in a 6 m × 5 m × 2 m room, as shown in Fig. 16.2.

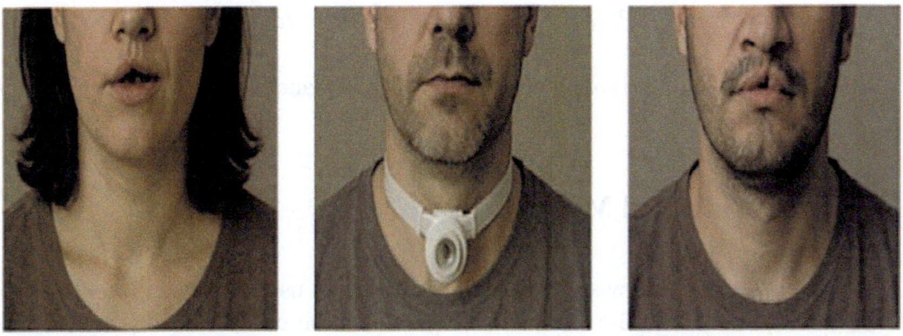

Fig. 16.1 Some cases of speech impairments: **a** Harelip **b** laryngectomy **c** dysglossia

Fig. 16.2 Room used in the tests to analyze the efficiency of command recognition

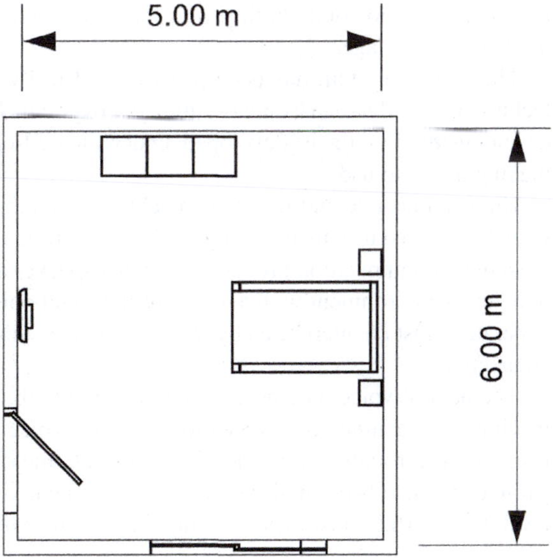

Evaluating the performance of a smart speaker is crucial. The processing systems of these devices may experience a decrease in their ability to distinguish the user's voice when the background noise level is close to or above 40 dB. The noise competes with the command in a masking effect. The user's voice loses intensity, increasing the likelihood of misinterpretation of the command. It is important to evaluate these limits to determine the extent to which their performance is reliable in everyday situations.

The implementation of a speaker with Bluetooth connectivity has been proposed. The inverse square law has been considered, which states that sound intensity decreases in proportion to the square of the distance from the source. In terms of sound pressure level (SPL), this implies a reduction of approximately 6 dB for every doubling of the distance. It can be estimated with the following Eq. (16.1):

$$\mathrm{SPL}_2 = \mathrm{SPL}_1 - 20 * \log\ 10(d_2/d_1) \tag{16.1}$$

SPL_1 and SPL_2 are the sound pressure levels at distances d_1 and d_2, respectively.

16.3 Materials and Methods

A computer with a Windows 10 operating system was used. It has an Intel Core i5, 8 GB RAM, and 256 GB SSD data storage. It can be considered a platform that sends the information generated in text and transforms it into voice. The acoustic signal is generated through a speaker with Bluetooth connectivity. A voice assistant interprets and executes the requested actions. The use of a Windows operating system is essential due to compatibility with the drivers and software necessary to operate the Python language.

The control system has been programmed in Python. It can integrate multiple technologies and has an extensive library ecosystem. This allows for efficient system development. Python is developed under an OSI-approved open-source license, making it free to use.

Human–machine and machine–machine communication are required between a speech-impaired user using the Pyttsx3 text-to-speech synthesizer, and the machine–machine communication process between a speaker and the voice assistant. This is done in an environment with a 40 dB background noise level. The voice parameters generated must be interpreted by the voice assistant through a speaker via Bluetooth connection.

The natural voice parameters are compared with the voice generated to achieve machine-to-machine communication, because voice assistants are designed to get instructions through natural speech. As a result, the speed, amplitude, and language parameters have been modified in an environment with a 40 dB background noise level. Figure 16.3 illustrates the setup diagram for voice generation.

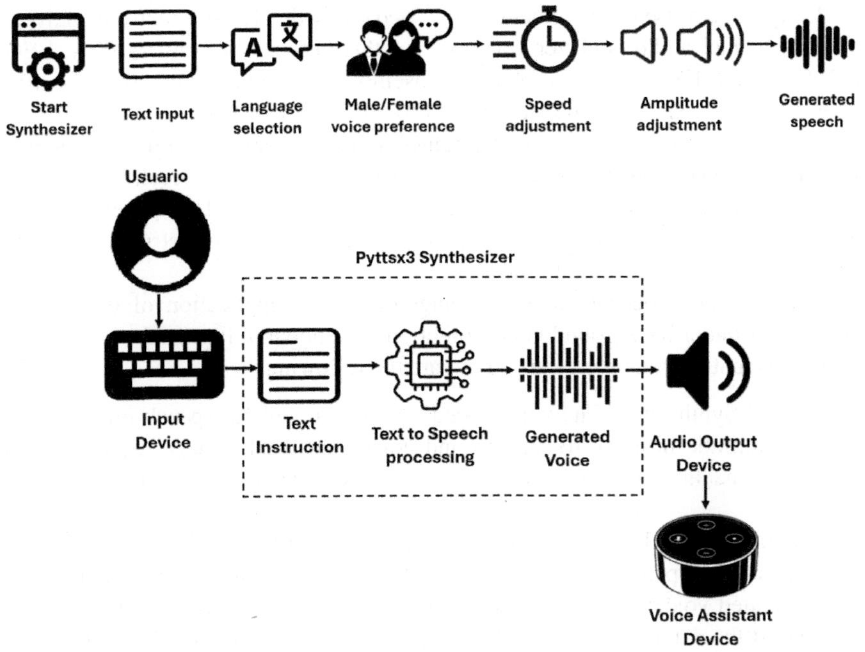

Fig. 16.3 Setup diagram of the Pyttsx3 synthesizer for the voice generation

In this case, the user gives a text instruction, and the program processes it. Then, it is played through a Bluetooth speaker. Finally, the voice assistant recognizes it, executing the initial instruction.

Coding a program in Python takes advantage of the capabilities of the pyttsx3 library. The library can generate a text-to-speech (TTS) environment, which is important for scripts with a synthetic voice. The developed code generates a voice file and saves it on the device. The voice generated has a level of 1.0. It is the maximum level Python allows for the playback of generated audio. At the same time, it provides a speed of 170 words per minute, which is a standard and manageable speed for the voice assistant. This is reproduced with a female voice.

A speaker generates the acoustic signal to achieve a greater connection distance and sound pressure level. The frequency response range is between 65 Hz and 20 kHz. Its sensitivity is 90 dB SPL (at 1 W/1 m). The Bluetooth range is 10 m, and it operates with a full-range driver.

A conventional voice assistant is required to receive and interpret the generated commands. It is complemented by 4 far-field microphones with active noise cancelation. It operates with integrated full-range driver speakers. Its frequency response range is between 60 Hz and 20 kHz. The connectivity characteristics are Wi-Fi 2.4 GHz/5 GHz, Bluetooth 5.0. Besides, temperature, proximity, and ambient light sensors have been integrated. Voice control of IoT devices is compatible with lights, plugs, locks, thermostats, cameras, and more.

Background noise measurement was carried out with a PAA6 spectrum analyzer. A dual-channel audio analyzer was used for this purpose. It features RTA, LEQ, RT-60, FFT, THD+N, polarity, phase, an oscilloscope, and a meter (dB SPL, dBu, dBV, and volts). SPL's can be measured between 30 and 130 dB.

The Pyttsx3 synthesizer was implemented as a text-to-speech engine in a control system developed in Python. The purpose is to generate artificial speech that interacts effectively with a voice assistant, without human intervention. The speech-impaired individual can type text on a user interface. Alternatively, the instructions can be written directly in the template shown in Fig. 16.4.

Below is the experimental block diagram for the application of the Pyttsx3 synthesizer under background noise conditions, as shown in Fig. 16.5.

The evaluations that were carried out are the following.

1. Pyttsx3 Synthesizer: The voice speed to a person without speech impairments, its amplitude in a 40 dB background noise, and the language (Spanish) of a human-machine communication were evaluated. It was done using text-to-speech input.
2. Natural Voice: The speed in words per minute with a natural female voice was evaluated in Spanish. This is an input parameter of a Pyttsx3 synthesizer.
3. Generated Voice: The characteristics of a female-generated voice were evaluated against the natural voice (female) in Spanish. It was done with the sentences in Spanish: "Set an alarm for 10 am," "Add butter to your shopping list," "Play Cadetes de Linares on Spotify"," What is 57,830 minus 10,234?".

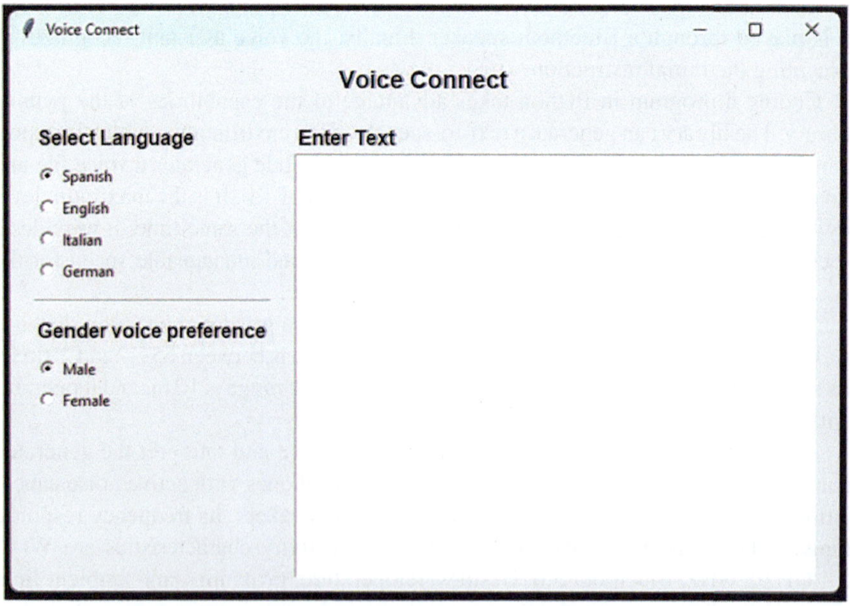

Fig. 16.4 Language selection and text input are done using the displayed communication template

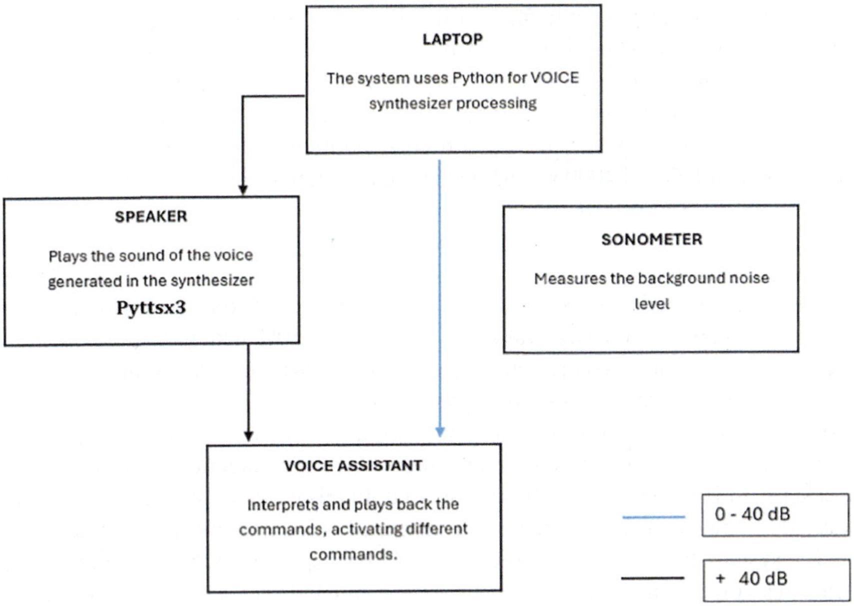

Fig. 16.5 Block diagram. The blue path is followed when the operation noise level is below 40 dB. Alternatively, the black path is followed when the noise is higher than 40 dB

4. Effectiveness tests: The commands of machine-to-machine communication were evaluated. A 40 dB background noise level and distances of 1, 2, 4, and 10 m were considered. A spectrogram displays the frequency components of the natural voice. The generated voice, involved in recognizing the instruction, was also considered. The similarity between the natural voice and the generated voice was evaluated with Pearson's correlation. The percentage of similarity with which the voice assistant system can interpret instructions in machine-to-machine communication was established.

16.4 Discussion of the Results

Command recognition efficiency was initially evaluated. The background noise level was measured at 40 dB at distances of 1, 2, and 4 m. Given a background noise level of 40 dB, the effectiveness of the voice assistant is limited to 2 m. The background noise interferes with the voice recognition accuracy as the sound of the command attenuates with distance.

According to this evaluation, the recommended level of voice assistance is 52–57 dB SPL. This exceeds 40–45 dB background noise with a good signal-to-noise ratio (SNR). Under these conditions, the voice assistance gets 52–57 dB SPL. The speaker output level was set to 52–57 dB SPL at 1 m. This allows instructions to be given 10 m away from the speaker and at least 11 m from the voice assistance device.

The harmonic frequencies in the natural voice have more energy during the recorded time history. On the other hand, the generated voice frequencies have less energy. In the natural voice, the highest concentration of energy was found in the range between 100 and 4000 Hz, while the higher frequencies of the generated voice have a uniform (robotic) distribution.

Figures 16.6 and 16.7 illustrate the spectrograms of the generated and natural voices, respectively.

The generated voice, developed with Python code, was compared with a natural voice. The Pearson similarity evaluation was close to 50% with the natural voice. It is enough for the voice assistant interpretation. The instruction recognition efficiency was evaluated in a room with a background noise level of 40 dB, at 1, 2, and 4 m distances. The recognition rates at 1 m, 2 m, and 4 m were 98%, 10%, and 0%, respectively. 100% efficiency was obtained in the range mentioned above when a speaker with Bluetooth connectivity was used. In this case, the sound pressure level was at least 50 dB, and the voice speed generated was 170 words per minute.

The system architecture is based on the Pyttsx3 speech synthesis engine, which generates voice commands from text. These commands are sent via Bluetooth to a speaker, whose acoustic signal is picked up by a virtual assistant. This approach was successfully validated in a home automation environment. In addition, an intuitive

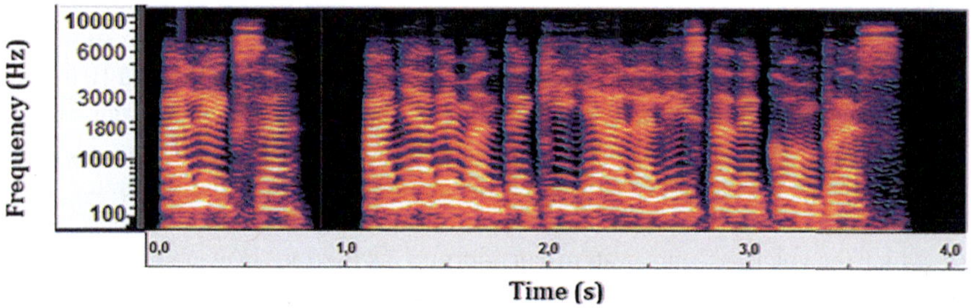

Fig. 16.6 Example of generated voice, phrase "Add butter to your shopping list"

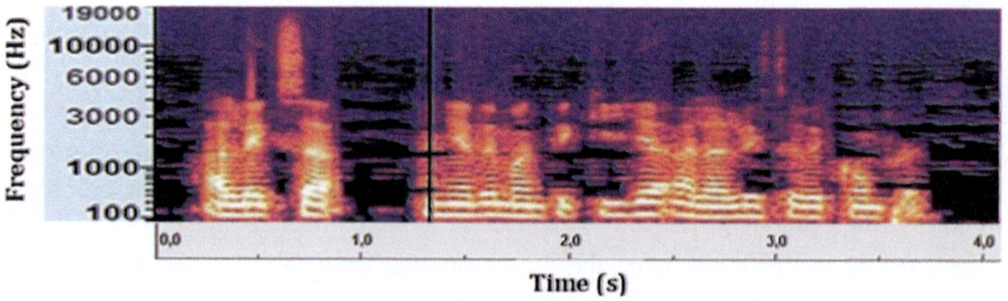

Fig. 16.7 Example of natural voice, phrase "Add butter to your shopping list"

interface was designed that allows for customizing the language and voice gender, thereby improving its adaptability.

16.4.1 Instruction "Speed"

Tests conducted with the synthetic voice at a speed below 90 words per minute resulted in inefficient interpretation of the voice assistant. There is instability in tests performed at speeds above 200 words per minute. A speed of 170 words per minute is proposed, based on the analysis of speed and efficiency in command recognition. This is very similar to a natural voice, and the voice assistant response remains stable.

16.4.2 Instruction "Language"

A configurable template, which can be in different languages (English, Spanish, French, German, Italian, Chinese, Japanese, Russian, Portuguese), was used. It allows the adjustment of the generated voice parameters for recognition by the voice assistant. During testing, the voice generated was compared with natural voice recordings. Although there are differences in formant frequencies, intelligibility was maintained.

Two critical factors were identified: playback speed and SPL. The system loses effectiveness if the speed is outside the range of 90–200 words per minute, or if the sound pressure level is below 50 dB.

16.5 Conclusions

Using the Pyttsx3 synthesizer with virtual assistants significantly enhances accessibility for individuals with speech disabilities. The differences between the frequencies of the natural voice and the generated voice do not affect the interpretation of instructions. Playback speed and sound pressure level impact on the system's efficiency. However, the quality of the voice generated can be improved. The voice assistants recognized up to a 50% Pearson similarity score. There are differences between the natural and generated voices. However, the instructions were correctly interpreted. The voice assistant interprets instructions at 170 words per minute. In noisy environments, a Bluetooth speaker with a sound pressure level of at least 50 dB is recommended. The user can be located 10 m from the voice assistant. This provides independence and mobility for sending instructions.

The results demonstrate that the Pyttsx3 implementation is a viable alternative for facilitating communication for people with speech disabilities.

Acknowledgments The authors kindly acknowledge the grant awarded by the Instituto Politécnico Nacional and SIP for the development of this research.

References

Beukelman DR, Mirenda P (2020) Augmentative and alternative communication: supporting children and adults with complex communication needs, 5th edn. Paul H. Brookes Publishing Co., Baltimore

Brumberg K, Pitt J, Guenther S (2018) Brain-computer interfaces for augmentative and alternative communication: a tutorial. Am J Speech Lang Pathol 27(1):1–12. https://doi.org/10.1044/2017_AJSLP-16-0244

Cuéntame de México (2025) Sección educativa. Instituto Nacional de Estadística y Geografía (INEGI): Discapacidad. https://beta.cuentame.inegi.org.mx/explora/poblacion/discapacidad/. Accessed on 21 May 2025

Lea T, Huang Z, Tooley L, Narain J, Yee D, Georgiou P, Tran TD, Bigham JP, Findlater L. From user perceptions to technical improvement: enabling people who stutter to better use speech recognition. Paper presented at the conference on human factors in computing systems is the premier international conference of human-computer interaction (CHI) 2023, Cornell University, Hamburg, Germany, 23–28 Apr 2023

Leung WZ, Cross M, Ragni A, Goetze S. Training data augmentation for dysarthric automatic speech recognition by text-to-dysarthric-speech synthesis. Paper presented at the 25th Interspeech conference 2024, Cornell University, Isla de Kos, Grecia, 1–5 Sept 2024

MacDonald T, Green S, Tomanek M et al (2024) Automatic speech recognition of conversational speech in individuals with disordered speech. Journal of speech. J Speech Lang Hear Res 67(11):4176–4185. https://doi.org/10.1044/2024_JSLHR-24-00045

Moses DA, et al. (2021) Neuroprosthesis for decoding speech in a paralyzed person with anarthria. N Engl J Med 385(3):217–227

Mujtaba D, Mahapatra NR, Arney M, Yaruss JS, Gerlach-Houck H, Herring C, Bin J. Lost in transcription: identifying and quantifying the accuracy biases of automatic speech recognition systems against disfluent speech. Paper presented at the annual conference of the North American Chapter of the Association for Computational Linguistics (NAACL) 2024, Cornell University, Mexico City, Mexico, 16–21 June 2024

United Nations (2006) Convention on the rights of persons with disabilities. United Nations, New York

Wilson BB, John J (2000) Acoustic variability in dysarthria and computer speech recognition. Clin Linguist Phon 14(4):307–327. https://doi.org/10.1080/02699200050024001

Zheng X, Phukon B, Hasegawa-Johnson M. Fine tuning automatic speech recognition for people with Parkinson's: an effective strategy for enhancing speech technology. Paper presented at the 25th interspeech conference 2024, Cornell University, Isla de Kos, Grecia, 1–5 Sept 2024

Chapter 17
IoT System for Estimation of pH and Electrical Conductivity in a Hydroponic Crop by Means of an Artificial Neural Network

Mario Antonio López-Pacheco, Mario Cesar Maya-Rodriguez, Mauricio Aarón Pérez-Romero, and Alejandra Armenta-Molina

Abstract This paper reports a prototype for pH and electrical conductivity monitoring of a hydroponic circuit of germinated spinach. Real-time monitoring has been implemented with a webcam. The data acquisition system is based on the Arduino UNO hardware structure. It is used in conjunction with a Raspeberry Pi 3. In the next step, this development is loaded into an IOT platform. It is hosted on Firebase for remote monitoring of the parameters of interest, and it is accessed in a mobile application developed in APK on Android. The collected data is processed and used for the offline training of a multi-layer neural network. This process was programmed in Python language. Parameters of interest can be estimated in the possible conditions of operation of the hydroponic system.

Keywords Artificial neural network · Hydroponics · IoT · Forecasting · pH monitoring · APK · Germinated spinach · Offline training

M. A. López-Pacheco · M. C. Maya-Rodriguez (✉) · M. A. Pérez-Romero
Instituto Politécnico Nacional. Escuela Superior de Ingeniería Mecánica y Eléctrica. Ingeniería en Control y Automatización, Edificio 2, Planta baja, Unidad Profesional Adolfo López Mateos "Zacatenco", Colonia Lindavista. Alcaldía Gustavo A. Madero, Mexico City, Mexico
e-mail: mmayar@ipn.mx

M. A. López-Pacheco
e-mail: mlaopezp@ipn.mx

M. A. Pérez-Romero
e-mail: maperezro@ipn.mx

A. Armenta-Molina
Instituto Politécnico Nacional. Escuela Superior de Ingeniería Mecánica y Eléctrica. Sección de Estudios de Posgrado e Investigación, Edificio 5, 2do Piso, Unidad Profesional Adolfo López Mateos "Zacatenco", Colonia Lindavista. Alcaldía Gustavo A. Madero, Mexico City, Mexico
e-mail: aarmentamo@ipn.mx

A. Öchsner (ed.), *Progress in Biomaterials and Biomedical Engineering*, Advanced Structured Materials 249, https://doi.org/10.1007/978-3-032-13551-3_17

17.1 Introduction

A hydroponic system is an irrigation system in which the roots of the crops receive the nutrients they need through a solution that dissolves in water and is absorbed by the roots, like soil-based cultivation (Perwiratama and Setidai 2019). In this system, water is the key factor, as it determines how many nutrients will reach the plant and in what form. It also considers factors such as water levels to prevent roots from tangling or rotting if the water and dissolved solutions are not in optimal conditions for cultivation. The nutrient solutions dissolved in water that plants receive contain various nutrients that must be monitored and regulated to ensure the best growing conditions. Some of the macronutrients in the solutions are nitrogen (N), phosphorus (P), and potassium (K). Secondary plant nutrients include calcium (Ca), magnesium (Mg), and sulfur (S). Other important components like oxygen and carbon are obtained from the atmosphere (Coleto Martinez 2006). Plant nutrients alter the pH of the nutrient solution as they are added. The pH of the nutrient solution changes as plants absorb secondary plant nutrients, directly affecting the composition of the aqueous solution. Additionally, the electrical conductivity in the solution also varies over time due to the absorption of nutrients by plants and the dissolved solids remaining in the water. In conclusion, when a plant absorbs nutrients from the solution, the values of electrical conductivity and pH will change, which is why hydroponic systems primarily monitor these two parameters. The multi-layer perceptron (MLP) is a feedforward neural network with one or more layers of neurons between its input and output layers (Haykin 2009). It is fully connected, meaning that each neuron in any layer is connected to all neurons in the previous and next layers. Due to this connection type, a MLP network propagates information from the input layer through the network from left to right, layer by layer, to provide a response in the output layer (Ljung 1999). In recent years, industrial sectors have progressively incorporated digital technologies to enhance efficiency, adaptability, and operational control (Peng et al. 2020). This shift, largely influenced by the advancement of industry 4.0, which focuses on integrating intelligent systems that can communicate with physical infrastructure via local or remote networks. Such a setup facilitates effortless remote configuration, improving user experience while minimizing the necessity for direct on-site adjustments, aligning with the broader objectives of digital transformation promoted by industry 4.0 initiatives (Hossain et al. 2024). Agriculture 4.0 originates from the fourth industrial revolution, where smart farms began integrating technological advancements into agriculture. Its goal is to enhance the adaptability of production systems, improve crop rotation for higher production levels, and optimize resource use efficiency—giving rise to what is known as precision agriculture (Wongpatikaseree et al. 2018; Kessler 2012). Precision agriculture uses monitoring and data analysis to help farmers make informed production management decisions. Furthermore, agricultural technology and practices enable the optimal use of resources such as water, fertilizers, and energy. This is accomplished by combining hardware, software, and communication services to measure and monitor agricultural variables through sensors, computers, and communication networks. Precision agriculture products also use various data management techniques to process information and provide insights to farmers and pest control agents (Herman and Surantha 2019; Lian and Matsushita 2025). This work focuses on predicting pH and electrical conductivity in a hydroponic crop, as both variables are interdependent. To achieve this prediction, a neural network is fed data from a pH sensor and an electrical conductivity sensor. By monitoring both variables, it is possible to adjust the plant's pH using a neutralizing solution, ensuring optimal acidity levels for plant growth. The prototype consists of a floating-root hydroponic system as the growth medium for spinach, along with a data acquisition system composed of the mentioned sensors connected to a microcontroller. This microcontroller processes the signals acquired by the sensors to monitor the studied variables.

17.2 Materials and Methods

17.2.1 Neural Network

The neural network topology used is shown in Fig. 17.1 and is formed by three layers. In all the layers, it is mandatory to define the nodes and neurons to reach the planned task, as in this case, the estimation of the variables (pH and electrical conductivity). The first one is the input layer where the quantity of information with which the NN will work is defined. The second one is the hidden layer that is responsible for making the performance. In this layer, each input is operated through multiple neurons on the hidden layer and through it gets an estimation at the output. The last one is the output layer, which contains the estimated data necessary for the testing process.

The MLP output equation according to Fig. 17.1 for the estimation of flow velocity profiles is given by,

$$\hat{y}(k) = g_j\left[\sum_{j=1}^{m} V_{j}f_j\left(\sum_{i=1}^{n} W_i X(k)_i + b_{Ii}\right)\right] + b_{Oj}, \tag{17.1}$$

where the vectors V_j and f_j are the weights of the MLP, the bias are given by b_{Ii} and b_{Oj}, the index n and m are the neurons number in each layer, and f_j are g_j the active functions. The input function is given by,

$$X(k) = \left[pH(k), CE(k)\right], \tag{17.2}$$

where $X(k)$ is the input vector; $pH(k)$ and $CE(k)$ are a series of time from the data acquisition storage.

The error equation is given by,

$$e(k) = \hat{y}_j(k) - y_j(k). \tag{17.3}$$

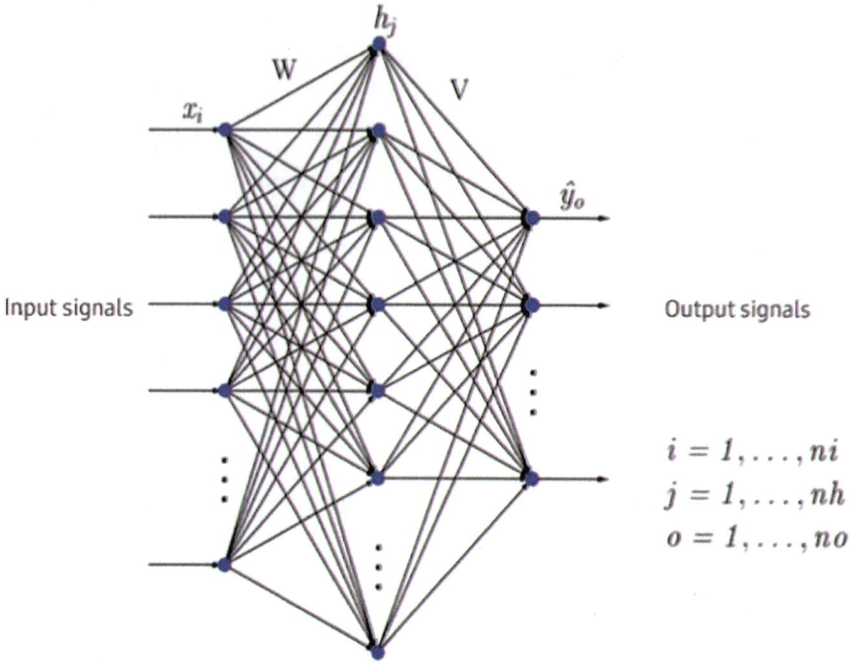

Fig. 17.1 Multi-layer perceptron topology

The index to minimize is,

$$J(k) = \frac{1}{n} \sum_{j=1}^{n} \left(\hat{y}_j(k) - y_j(k)\right)^2. \quad (17.4)$$

and the method to update the weights of the MLP is the backpropagation equation given by,

$$w(k+1) = w(k) + \eta \frac{\partial J(k)}{\partial w(k)}, \quad (17.5)$$

and the gradient is defined by,

$$\Delta w(k) = w(k+1) - w(k) = \eta \frac{\partial J(k)}{\partial w(k)}, \quad (17.6)$$

where η is the learning rate (Shibble et al. 2009).

17.2.2 Data Acquisition System

The spinach plant was selected for this project due to its high-water dependency, with 90.7% of its composition being water. This characteristic makes it an ideal subject for study, as its quality, health, and appearance are highly sensitive to variations in water conditions. Given the nature of hydroponics, very specific pH and electrical conductivity ranges are required to maintain an optimal environment. For spinach, the pH must remain between 5.5 and 6.5, while the dissolved salts should stay within 1.8–2.4 parts per million (ppm) to ensure a healthy plant with a nutritional value comparable to traditionally cultivated spinach grown in solid substrate environment. The input vector $X(k)$ is constructed by the acquisition data system, Fig. 17.2 shows the hardware used to fulfill this objective.

The pH-4502C module provides an analog voltage output ranging from 0 to 5 V, making it compatible with TTL-based technologies such as Arduino and Raspberry Pi. Ideally, a pH of 0 should correspond to 0 V, while a pH of 14 should generate 5 V. The term total dissolved solids (TDS) refers to the amount of dissolved solid particles per liter of water. Generally, a higher TDS value indicates a greater concentration of dissolved solids, which means the water is less pure. Therefore, TDS can be used as a reference parameter to assess the water cleanliness. TDS probes must not be used in water above 55 °C, and they should not be positioned too close to the container's edge, as this may affect readings. While the probe head and cable are waterproof and

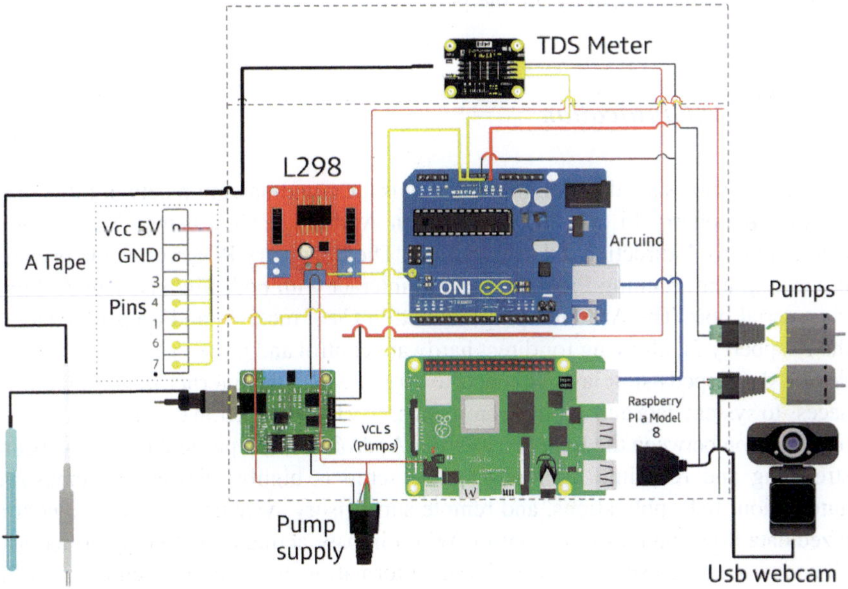

Fig. 17.2 Data acquisition system

can be fully submerged, the signal adapter board and connection interface are not waterproof and should be kept dry.

The electrical conductivity sensor consists of a TDS probe and a signal adaptation board to process measurements.

The monitoring system to monitor pH and electrical conductivity utilizes a Raspberry Pi microcomputer and an Arduino Uno microcontroller. Their roles are as follows:

- Microcontroller (Arduino Uno):
  - Controls the water pump.
  - Manages sensor data collection.
  - Sends data to the microcomputer via serial communication.
- Microcomputer (Raspberry Pi):
  - Functions as a server, transmitting measurement data via TCP/IP protocol to a cloud-based web platform.
  - Enables remote monitoring from any computer.

This combination leverages the wireless capabilities and computing power of a low-cost system-on-chip (SoC) computer such as Raspberry Pi, alongside the extensive module support and analog/digital input/output capabilities of Arduino Uno, resulting in a versatile and efficient hydroponic monitoring system. The USB-webcam provides the image on real time of the hydroponic system and allows the supervision of the system by remote personal.

17.2.3 Communication

Figure 17.3 shows the diagram that represents the communication network that integrates a Raspberry Pi, an Arduino, and an Android device, using Firebase as a central hub for bidirectional data exchange. The Raspberry Pi serves as the primary processing unit, running Python scripts to interact with both Firebase and Arduino via a serial port. The Arduino, programmed in C++, receives and transmits data to the Raspberry Pi, allowing for direct hardware control and monitoring. The Android device, developed using Java, connects to Firebase over the internet, enabling remote access to system data and control commands. A VPN connection ensures secure data transmission between the Raspberry Pi and Android device, particularly for webcam streaming and real-time monitoring. The setup is highly relevant for industrial automation, IoT applications, and remote supervisory systems, providing synchronized data flow and real-time control. With Firebase acting as a cloud intermediary, all components can seamlessly exchange information, making this architecture efficient and scalable. Given our expertise in control systems, this configuration could be refined or expanded for advanced automation solutions.

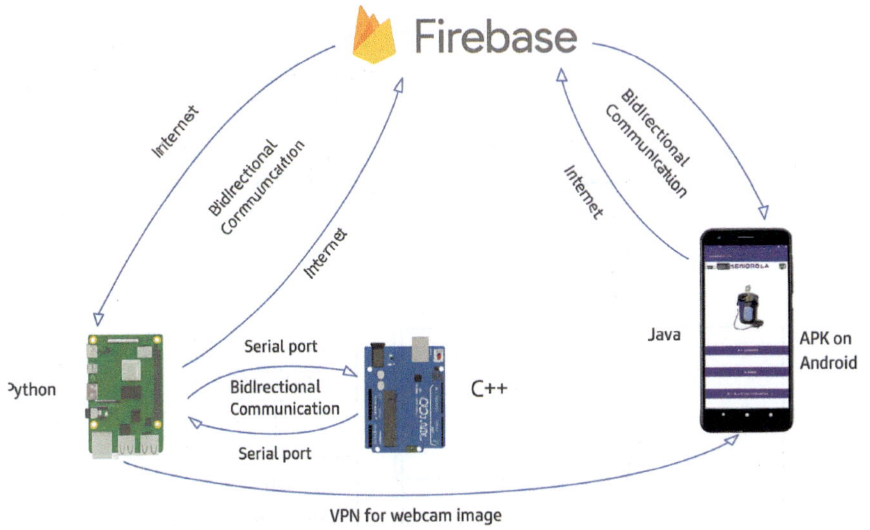

Fig. 17.3 Scheme of communication

17.2.4 Training Process

The diagram in Fig. 17.4 illustrates an automated training and update system utilizing Firebase and Android. The training process begins with the generation of reports based on data collected from both sources. This data undergoes iterative processing through a loop that operates over a set number of epochs, where forward processing transforms the data and backward processing adjusts parameters accordingly. As the loop runs, a decision mechanism determines whether the process should continue or conclude. Upon completion, the results are recorded in a report and sent to Firebase for further use.

Meanwhile, the update process ensures real-time monitoring using Firebase controls. Initially, the system retrieves parameters from Firebase and listens for active commands. If no commands are detected, the system proceeds to measure pH and electrical conductivity. Otherwise, it loops back to Firebase controls. Following measurement, the system performs a forward prediction, after which newly collected data is transmitted to Firebase, and the process repeats. Ultimately, this system integrates an adaptive training mechanism with real-time data collection, facilitating continuous improvement and efficient monitoring. Firebase acts as the central hub, storing results while managing dynamic updates to optimize predictive accuracy and decision-making.

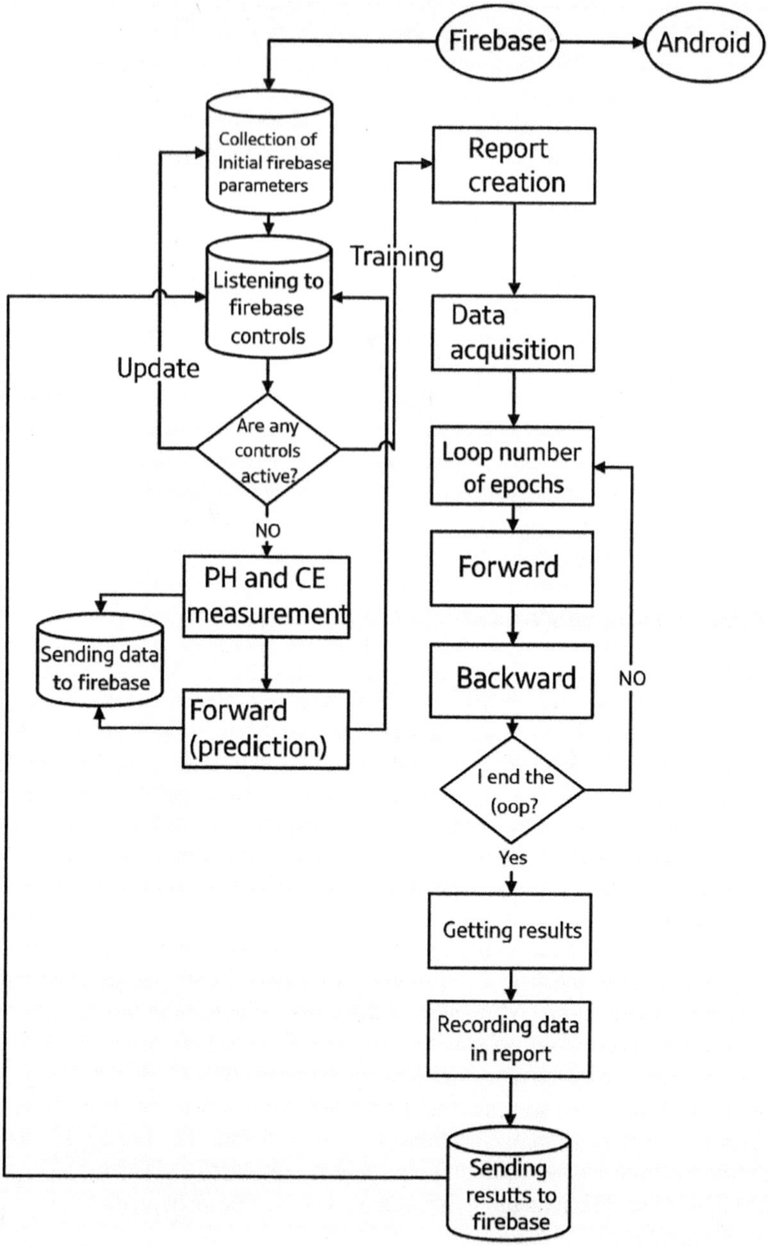

Fig. 17.4 Training flow chart

17.3 Results and Discussion

The estimation of pH and EC variables depends on many factors. The hyperparameters of a neural network are essential for achieving good results. A single-hidden-layer MLP was used, where the initial weights were selected within a range of $[-1, 1]$. A learning rate constant was set between $[0, 1]$. The number of epochs depends on the amount of available data for training.

The estimated value of pH and EC are presented in Fig. 17.5. The following presents the results obtained from an experiment, considering a single-event estimation of the future according to Eq. (17.1).

The obtained results serve to illustrate the effectiveness of the system. To improve them, it is necessary to work on generating sufficiently large databases, considering various climatic and process-related factors. This is essential for observing the dynamic behavior of the hydroponic cultivation system. Subsequently, it is necessary to adjust and configure the system's hyperparameters according to the stored data conditions. However, care must be taken to avoid overfitting the network and to account for local minima during the training phase. For future work, it is proposed to implement meta-heuristics to reduce dependence on the selection of initial conditions in the estimation system.

17.4 Conclusions

This work presents the estimation of key variables for hydroponic cultivation, such as pH and electrical conductivity, through a mobile application with IoT services. The estimation is carried out using artificial neural networks of the MLP type, which, through training stages, improve precision and accuracy by considering different environmental and operational conditions. This allows timely decision-making regarding the crops to maximize the benefits of hydroponic cultivation.

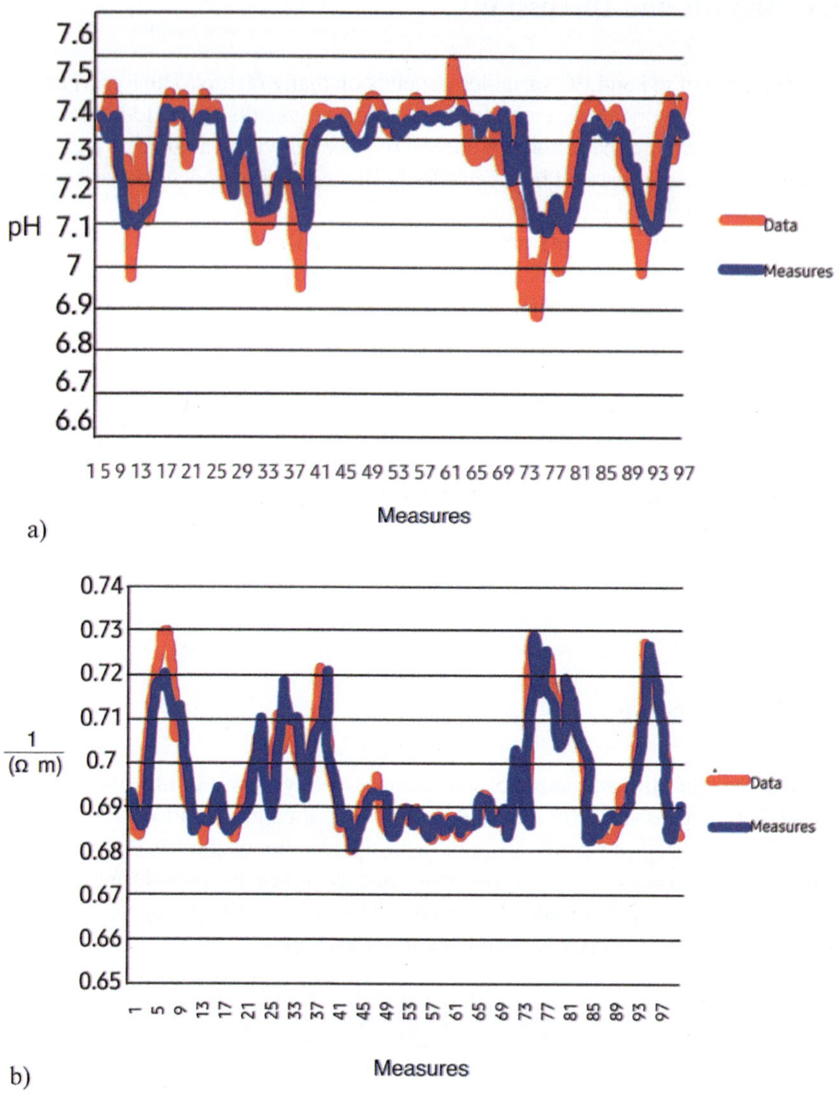

Fig. 17.5 pH (**a**) and CE (**b**) estimations by means of MLP

Acknowledgments The authors kindly acknowledge the support provided by the Instituto Politécnico Nacional through projects SIP/IPN 20252370 and 20251381.

References

Coleto Martinez JM (2006) Agricultura Convencional y Agriculturas Alternativas

Haykin S (2009) Neural networks and learning machines. Pearson, USA

Herman, Surantha N (2019) Intelligent monitoring and controlling system for hydroponics precision agriculture. In: Proceedings of the 7th international conference on information and communication technology (ICoICT). Indonesia

Hossain M, Kayas G, Hasan R, Skjellum A, Noor S, Islam SMR (2024) Fut Int 16: 40. https://doi.org/10.3390/FI16020040

Kessler GC (2012) Computer security handbook, pp 6.1–6.31. https://doi.org/10.1002/9781118851678.ch6

Lian S, Matsushita F (2025) Rapid development of a construction data dashboard using low-code programming. Lect Notes Civ Eng 591:1339–1346. https://doi.org/10.1007/978-981-96-4051-5_128

Ljung L (1999) System identification: theory for the user. Prentice Hall PTR, Upper Saddle River, NJ

Peng S-L, Pal S, Huang L (eds) (2020) Principles of internet of things (IoT) ecosystem: insight paradigm, vol 174. https://doi.org/10.1007/978-3-030-33596-0

Perwiratama R, Setidai YK Smart hydroponic farming with IoT-based climate and nutrient manipulation system (2019)

Shibble Md, Kalra PK, Chandra B (2009) Time series prediction with multilayer perceptron (MLP): a new generalized error based approach. In: Advances in neuro-information processing, part II. Springer, pp 37–44

Wongpatikaseree K, Hnoohom N, Yuenyong S (2018) Machine learning methods for assessing freshness in hydroponic produce. Thailand

Chapter 18
Computational Non-Premixed Combustion and Conjugate Heat Transfer Analysis for a Poultry Scalder

Brandon Oropeza-Oropeza, Jesús Mares-Carreño, Griselda Stephany Abarca-Jiménez, Juan Cruz-Castro, Yunuén López-Grijalba, and Manuel Vladimir Vega-Blanco

Abstract Technology has contributed to the modernization of poultry processing plants with specialized machinery to meet this ever-increasing market demand and generate efficient, healthy, safe, and profitable production. In such facilities, scalding is an essential stage in chicken processing, as it is a factor that significantly influences the quality of the product. Technology has contributed significantly to the efficient execution of this process and offered added value in reducing resource consumption, such as electricity, water, and fuel. Despite the existence of this innovative technology, it is not achievable for all establishments, especially small-scale producers, since it is expensive considering the production-investment in machinery-sales ratio. This work focuses on studying the thermal behavior of a scalder by analyzing the combustion and heat transfer processes that occur during the scalding process. A non-premixed combustion analysis and a conjugate heat transfer analysis were performed using computational fluid dynamics. Experimental measures were taken in an existing scalder machine to validate the numerical results. The results are used to generate

B. Oropeza-Oropeza · J. Mares-Carreño · G. S. Abarca-Jiménez (✉) · J. Cruz-Castro · Y. López-Grijalba · M. V. Vega-Blanco
Instituto Politécnico Nacional, Unidad Profesional Interdisciplinaria de Ingeniería Campus Hidalgo, San Agustín Tlaxiaca, Hidalgo, México
e-mail: gabarcaj@ipn.mx

B. Oropeza-Oropeza
e-mail: boropezao1500@alumno.ipn.mx

J. Mares-Carreño
e-mail: jmaresc@ipn.mx

J. Cruz-Castro
e-mail: jucruzc@ipn.mx

Y. López-Grijalba
e-mail: ylopezg@ipn.mx

M. V. Vega-Blanco
e-mail: mvvegab@ipn.mx

A. Öchsner (ed.), *Progress in Biomaterials and Biomedical Engineering*, Advanced Structured Materials 249, https://doi.org/10.1007/978-3-032-13551-3_18

an improved design for this type of scalder used in small-scale producers with a sustainable approach.

Keywords Computational fluid dynamics · Heat transfer processes · Scalding process · Sustainability

18.1 Introduction

Sustainability is defined as the efficient and equitable distribution of resources over time. Sustainable development, on the other hand, is a form of development that meets the needs of the present generation without compromising the ability of future generations to meet their own needs. Although there are two similar concepts, sustainability is the goal or objective of a process called sustainable development (Mensah, 2019).

Poultry meat is a nutritious and affordable source of protein for most people worldwide. Its consumption has grown steadily for many years due to the increase in population and the economic capacity to acquire it, resulting in a shift in consumption patterns from grains to meat products (Tondeur and Simons, 2020).

The poultry industry has consolidated over time by developing processes, from food processing to the distribution of chicken meat, making it more accessible to consumers. Processing plants play a crucial role in transforming meat for human consumption, where the scalding process within these establishments is a vital factor in maintaining product quality.

Technological advancements have enhanced the performance of scalding systems by improving process reliability and contributing to resource optimization, particularly in the use of electricity, water, and fuel. For example, Meyn's ® commercial equipment operates using an airless water flow system, which helps to maximize heat transfer between the hot water and the birds' feather follicles, eliminating thermal energy loss due to agitation and air injection (Meyn-Specialist in Poultry Processing Solutions, 2025). Marel®, on the other hand, offers a design that involves injecting hot, humid air, promising a water reduction of up to 75% and energy savings of 50% (Marel|Food processing solutions, 2025). However, despite these improvements, such advanced systems remain inaccessible to many small-scale producers due to high capital costs and a relatively low return on investment.

In many of these facilities, equipment continues to be used without knowing its actual efficiency, resulting in high operating costs and excessive resource consumption, such as water and fuel. Therefore, analyzing its performance is essential to identify opportunities for technical improvement, increase profitability, and promote more sustainable design.

Therefore, this work focuses on the thermal analysis of a scalder using computational fluid dynamics (CFD) tools to evaluate temperature distribution, explore design alternatives that minimize energy consumption, and improve process uniformity. This approach enables the analysis of thermal behavior without the need to build a physical prototype, thereby streamlining the development of viable designs and resource-efficient technologies for the poultry processing plant sector.

18.2 Statement of the Problem

In small-scale poultry processing facilities, the thermal performance of scalders has often not been formally evaluated. As a result, their efficiency remains uncertain, and opportunities for optimization are limited.

This study aims to investigate the thermal behavior of this type of equipment through numerical simulation, focusing on analyzing temperature distribution and water heating efficiency. To ensure the reliability of the simulation results, a validation process is carried out by comparing the numerical data with actual physical measurements obtained from the existing system. This comparison allows the adjustment and calibration of the computational model.

Once validated, the simulation results are expected to provide a deeper understanding of the thermal behavior of current scalder designs. This insight will serve as a foundation for proposing technical improvements to enhance efficiency and optimize thermal performance in small-scale operations.

18.3 Materials and Methods

This study focuses on thermal analysis during the water heating process in a scalder used in a small-scale poultry processing plant. The methodology outlined below was employed:

1. A physical inspection of the existing scalder model was conducted to obtain its dimensional and structural characteristics.
2. The geometric configuration of the system was modeled using simplification criteria to reduce computational cost.
3. Numerical simulations were performed using computational analysis tools to evaluate the heat transfer behavior within the system.
4. The simulation results were validated by comparing the computational output with experimental measurements obtained through instrumentation.

The physical inspection was conducted at a small-scale production facility to determine the actual operating conditions of the scalder. Figure 1 presents an image of the equipment observed, along with the main components of interest for the analysis.

Figure 2 includes their overall dimensions, and Fig. 3 shows the general components modeled. Special attention was paid to the water heating process, with the time required to reach an operating temperature of 80 °C being recorded on average.

Heating is achieved through a non-premixed combustion system consisting of a linear burner located at the base of the structure (see Fig. 3, element (4). This system

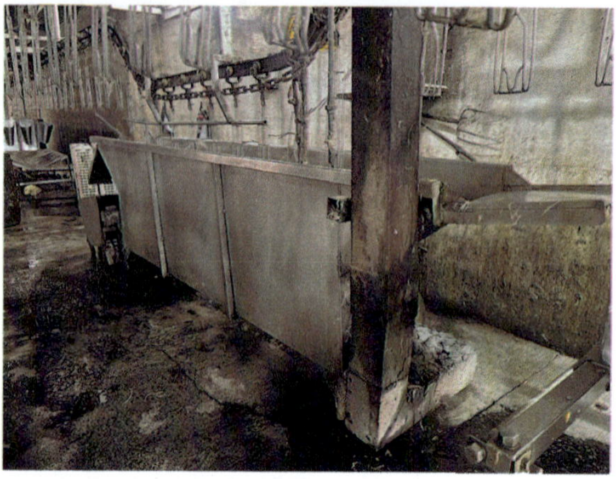

Fig. 1 Physical poultry scalder

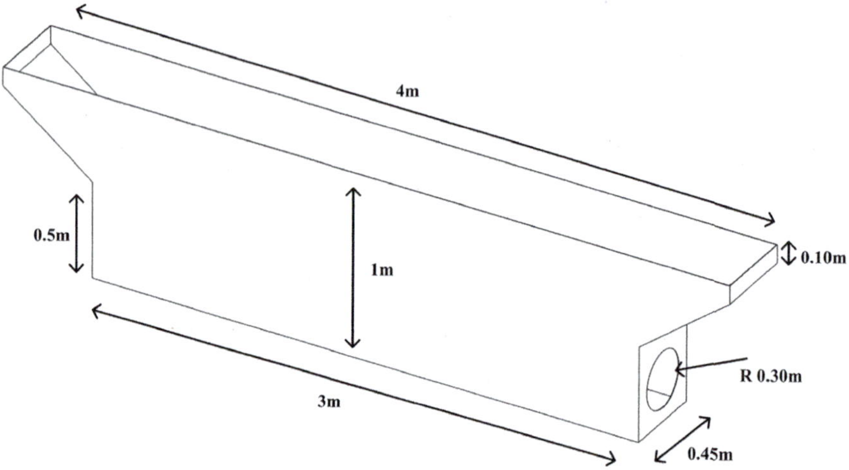

Fig. 2 Physical poultry scalder dimensions

injects a mixture of LP gas and air into a circular tube, where combustion generates heat that is transferred to the water through the tube walls.

The information gathered during the inspection was general, as several parameters could not be precisely determined. For example, the scalder's construction materials were identified, although its specifications could not be confirmed. Based on the visual characteristics, it was determined that the water tank was made of stainless steel, while the combustion tube was made of carbon steel. Furthermore, the operating parameters of the combustion system such as the injection speed and pressure of air and LP gas were approximated due to the system's lack of technical documentation and complex configuration. For this reason, initial representative values for

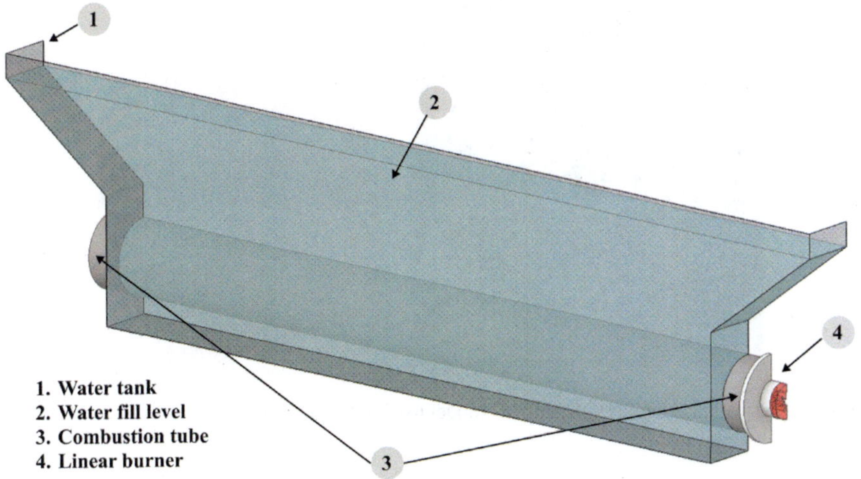

Fig. 3 Schematic representation of the poultry scalder

these parameters were assumed and subsequently adjusted during the analysis and simulation process.

The scalder geometry was modeled in three dimensions (Fig. 4) using the ANSYS® SpaceClaim software and to reduce the computational cost of the analysis, geometric simplification criteria were applied, considering only the essential domains of the system: the volume of water contained in the tank, the combustion tube, and the region occupied by the gases resulting from combustion. Moreover, because the equipment exhibits symmetry in its geometry and operating conditions, only half of the system was modeled.

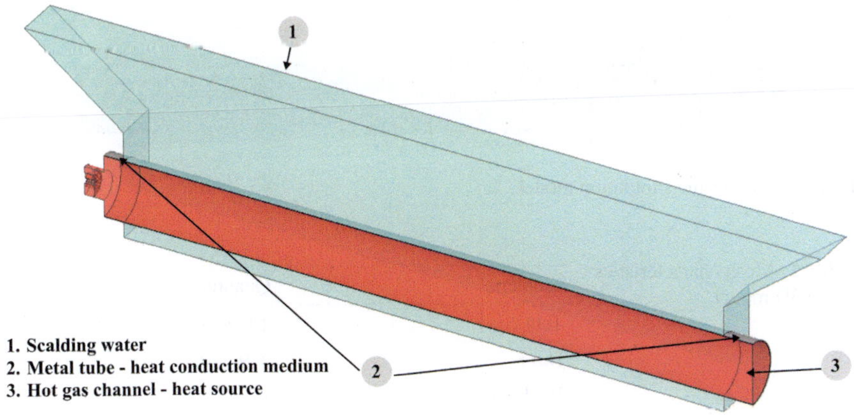

Fig. 4 Simplified geometry used for conjugated simulation

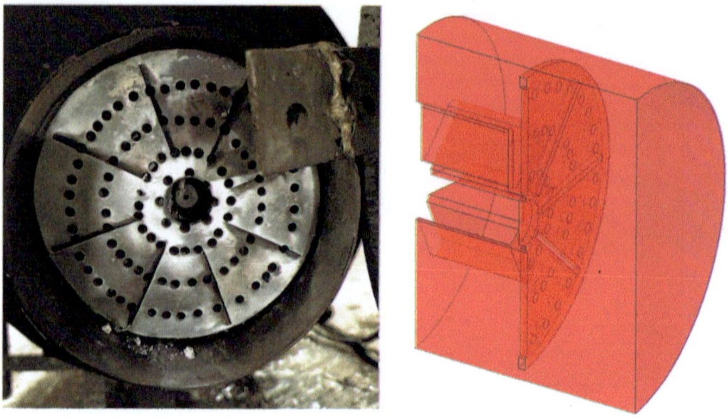

Fig. 5 Physical head burner (left) and 3D model used in the scalder (right)

Regarding the combustion system, only the burner head was included, as it represents the region where the initial mixing of air and LP gas occurs (Fig. 5). This part features a diffuser with complex geometry that, for simulation purposes, was also simplified while maintaining the functional characteristics necessary to adequately represent the physical phenomenon.

The model was discretized using a mesh composed primarily of low-order tetrahedral elements, comprising a total of 773,122 elements (Fig. 6). The element types used in the mesh are detailed in Table 1.

To evaluate the discretization quality, the orthogonal quality and skewness parameters were analyzed, yielding minimum and maximum values of 0.24 and 0.96, respectively, for orthogonal quality, and 0.004 and 0.76, respectively, for skewness.

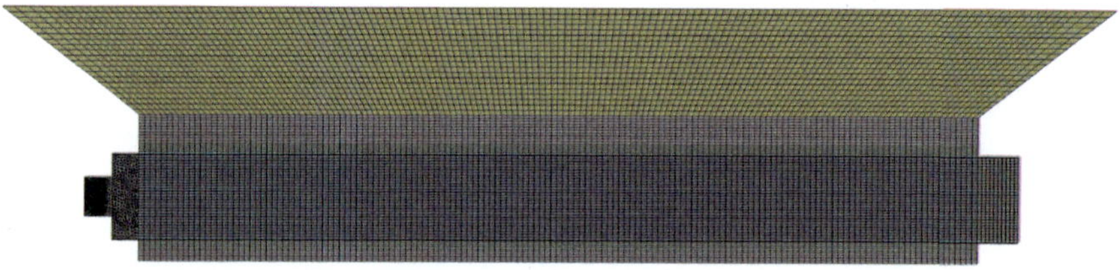

Fig. 6 Mesh for the simulation model

Table 1 Mesh characteristics of the 3D model

Element	Quantity
Tet4	491 848
Hex8	279 390
Wedge6	1 500
Pyramid5	384
Total	**773 122**

The distribution of these parameters is presented in Fig. 6. These results indicate that the mesh quality falls within the ranges recommended in the literature (6.2. Mesh Requirements and Considerations, 2025), making it suitable for numerical simulation purposes.

The numerical simulation was carried out in two stages. The first consisted of a steady-state analysis of the combustion process, intending to obtain the temperature profile generated by the flame, without exploring the details of the chemical reactions. For this purpose, the species transport combustion model was used, which allows modeling the mixing and transport of chemical species, as well as the release of energy by combustion, without requiring detailed reaction mechanisms. Figure 7 shows the geometric model used for this simulation, the boundary conditions including an inlet velocity of 32 m/s for the air, and two different velocities for the LP gas: 1 m/s corresponding to the fuel exit through the injector (nozzle), and 5 m/s for the peripheral nozzles. These values were estimated based on the characteristics of the existing system and adjusted to obtain a representative temperature profile useful for the subsequent stage of the thermal analysis. For air, the ideal outlet velocity was calculated based on the characteristics of the burner blower, including rotation speed, impeller type, and outlet diameter. For the gas outlet, a numerical simulation was performed considering the branching of the burner pipes and the operating pressure of the gas valve.

The second stage consisted of a transient flow analysis of the water heating process using conjugate heat transfer (CHT) analysis. The model used is shown in Fig. 8. The previous combustion stage was solved in a steady state to obtain a representative thermal profile in the flue gas domain. This made it possible to avoid detailed transient modeling of the chemical reactions, which would have required very small-time steps to properly capture flame behavior.

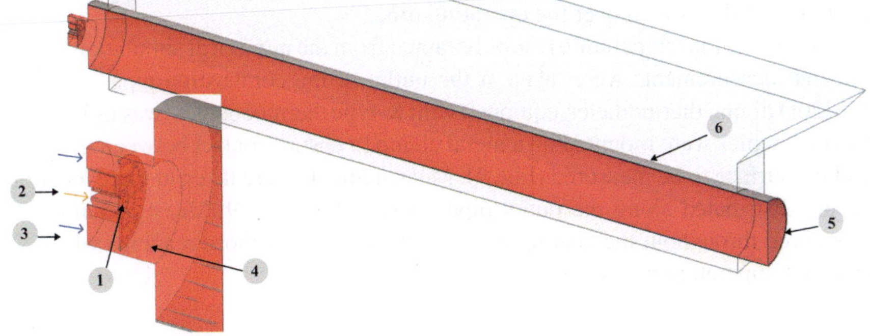

Fig. 7 Schematic diagram of the combustion simulation domain

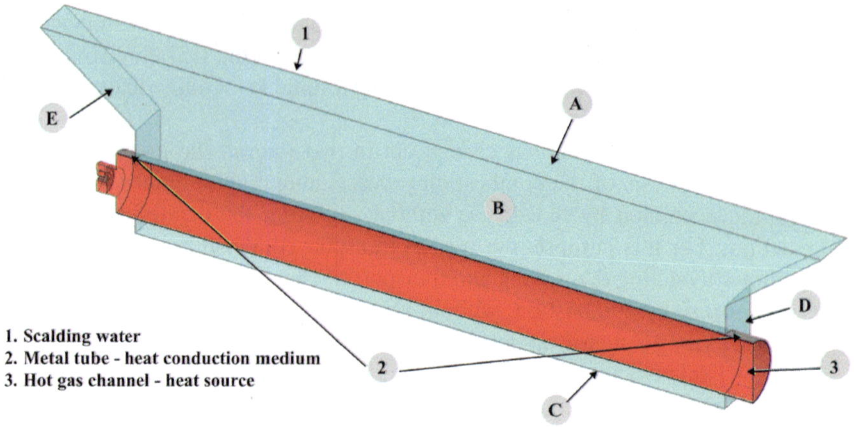

Fig. 8 Schematic diagram of the CHT simulation domain

Table 2 Convection heat transfer coefficients on walls

Wall	Heat transfer coefficient (W/m^{2}K)
A	5.85
B	5.08
C	2.74
D	7.39
E	5.81

This temperature profile obtained was kept fixed and used as an initial condition in the gas region, allowing the transient simulation of water heating to be carried out with a time step of one second. To represent thermal losses to the environment, boundary conditions with natural convection heat transfer coefficients on the walls were applied. The values assigned to each surface are detailed in Table 2.

Numerical analysis began with a uniform temperature of 25 °C in the water domain and was conducted for a total of 80 min, allowing for the observation of the thermal evolution of the system over the operating time.

To validate the temperature results obtained from the numerical simulation, experimental measurements were taken at the outlet of the combustion pipe. A UNI-T UT320D digital thermometer, equipped with K-type thermocouples, was used. These thermocouples were mounted on a metal clamp to ensure contact between the probe and the surface to be measured (Fig. 9). Measurements were taken at three locations evenly distributed along the outlet pipe, as shown in Fig. 9. Measurements were monitored throughout the heating process, capturing only those readings where the surface temperature was stable.

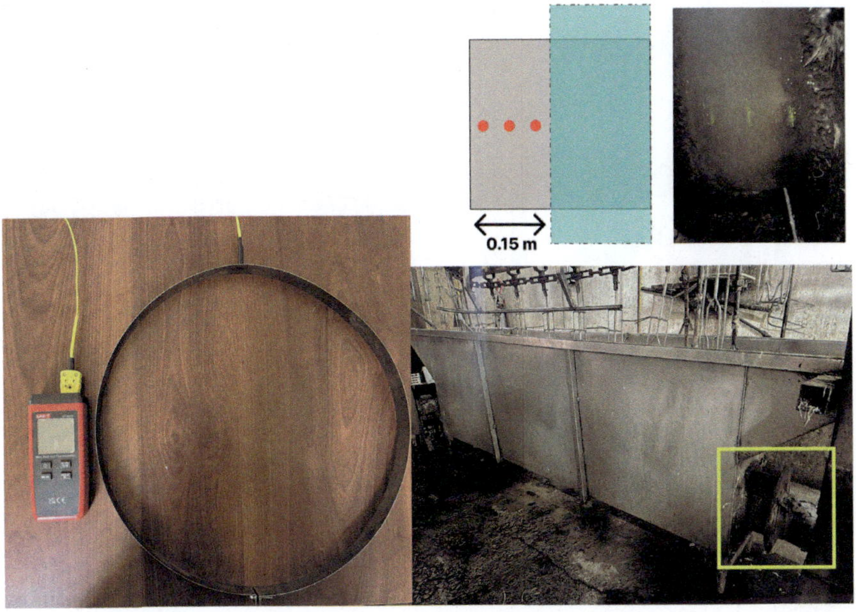

Fig. 9 Photograph of the measurement device with K-type thermocouple (left) and location of the temperature measurements on the scalder wall (right) used for validation

18.4 Results

The results obtained from the numerical simulation, focusing on the temperature distribution in the scalder's water volume, are presented in Fig. 10. This figure shows three views corresponding to cross-sections taken at different positions along the scalder's length: specifically at 0.5, 1.5 and 2.5 m from the inlet end. These sections allow us to visualize how the water temperature varies along the longitudinal axis of the equipment.

To evaluate the temperature distribution (Fig. 10), the average temperature value and standard deviation were analyzed, obtaining 81.83 °C and 0.58 °C, respectively, for section (a), 81.88 °C and 0.7 °C, for section (b), 81.11 °C and 0.69 °C, respectively, for section (c). As can be seen, the temperature variation within each cross-section is generally less than 0.7 °C, indicating a homogeneous distribution. In addition, the average temperature variation between the different sections does not exceed 1 °C, indicating that the heating system provides relatively uniform heat transfer throughout the scalder.

The results presented in Figs. 11, 12, and 13 correspond to experimental measurements performed to compare and validate the results obtained from the numerical simulation. Three images are included for each measurement point: on the left, a photograph showing the location of the thermocouple in the actual equipment; in

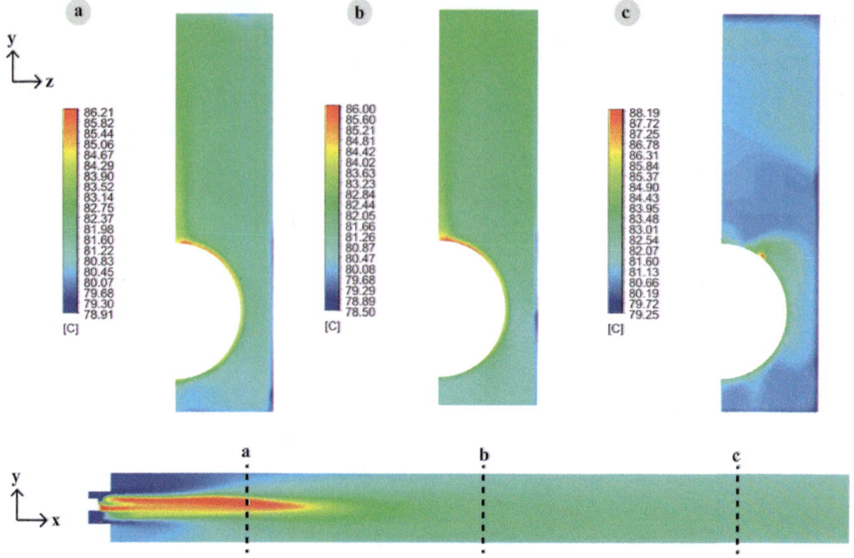

Fig. 10 Temperature contours in cross sections a-c located at 0.5 m, 1.5 m, and 2.5 m, respectively, along the scalder

the center, the reading recorded by the digital thermometer; and on the right, the temperature obtained in the numerical simulation at the same location.

The relative differences between the experimentally measured and simulated temperatures were 8.84% at point 1, 2.43% at point 2, and 15.27% at point 3. Overall, the observed differences are considered acceptable for initial validation of the thermal model. However, a higher difference was obtained at point 3, which was expected, since in that area, close to the combustion tube outlet, there is a reduction in the

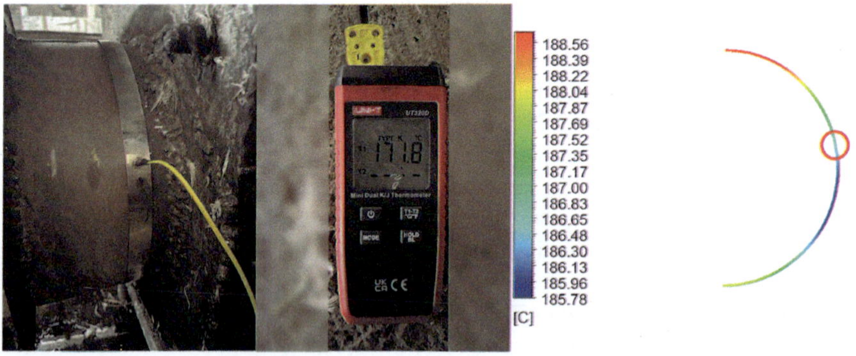

Fig. 11 Validation at position 1. Left: thermocouple placement; center: recorded temperature; right: simulation result

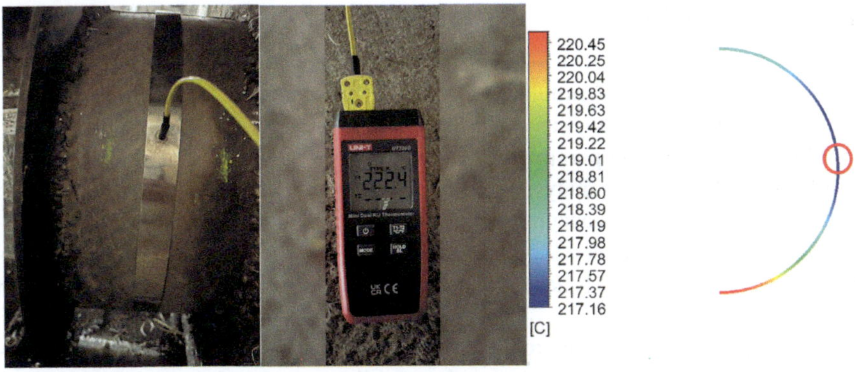

Fig. 12 Validation at position 2. Left: thermocouple placement; center: recorded temperature; right: simulation result

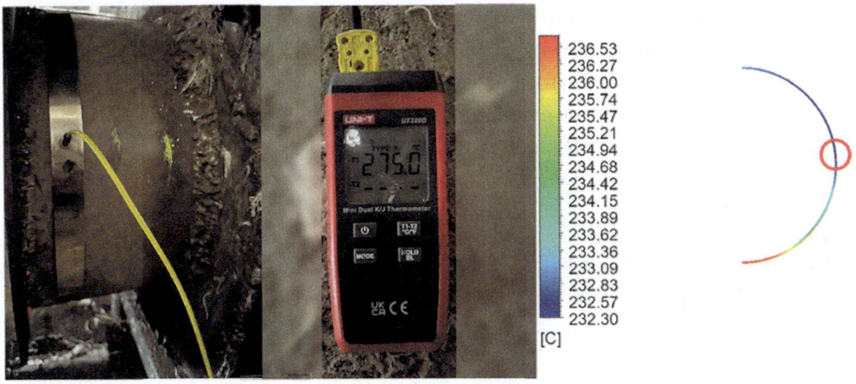

Fig. 13 Validation at position 3. Left: thermocouple placement; center: recorded temperature; right: simulation result

system's cross-section, which generates a restriction on the gas outlet and, consequently, a higher concentration of thermal energy. This geometric characteristic was not included in the simplified model used for the simulation, which explains the discrepancy observed at that point.

In summary, the comparison between simulated and experimental data indicates that the computational model provides an adequate representation of the real system's thermal behavior. The correspondence between simulated temperature profiles and measured surface temperatures supports the model's reliability and its potential use in further optimization efforts.

18.5 Conclusion

In this study, a numerical simulation of the thermal behavior of a scalder used in a chicken processing facility was carried out to analyze the water heating process.

Measurements in an operating environment have made it possible to validate the results of CFD numerical analysis. This allowed the model to be adjusted and ensured that the numerical results accurately represented the equipment's behavior.

The comparison between the simulated results and the experimental data shows that the developed model is acceptable, reliable, and can be used to propose design improvements.

One relevant finding is that reducing the equipment's dimensions could be beneficial. This would involve working with a smaller volume of water, which in turn would reduce heating time and energy consumption.

Regarding the variation of the experimental and numerical results, it is important to notice that the actual material conditions can contribute to these discrepancies. The equipment evaluated has been working for seven years, only basic maintenance has been applied, and these promote phenomena like pipe wall thinning, among others, that contributed to a poor performance in the scalder.

In future work, we propose evaluating new heating alternatives, such as immersion electric heaters, to more efficiently utilize the energy supplied to the system and improve the scalder's thermal performance.

Acknowledgements The grant for the development of the Projects SIP2025B068, SIP20253567, SIP20254472, SIP20254020, and SIP 20254415 was awarded by the National Polytechnic Institute (IPN). It is kindly acknowledged.

References

Mensah J (2019) Sustainable development: Meaning, history, principles, pillars, and implications for human action: Literature review. Cogent Social Sciences. https://doi.org/10.1080/23311886.2019.1653531

Tondeur W, Simons P (2020) Señales de la Carne de Pollo: una guía práctica para mejorar la calidad de la carne de ave. Roodbont Publishers B. V, Países Bajos

Meyn-Specialist in Poultry Processing Solutions (2025). https://www.meyn.com/. Accessed 17 May 2025.

Marel|Food processing solutions (2025). https://marel.com/en/. Accessed 4 Apr 2025.

6.2. Mesh Requirements and Considerations (2025). https://ansyshelp.ansys.com/public/account/secured?returnurl=/Views/Secured/corp/v242/en/flu_ug/flu_ug_GridQuality.html. Accessed 24 May 2025.

Chapter 19
Biomechanical Study for the Development of Personalized Hand Prostheses

Gabriel Josué Reyes-Morales, Juan Alfonso Beltrán-Fernández, Alejandro Tonatiu Velázquez-Sánchez, Verónica Guzmán-Mercado, and Karen Pamela Vázquez-Thierry

Abstract Upper-limb amputations constitute a clinical condition with a profound impact on patients' quality of life, limiting functional autonomy and social integration. Over the past decades, various types of hand prostheses have been developed to compensate for anatomical loss and to partially restore motor function. However, highly personalized prosthetic models often require considerable financial investment, which in most cases is not affordable for the affected population. In this context, the present study proposes the development of a personalized mechanical hand prosthesis fabricated through three-dimensional printing, aiming to achieve reduced cost while maintaining anatomical precision and functional reliability. The design of the prosthesis is based on the segmentation of computed tomography images, which ensures an individualized adaptation to the patient's morphology. Subsequently, the digital models are optimized using a computer-aided design software, enabling the evaluation of structural and functional parameters as well as durability testing prior to manufacturing. This approach integrates medical image segmentation, digital modeling, and additive manufacturing to provide an accessible and scalable strategy

G. J. Reyes-Morales · J. A. Beltrán-Fernández (✉) · A. T. Velázquez-Sánchez · V. Guzmán-Mercado · K. P. Vazquez-Thierry
Instituto Politécnico Nacional, Sección de Estudios de Posgrado e Investigación, Escuela Superior de Ingeniería Mecánica y Eléctrica, Unidad Zacatenco, "Unidad Profesional Adolfo López Mateos", Edificio 5, Segundo Piso, Colonia Lindavista, Alcaldía, Gustavo A. Madero, Mexico City, Mexico
e-mail: jbeltran@ipn.com

G. J. Reyes-Morales
e-mail: greyesm1100@alumno.ipn.mx

A. T. Velázquez-Sánchez
e-mail: atvelazquezs@ipn.mx

V. Guzmán-Mercado
e-mail: vguzmanm0900@alumno.ipn.mx

K. P. Vázquez-Thierry
e-mail: kvazquezt2200@alumno.ipn.mx

A. Öchsner (ed.), *Progress in Biomaterials and Biomedical Engineering*, Advanced Structured Materials 249, https://doi.org/10.1007/978-3-032-13551-3_19

for hand prosthesis development. It is anticipated that this workflow will contribute both to the clinical management of amputee patients and to the advancement of applied research in biomechanics and rehabilitation.

Keywords Prosthesis · Hand · Customized · Biomechanics · Amputation

19.1 Introduction

The upper-limb constitutes one of the most functionally complex anatomical regions, owing to the wide range of hand movements and the large amplitude of joint motion. When an amputation of this extremity occurs, patients are compelled to adapt to a new lifestyle and are often at risk of developing psychological sequelae associated with the loss and the traumatic experience (González 2009; Lamandé et al. 2014).

The leading causes of upper-limb amputations are associated with occupational accidents and pyrotechnic-related injuries (Bustamante Carvallo 2018). It is estimated that between 5 and 10% of all amputations correspond to upper extremities. In Mexico, during 2023, the Instituto Mexicano del Seguro Social (IMSS) reported approximately 201,000 work absences due to hand-related accidents, equivalent to an average of 550 daily cases (González 2009; Instituto Mexicano del Seguro Social 2022—2023).

Currently, prostheses for partial or complete hand and finger amputations are generally classified as either cosmetic or functional. Cosmetic devices primarily serve an aesthetic purpose, whereas functional prostheses may be actuated either by residual body movements or through external power sources (Rodríguez et al. 2022). However, patient–prosthesis adaptation often remains challenging, as affordable models are typically standardized and fail to achieve precise fitting between the residual limb and the artificial implant.

The development of a prosthesis that combines functionality, ergonomics, and affordability represents a considerable challenge. To address this, various prosthetic design techniques were examined to identify a method capable of accurately reproducing amputation geometry and establishing a reliable anchoring system for direct contact with the residual limb. In parallel, prototypes are being produced through 3D printing using different materials to determine the option that ensures optimal mechanical performance, efficient manufacturability, and reduced cost.

19.2 Development

A mixed methodological approach was adopted for this study, combining Quality Function Deployment (QFD) and Cross Industry Standard Process for Data Mining (CRISP-DM). The application of QFD, specifically through the construction of the "house of quality," allowed patient requirements to be systematically identified and subsequently translated into technical design parameters for the prosthesis. In this way, user expectations were linked directly to objective engineering criteria.

In parallel, the CRISP-DM framework provided a structured process encompassing the stages of design, modeling, and prototype evaluation. This methodology ensured consistent integration between clinical needs, digital modeling procedures, and additive manufacturing processes, thereby maintaining traceability from the patient's initial requirements to the technical validation of the device.

Figure 19.1 presents the diagram of the overall research methodology applied in this work. At this stage, the focus was placed on the phases of "Understanding patient requirements," "Defining design parameters," and "Design and modeling."

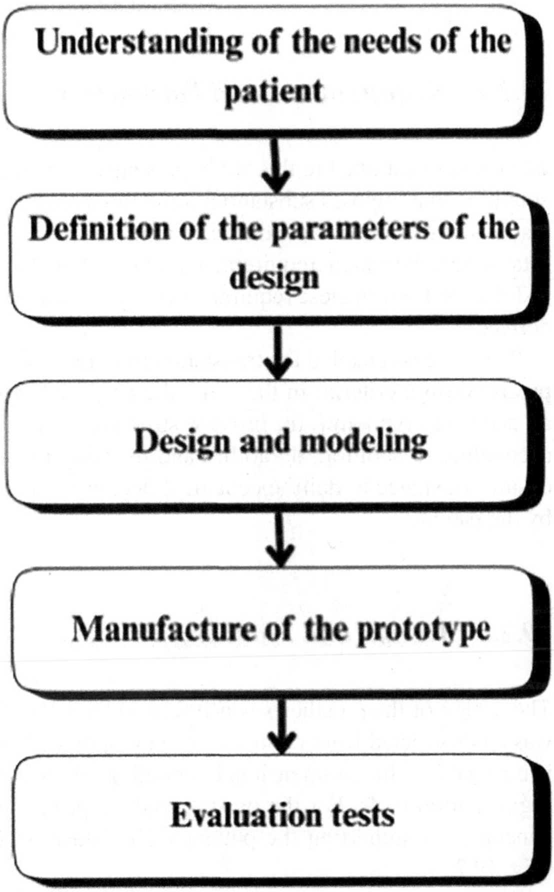

Fig. 19.1 Methodology

Table 19.1 Patient requirements for the design of a personalized hand prosthesis

Patient requirement	Description	Category
Restoration of gripping function	Ability to hold and manipulate objects	Functional
Comfort of prosthetic socket	Prevention of pressure points or pain at the residual limb during prolonged use	Ergonomic
Device lightness	Reduction of overall prosthesis weight	Ergonomic
Customized residual-limb fitting	Stable and anatomically adapted attachment system	Ergonomic
Low cost	Economic accessibility, particularly in the absence of medical coverage	Ergonomic
Material durability	Resistance to daily use without fractures or permanent deformation	Functional

19.2.1 Requirements and Parameters

The patient examined in this study presents a partial amputation of the right hand, a condition that imposes substantial limitations on the execution of daily activities and restricts functional independence. Within the methodological framework previously established, the patient requirements were systematically identified and are presented in Table 19.1. From these requirements, the corresponding design specifications were derived.

This process enabled the translation of clinical and functional considerations into precise design criteria. In this way, the proposed prosthesis is expected to achieve an accurate ergonomic fit, provide structural reliability, and remain economically accessible. In addition, durability and usability requirements were incorporated to ensure resistance to daily mechanical demands and to facilitate practical operation by the patient.

19.2.2 Design and Modeling

The design of the prosthesis was based on the patient's specific morphology, which was reconstructed from computed tomography (CT) data using ScanIP®. This software enables three-dimensional modeling of medical images through advanced segmentation tools. For the present study, a projection of the amputated hand was generated by importing the patient's CT dataset in DICOM format into ScanIP® (Fig. 19.2).

The segmentation process began with the creation of a binary mask that delimited the region of interest (ROI). Successive tomographic slices were then analyzed,

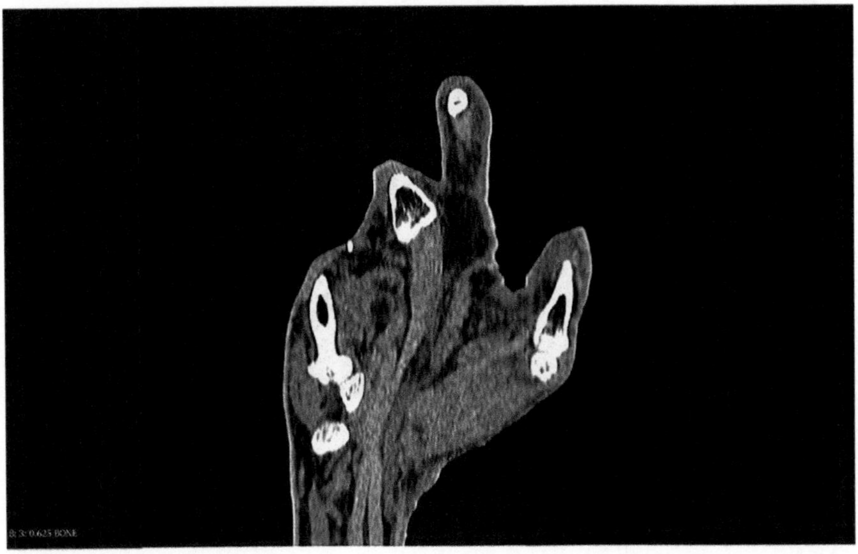

Fig. 19.2 Computed tomography scan of the patient's partial hand amputation

and the individual bones of the residual limb were manually selected and reconstructed to generate a volumetric representation (Fig. 19.3). The segmentation workflow employed semi-automatic methods, complemented by manual correction, to ensure fidelity of the anatomical boundaries (Fig. 19.4).

Once the segmentation was completed, the three-dimensional reconstruction of the extremity was visualized within the ScanIP® interface to confirm the accuracy of the generated geometry (Fig. 19.5). After validation, the model was exported in STL format, enabling its integration into CAD environments and subsequent mechanical and functional evaluations (Fig. 19.6).

19.2.3 Mesh Refinement with Meshmixer®

Following segmentation and STL export, the model was refined using Meshmixer®, a computational tool designed for editing and optimizing three-dimensional meshes. This stage included procedures such as geometry repair, surface refinement, and mesh editing to enhance the accuracy and manufacturability of the prosthetic model.

In this specific case, the software was employed to remove external elements unrelated to the hand anatomy (Fig. 19.7) and to smooth irregular surface areas so that the model would not present a coarse or fragmented appearance (Fig. 19.8). These refinements contributed to achieving a prosthetic model with adequate surface quality for subsequent mechanical analysis and 3D printing.

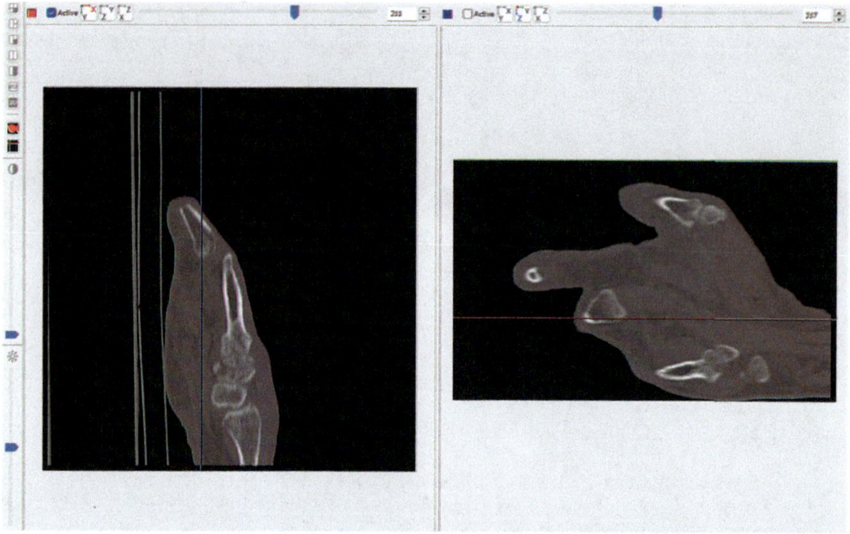

Fig. 19.3 Import of the computed tomography dataset into the ScanIP® software environment for subsequent segmentation

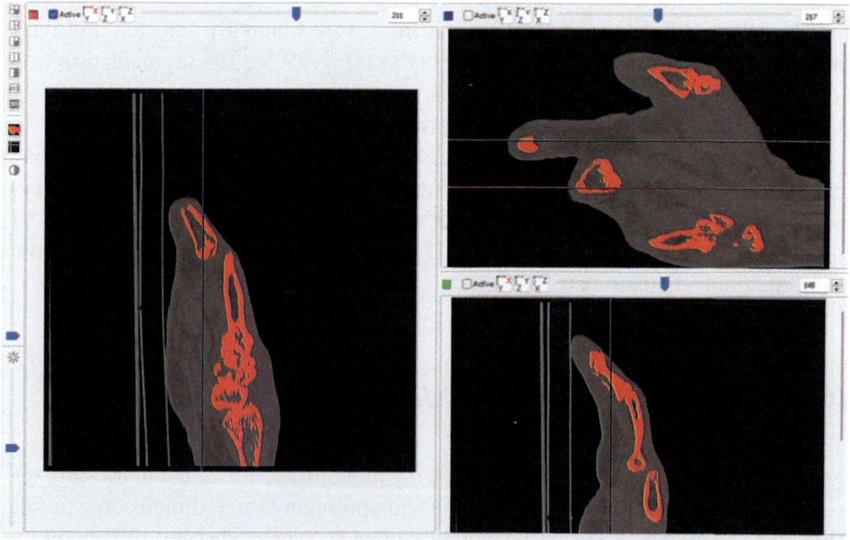

Fig. 19.4 Segmentation of the computed tomography dataset in ScanIP®, showing the selection of individual bone structures for volumetric reconstruction

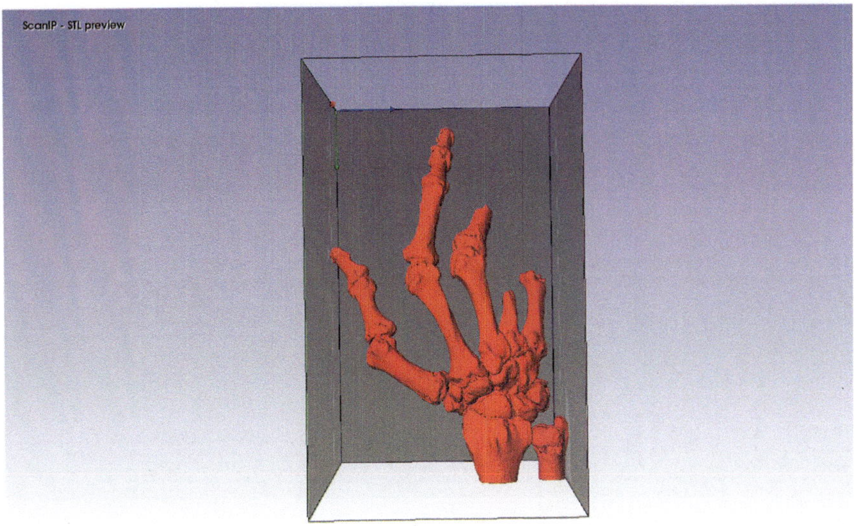

Fig. 19.5 Three-dimensional reconstruction of the patient's residual limb obtained from segmented tomographic data

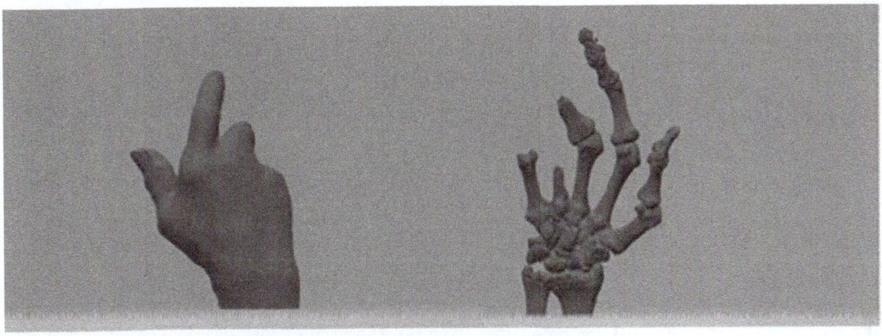

Fig. 19.6 Exported model in STL format, suitable for integration into CAD environments and subsequent analysis

Following the removal of non-anatomical external components (Fig. 19.7), the model was subjected to a refinement stage aimed at improving surface quality. This process was necessary to eliminate irregularities introduced during segmentation and to prepare the geometry for subsequent CAD processing and additive manufacturing. Through surface smoothing and localized corrections performed in Meshmixer®, a continuous and uniform model was obtained, as illustrated in Fig. 19.8.

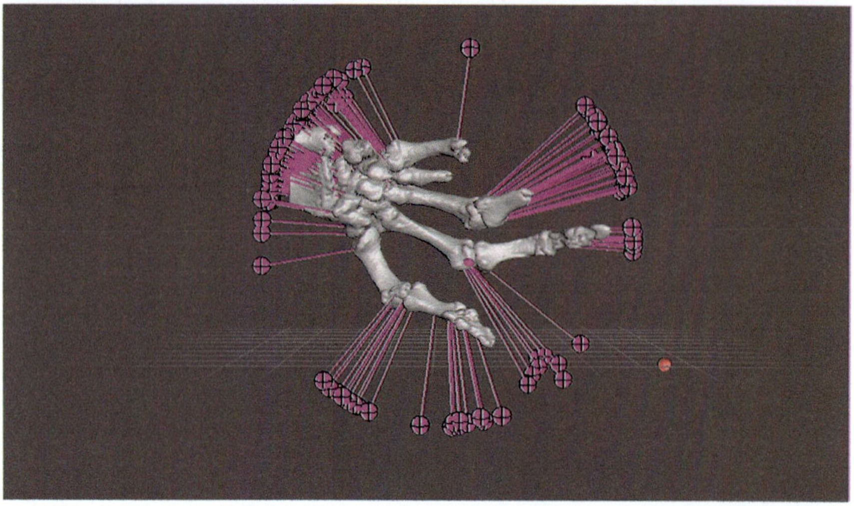

Fig. 19.7 Removal of external, non-anatomical components from the STL model using Meshmixer®

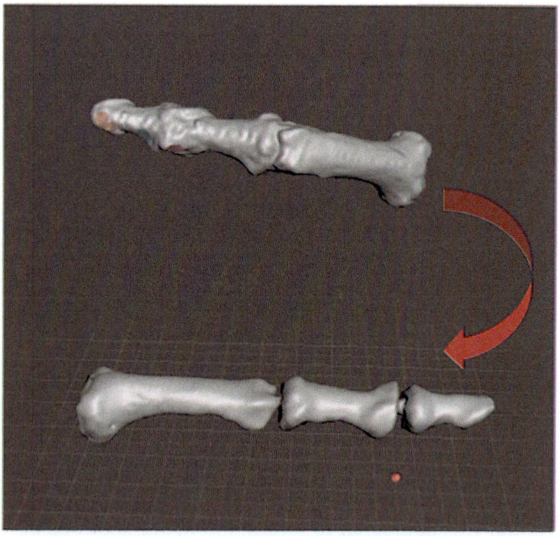

Fig. 19.8 Refinement of the STL model in Meshmixer®, improving surface continuity and overall geometric quality

19.2.4 CAD Design with Onshape®

The final model obtained after refinement was processed in Onshape®, a cloud-based platform for computer-aided design (CAD). This tool enabled the creation and editing of three-dimensional geometries with sufficient precision for prosthetic applications. Within this environment, the prosthetic concept was further developed,

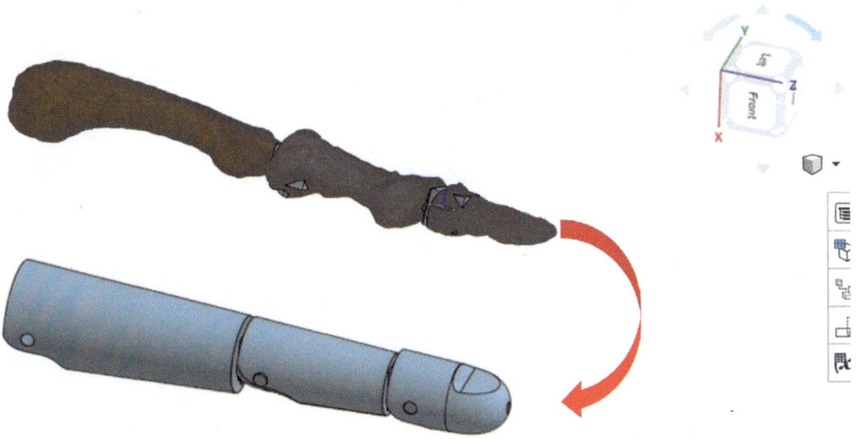

Fig. 19.9 Development of the prosthetic model within the Onshape® CAD environment

allowing adjustments to the structure and the addition of design features that facilitate its functional evaluation (Fig. 19.9).

19.2.5 Finger Design

The prosthetic design was developed through the construction of independent phalanx segments (Fig. 19.10). Each segment incorporated hinge-type connection elements, allowing relative motion between phalanges. This configuration was considered to enable controlled finger articulation through the use of an external harness system.

The model integrates independent phalanx segments connected by hinge elements, adapted to the patient's residual limb anatomy. The design was generated from CT-based segmentation, refined through Meshmixer®, and finalized in Onshape® prior to additive manufacturing and subsequent numerical validation.

The hinge–harness configuration was selected because it combines simplicity, mechanical reliability, and low manufacturing cost. Previous studies have reported that cable-driven prostheses often require frequent adjustments and present long-term maintenance challenges due to cable fatigue and tension loss (Carey et al. 2015). Electrically actuated prostheses, while capable of providing higher dexterity, are associated with increased weight, dependence on external power sources, and higher overall costs, which limit their accessibility in low-resource contexts (Brack et al. 2020; Hashim 2018). In contrast, harness-driven systems provide a lightweight and economically feasible option, making them suitable for patients requiring functional restoration without the financial burden of advanced myoelectric devices. This choice therefore balances functional recovery with affordability, while maintaining sufficient durability for daily use.

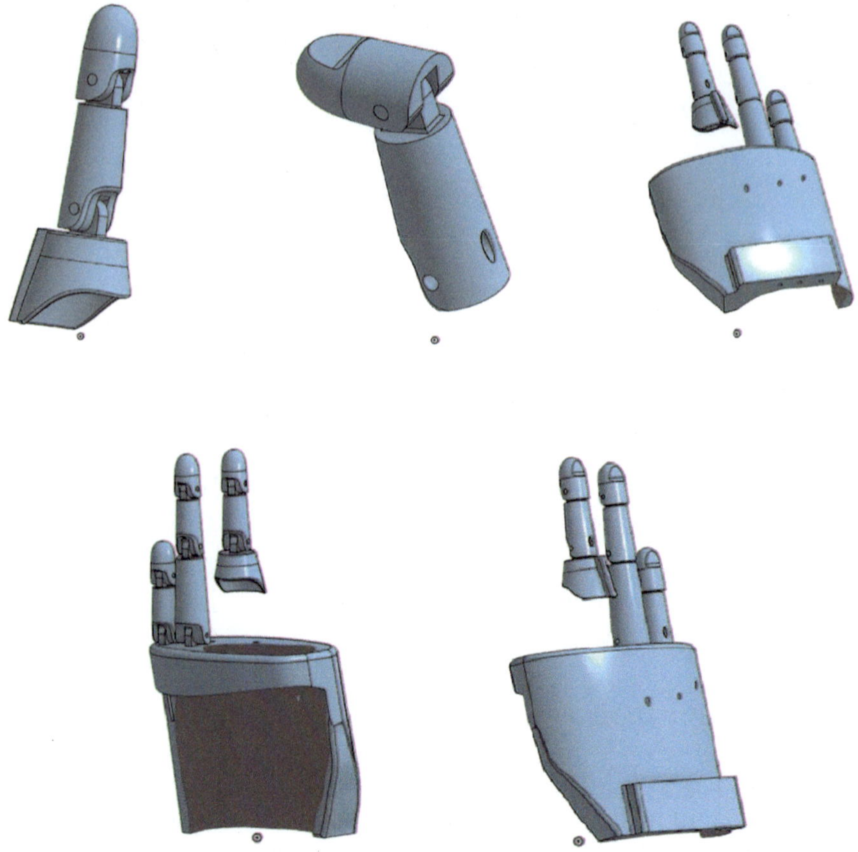

Fig. 19.10 Final CAD design of the personalized mechanical hand prosthesis

By employing clinical imaging data as the foundation for model generation, the prosthetic design achieves a high degree of anatomical fidelity. This approach ensures an accurate and ergonomic fit of the device to the patient's residual limb, thereby improving comfort during prolonged use and reducing the risk of pressure points or maladaptation. The direct support of tomographic information also minimizes subjective approximations in the modeling process, allowing for reproducibility and precision across different clinical cases.

The integration of three-dimensional (3D) printing technologies with readily available polymers offers a practical pathway for producing functional devices in a short time frame. Additive manufacturing not only accelerates the prototyping stage but also reduces production costs, making the prosthesis accessible to a broader patient population (Figs. 19.11 and 19.12).

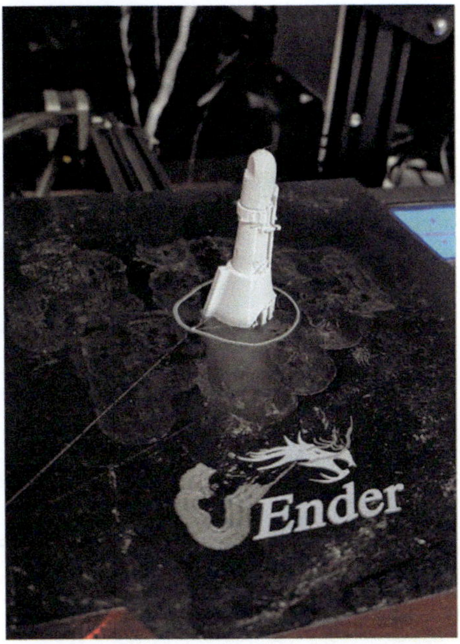

Fig. 19.11 Printing process

The fabrication of a physical model of the patient's amputated hand served as a critical step for verifying the digital design. Through this stage, geometric discrepancies could be detected and corrected, ensuring that the final version of the prosthesis preserved both functional and morphological accuracy. With these refinements completed, the next phase of the project involves the implementation of a numerical analysis. This simulation will evaluate the distribution of stresses generated during routine daily activities and verify that they remain within the mechanical resistance limits of the selected material, thereby validating the structural reliability of the proposed prototype before clinical use.

19.3 Conclusions

The final prosthetic design fulfilled both the requirements established during the design stage and the patient-specific anatomical needs. The model demonstrated an adequate adaptation to the patient's residual limb, ensuring ergonomic integration and user comfort.

The use of medical image segmentation enabled the creation of a personalized prosthesis with high anatomical fidelity. By employing 3D printing, it is possible not only to fabricate functional prototypes of the prosthesis but also to produce a full-scale replica of the patient's partially amputated hand. This replica serves as a test

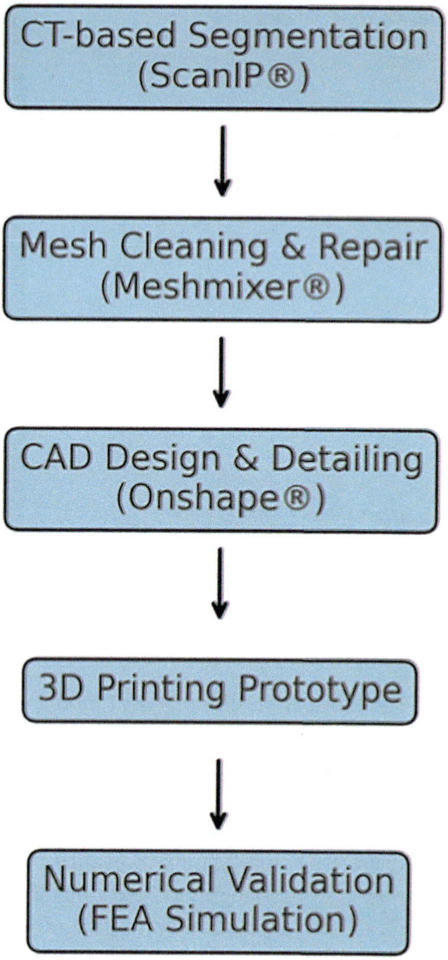

Fig. 19.12 Workflow for the development of the personalized hand prosthesis, illustrating the sequential stages from CT-based segmentation in ScanIP® through mesh refinement in Meshmixer®, CAD detailing in Onshape®, additive manufacturing, and finite element validation

platform for evaluating the fit of the device and verifying its mechanical compatibility prior to clinical use.

The integration of computational tools throughout the workflow contributed to a substantial reduction in design and development time. The availability of clinical imaging allowed the reconstruction of the missing phalanges and facilitated the efficient design of the prosthesis with minimal iterations. This streamlined process highlights the potential of image-based workflows to accelerate prosthetic development while maintaining precision.

In addition, the implementation of 3D models provides a robust framework for mechanical validation. Durability and performance tests can be carried out using digital image correlation and finite element simulations, ensuring that the stresses generated during daily activities remain below the mechanical resistance of the selected materials.

Overall, the study demonstrates the feasibility of producing low-cost, patient-specific hand prostheses by combining medical image segmentation and additive manufacturing. Beyond clinical application, the methodology establishes a reproducible framework that supports biomedical research, educational training, and the advancement of personalized rehabilitation technologies within healthcare institutions.

Acknowledgments This study was made possible through the institutional support of the:
• Instituto Politécnico Nacional (IPN).
• Comisión de Operación y Fomento de Actividades Académicas (COFAA).
• Secretaría de Investigación y Posgrado (SIP).
• Secretaría de Ciencia, Humanidades, Tecnología e Innovación (SECIHTI).
• Programa Institucional de Formación de Investigadores (PIFI), whose contributions were fundamental to the successful development of this research.

References

Brack T, Rombach I, Aldington D, Metcalf O (2020) Cost-effectiveness of upper-limb prostheses: a review of the literature. Prosthetics Orthot Int 44(1):3–15. https://doi.org/10.1177/0309364619878594

Bustamante Carvallo MM (2018) Malky: Diseño e implementación de una prótesis parcial de mano personalizada

Carey SL, Lura DJ, Highsmith MJ (2015) Differences in myoelectric and body-powered upper-limb prostheses: systematic literature review. J Rehabil Res Dev 52(3):247–262. https://doi.org/10.1682/JRRD.2014.08.0192

González A (2009) Prótesis en amputaciones de mano y antebrazo. In: Zambudio R (ed) Prótesis, órtesis y ayudas técnicas, pp 143–154

Hashim NA (2018) Advantages and disadvantages of body-powered upper limb prostheses: a review. Malays J Med Health Sci 14(3), 51–57. https://pubmed.ncbi.nlm.nih.gov/29199518

Instituto Mexicano del Seguro Social. Informe de Labores y Programa de Actividades 2022–2023: Capítulo III. Seguro de Riesgos de Trabajo. https://www.imss.gob.mx/sites/all/statics/pdf/informes/20222023/07-Cap03.pdf. Accessed 3 Sept 2025

Lamandé F, Dupré JC, Talbot P, Gillet M, Januscevics T, Dréjas-Zielinska M (2014) Amputación del miembro superior. EMC Kinesiter Med Física 35(2):1–20

Rodríguez EG, Cano LG, Pastor BS (2022) Actualización en prótesis para amputaciones parciales de mano y dedos. Rehabilitación 56(4):375–382. https://doi.org/10.1016/j.rh.2022.03.004

Chapter 20
3D Segmentation and Modeling of Thoracic Organs for Surgical Planning and Medical Research

Carlos Uriel Castelán-Sánchez, Juan Alfonso Beltrán-Fernández, Mauricio González Rebattú y González, Alejandro Gónzalez-Rebattú, Elías Humberto Hermida-Ochoa, Alejandro Tonatiu Velázquez-Sánchez, Erik Omar Alvarado-Alcántara, Karen Pamela Vázquez-Thierry, and Pablo Moreno-Garibaldi

Abstract A methodology for the segmentation and three-dimensional (3D) modeling of thoracic organs from computed tomography scans is described. The process employs specialized software tools that enable the accurate delineation of anatomical structures and the generation of detailed volumetric reconstructions. The resulting 3D models provide anatomically faithful representations that can be integrated into surgical planning workflows, offering surgeons enhanced spatial understanding of patient-specific anatomy and supporting more precise preoperative strategies. Beyond clinical applications, these models constitute valuable resources for medical research, allowing detailed investigation of thoracic organ morphology and function under reproducible conditions. The findings highlight the potential of 3D segmentation and modeling to strengthen decision-making in surgical planning, advance anatomical research, and improve the quality of medical education.

Keywords 3D segmentation · Thoracic organs · Surgical planning · Medical research · Computed tomography (CT)

C. U. Castelán-Sánchez · J. A. Beltrán-Fernández (✉) · A. T. Velázquez-Sánchez · E. O. Alvarado-Alcántara · K. P. Vázquez-Thierry · P. Moreno-Garibaldi
Instituto Politécnico Nacional, ESIME Unidad Zacatenco. Sección de Estudios de Posgrado E Investigación, Unidad Profesional Adolfo López Mateos. Col. Lindavista, Mexico City, Mexico
e-mail: jbeltran@ipn.mx

A. T. Velázquez-Sánchez
e-mail: atvelazquezs@ipn.mx

M. G. Rebattú y González · A. Gónzalez-Rebattú
ISSSTE Hospital Regional 1° de Octubre, Av. Instituto Politécnico Nacional 1669, Mexico City, Mexico

E. H. Hermida-Ochoa
Hospital de Ortopedia Dr. Germán Díaz Lombardo, CILAB, Mexico City, Mexico
e-mail: drelias@hermidagroup.com

A. Öchsner (ed.), *Progress in Biomaterials and Biomedical Engineering*, Advanced Structured Materials 249, https://doi.org/10.1007/978-3-032-13551-3_20

20.1 Introduction

The thoracic cage constitutes a complex osteocartilaginous framework that protects vital organs such as the heart and lungs while also supporting the musculature involved in respiration and upper limb mobility. Its anatomical configuration integrates several bones of critical biomechanical importance, including the clavicle, humerus, and ribs. The morphology and mechanical behavior of these elements play a decisive role in maintaining trunk stability, transmitting forces between the upper limbs and the axial skeleton, and ensuring functional integrity during daily activities (Kani et al. 2019; Granacher et al. 2013).

In this study, segmentation of three representative anatomical structures—clavicle, humerus, and rib—was carried out using computed tomography (CT) imaging. The methodological workflow employed specialized software platforms, including ScanIP for precise image segmentation, Meshmixer for digital model refinement, and ANSYS for biomechanical evaluation. This combination enabled the transformation of medical images into anatomically accurate three-dimensional models and their subsequent analysis under controlled flexion conditions.

The application of such approaches holds particular relevance in both clinical and scientific contexts. In the clinical domain, patient-specific anatomical reconstructions provide surgeons with enhanced spatial understanding and serve as complementary tools for preoperative planning, thereby reducing intraoperative uncertainty. In the scientific field, these methods allow for a more accurate characterization of human anatomy, support the development of new research lines in biomedical engineering, and contribute to the design of safer and more efficient surgical techniques and implants (Oliveira et al. 2011).

20.2 Materials and Methods

The study was structured into four stages: image acquisition, anatomical segmentation, mesh refinement, and finite element analysis. Each stage is described below.

20.2.1 Image Acquisition

Computed tomography datasets were obtained in digital imaging and communications in medicine (DICOM) format from clinical sources. All procedures complied with institutional ethics committees and national regulations governing the use of patient imaging for research. Written informed consent was obtained before including the data, in accordance with legal and ethical standards.

The CT scans had a slice thickness of 1.0 mm, a resolution sufficient to reproduce the geometry of the long bones and thoracic structures while maintaining manageable file size. These datasets constituted the material used for segmentation and subsequent modeling.

20.2.2 Anatomical Segmentation

Segmentation of thoracic bones was carried out using ScanIP (Simpleware, Synopsys Inc.), a medical image processing platform designed for DICOM data. A semi-automatic approach based on intensity thresholds was combined with manual refinement to improve accuracy.

The full thoracic dataset was imported into the software, and the Confidence Connected Region tool was applied to isolate the humerus, clavicle, and rib. This algorithm grouped voxels with similar intensities, allowing selective extraction of osseous structures. Threshold parameters were adjusted iteratively to exclude artifacts and preserve cortical bone.

Manual refinement was then performed slice by slice to correct irregular boundaries and improve continuity in regions of complex morphology, such as the humeral head and the sternal joints. The resulting segmentations were exported in STL (stereolithography) format, producing individual models for each bone.

Validation was carried out by comparing the segmented masks against the original CT images in axial, sagittal, and coronal views. This process confirmed that the segmented structures maintained their geometry and reproduced the anatomical detail required for subsequent biomechanical analysis (Figs. 20.1 and 20.2).

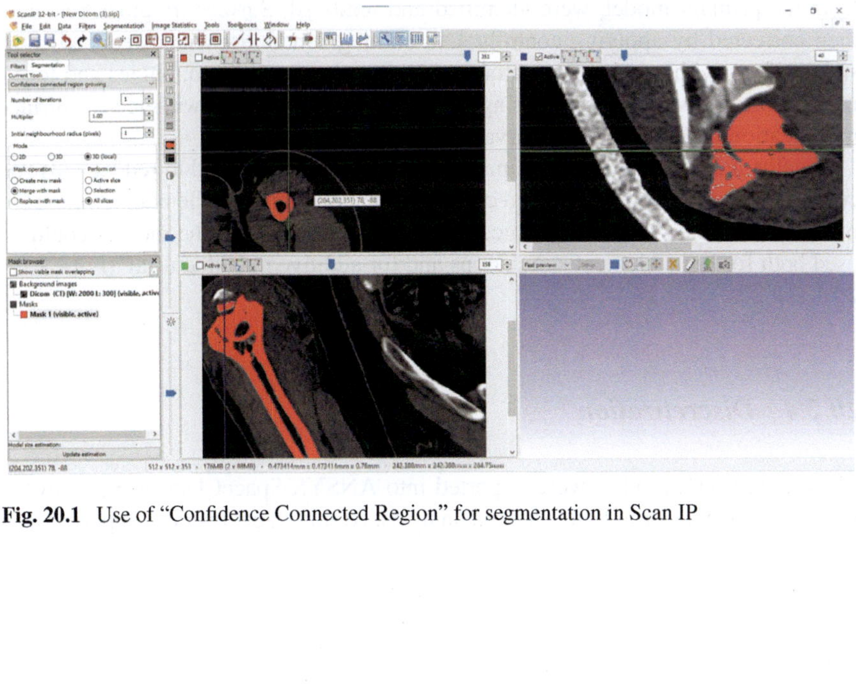

Fig. 20.1 Use of "Confidence Connected Region" for segmentation in Scan IP

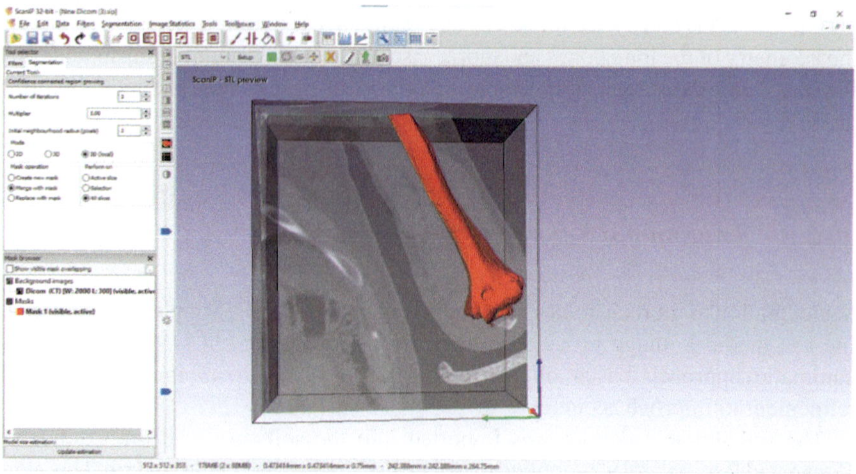

Fig. 20.2 Humerus STL file generated from Scan IP

20.2.3 *Mesh Refinement*

The STL models obtained from the segmentation stage were imported into Meshmixer (Autodesk Inc.) for refinement and optimization. This stage was necessary to ensure that the digital models achieved the geometric accuracy and surface continuity required for subsequent biomechanical analyses.

Several corrective operations were applied. First, discontinuities and open surfaces generated during segmentation were repaired through automated mesh-filling algorithms. Floating artifacts, consisting of small non-anatomical fragments disconnected from the primary model, were identified and removed. Surface irregularities were then corrected by applying controlled smoothing functions, which reduced stair-step artifacts without altering anatomical landmarks. In addition, bulges and localized distortions were corrected using the Sculpt tool, which allows selective surface modification to restore natural curvature.

Finally, a controlled mesh decimation process was performed to reduce polygon count. This optimization improved computational efficiency while maintaining sub-millimetric fidelity of the anatomical geometry, ensuring that the models could be used both for finite element simulations and for additive manufacturing (Figs. 20.3, 20.4 and 20.5).

20.2.4 *Discretization*

The cleaned STL models were imported into ANSYS SpaceClaim to perform the final refinement prior to finite element analysis. At this stage, residual imperfections

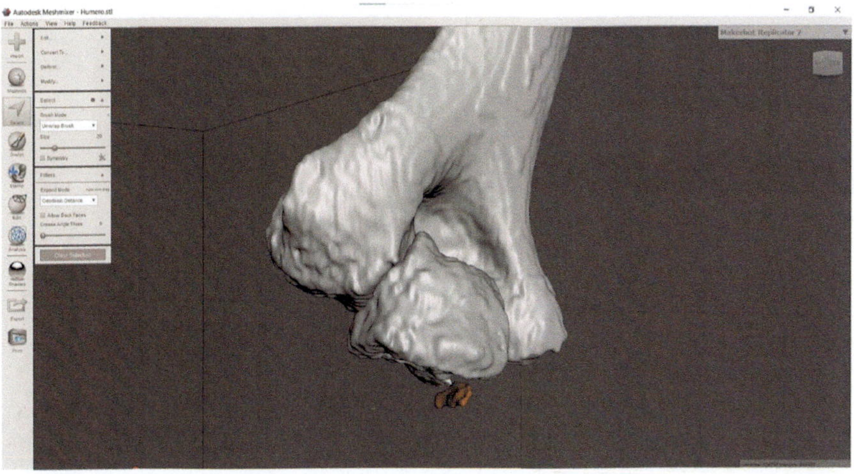

Fig. 20.3 Removal of floating fragments in Meshmixer to clean the STL model of the humerus

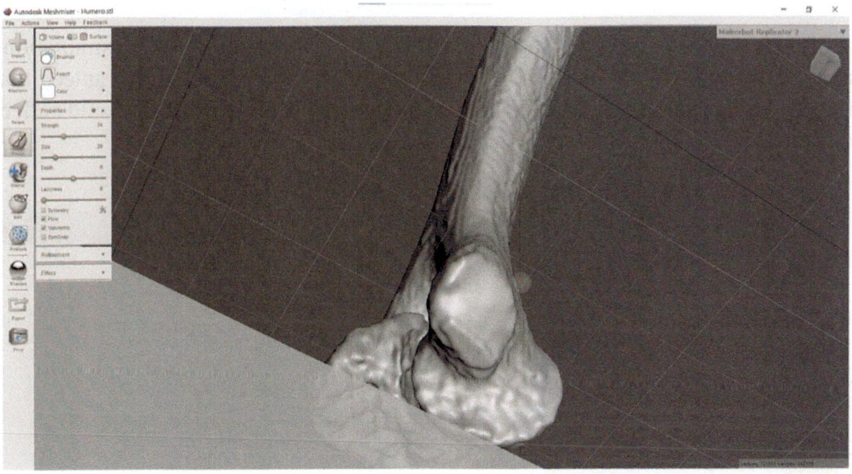

Fig. 20.4 Local surface correction of the humerus model using the "Sculpt" tool in Meshmixer

such as surface irregularities, small gaps, or intersecting facets were corrected to ensure that the digital geometry could be meshed without numerical instabilities.

Following this preparation, the models were discretized into finite elements using the meshing tools provided in the ANSYS Workbench environment. The discretization process divided the anatomical volumes into an optimal number of tetrahedral elements, balancing computational cost with the level of geometric detail required. A mesh convergence criterion was applied to verify that the results of subsequent simulations would not be affected by further refinement.

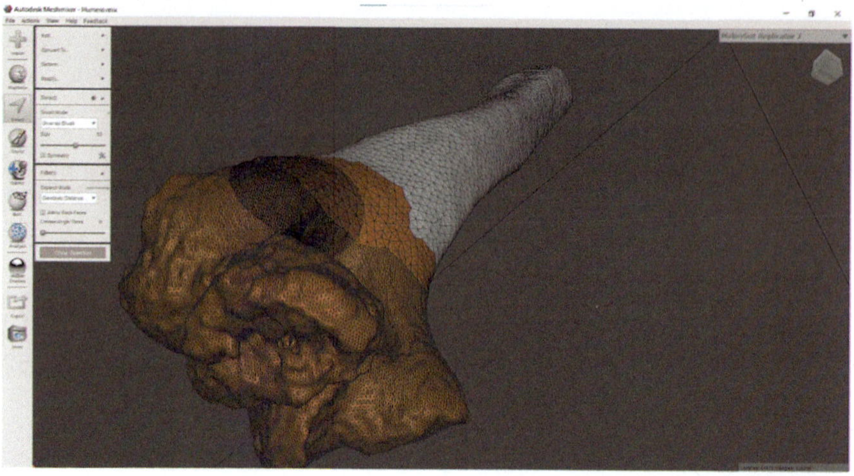

Fig. 20.5 Mesh decimation process applied in Meshmixer to reduce polygon count while preserving anatomical fidelity

This step was essential for ensuring both the numerical stability of the simulations and the anatomical fidelity of the models. Properly defined meshes guaranteed that the stress distribution patterns generated under mechanical loading would reflect realistic anatomical behavior (Fig. 20.6).

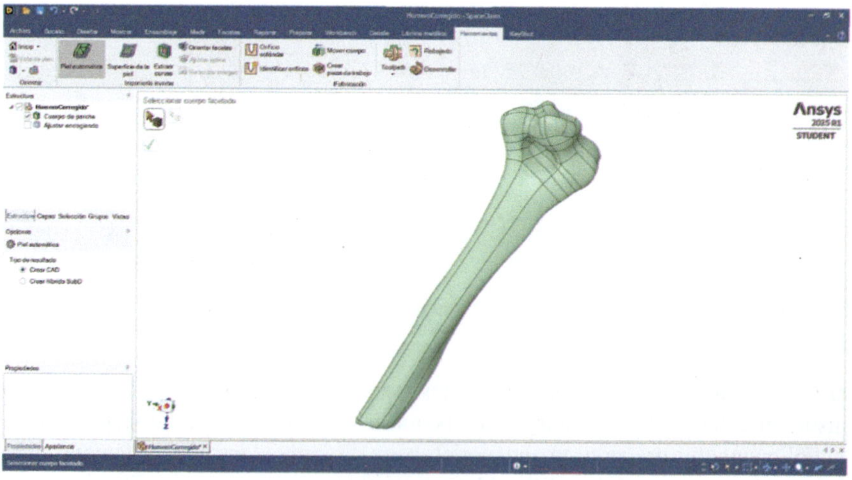

Fig. 20.6 Humerus model refined and discretized in ANSYS SpaceClaim, showing the final finite element mesh generated from the segmented STL geometry

20.2.5 Finite Element Analysis

The refined meshes were transferred into ANSYS Workbench for biomechanical simulation. Controlled flexural loading conditions were defined for each anatomical model, with forces ranging from 10 to 100 N to approximate physiologically relevant magnitudes. The boundary conditions were established by fixing anatomical regions corresponding to articular constraints while applying loads to regions typically subjected to functional stresses.

In the case of the humerus, the olecranon fossa was constrained to represent elbow articulation, and forces were applied to the humeral head to replicate joint loading. This configuration allowed the evaluation of bending response under conditions consistent with daily activities and clinical testing protocols.

The analysis focused on three primary outputs:

- Von Mises stress distributions, to identify regions of concentrated stress that could indicate susceptibility to mechanical failure.
- Maximum principal stress values, to distinguish tensile and compressive loading zones within the cortical and trabecular structures.
- Unitary deformation, to assess global displacement and localized strain patterns under increasing load magnitudes.

These outputs provided quantitative insight into the mechanical response of the bones under controlled loading scenarios, thereby establishing a framework for future applications in computational biomechanics, implant design, trauma analysis, and preoperative surgical planning (Fig. 20.7).

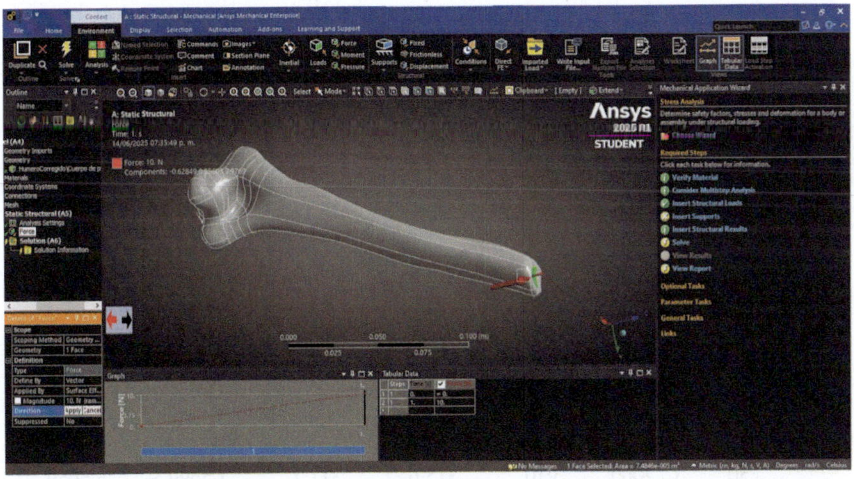

Fig. 20.7 Simulation of applied force to humerus STL model performed in ANSYS Workbench

20.3 Discussion

The finite element simulations revealed marked differences in the mechanical response of the clavicle, humerus, and rib when subjected to flexural loads ranging from 10 to 100 N (Table 20.1). In all cases, the relationship between applied load, stress, and deformation followed a nearly linear trend, confirming that the bone tissue behaved elastically within the studied range of forces.

For the clavicle, the von Mises stress increased from 2.49 MPa under a 10 N load to 24.86 MPa at 100 N. Maximum deformation rose correspondingly from 1.03 mm to 10.31 mm. The proportional increase in strain with load magnitude indicated a relatively uniform distribution of stress across the bone. These findings are consistent with the clavicle's anatomical role as a slender structure responsible for transmitting forces between the upper limb and the thorax, undergoing significant displacements while maintaining structural integrity (Kemper et al. 2009) (Fig. 20.8).

The humerus demonstrated the lowest stress values among the three bones. At 100 N, the von Mises stress reached only 7.07 MPa, with a maximum deformation of 2.55 mm. The modest strain levels and limited displacement reflect the humerus' greater cross-sectional area and cortical thickness, which confer structural robustness. The results indicate that the humerus can accommodate functional loading

Table 20.1 Results of finite element simulations for clavicle, humerus, and rib under flexural loads ranging from 10 to 100 N

Bone	Applied load (N)	Number of nodes	Number of elements	Von-Mises Stress (MPa)	Maximum principal stress (MPa)	Unitary strain (mm/mm)	Total deformation (mm)
Clavicle	10	1322	627	2.486	2.4674	8.6761×10^{-4}	1.0312
	50	1322	627	12.43	12.337	4.338×10^{-3}	5.1561
	100	1322	627	24.86	24.674	8.6761×10^{-3}	10.312
Humerus	10	2319	1180	0.70695	0.71301	2.4751×10^{-4}	0.25488
	50	2319	1180	3.5347	3.565	1.2376×10^{-3}	1.2744
	100	2319	1180	7.0695	7.1301	2.4751×10^{-3}	2.5488
Rib	10	2000	910	63.12	62.339	3.1399×10^{-4}	1.3012
	50	2000	910	315.6	311.7	1.5699×10^{-3}	6.5059
	100	2000	910	631.2	623.39	3.1399×10^{-3}	13.012

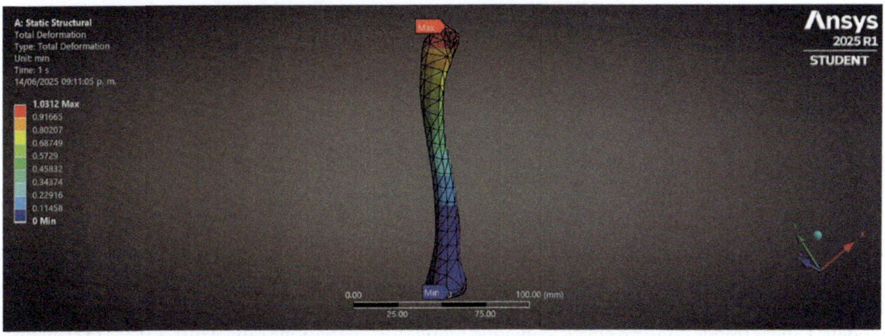

Fig. 20.8 FEM clavicle results in ANSYS workbench

with minimal elastic deformation, consistent with its role as a primary load-bearing element of the upper limb (Sumner and Andriacchi 1996).

In contrast, the rib exhibited the most pronounced mechanical response. At 100 N, the von Mises stress rose sharply to 631.2 MPa, with maximum deformation exceeding 13 mm. These high stress and strain values suggest a limited resistance to localized flexural loading. This observation corresponds to the rib's anatomical characteristics, which include thin cortical walls and a curved geometry that favors compliance and mobility rather than resistance to high mechanical forces. Functionally, this flexibility is necessary to accommodate respiratory movements but implies increased susceptibility to fracture under concentrated loads (Liebsch and Wilke 2018).

The comparative analysis of these three bones indicates that geometry and anatomical function directly influence their mechanical behavior. The clavicle displayed high displacements under moderate stresses, the humerus exhibited stability and load-bearing capacity, and the rib showed mechanical fragility under localized loading. From a biomedical standpoint, such results are essential to support surgical planning, implant development, and the assessment of fracture risk. Furthermore, the data confirm the value of patient-specific finite element simulations for predicting biomechanical performance under clinically relevant conditions.

The graph presented in Fig. 20.9 illustrates the relationship between applied load, von Mises stress, and maximum deformation for the analyzed bones. In all cases, the curves display a proportional increase in both stress and deformation with rising load magnitudes, confirming that the mechanical response remained within the elastic regime for forces between 10 and 100 N. No evidence of nonlinearities, plastic behavior, or failure thresholds was observed within this loading range.

The slope of each curve reflects the intrinsic structural resistance of the bone. Steeper slopes correspond to geometries that are less capable of sustaining external forces without deformation, while gentler slopes indicate greater stiffness and resistance to flexural loading. In this context, the humerus exhibited the lowest gradients, consistent with its robust morphology and function as a load-bearing element. The clavicle showed intermediate values, reflecting its role as a slender structural

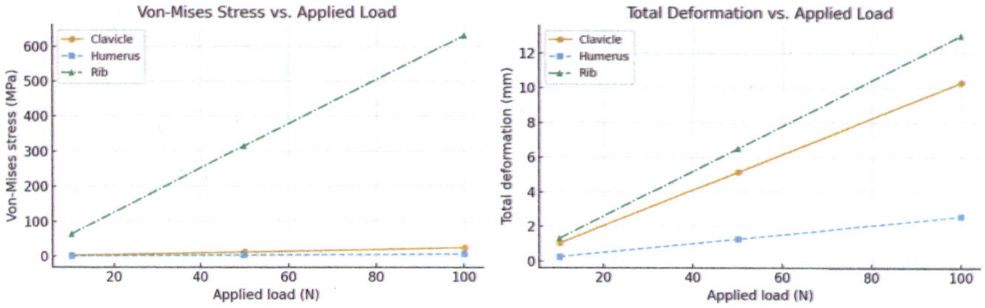

Fig. 20.9 Stress and deformation as functions of applied load for clavicle, humerus, and rib models. Linear trends confirm elastic behavior, while slope variations reflect differences in structural resistance

connector, whereas the rib presented the steepest slopes, indicating high susceptibility to deformation under concentrated loading.

These results confirm that bone geometry and anatomical function govern mechanical performance under physiological conditions. Linear elastic trends suggest that, within the studied range, the bones maintain structural integrity, but their distinct responses emphasize the importance of geometry-specific analyses when evaluating fracture risk, implant design, or load-sharing behavior in surgical contexts.

20.4 Discussion

The simulation results highlight clear differences in the mechanical performance of the three bones studied. The clavicle demonstrated a capacity to undergo relatively large displacements under moderate stresses, reflecting its anatomical role in transmitting forces between the upper limb and the thoracic cage. The proportional increase in strain indicated uniform load distribution across the structure, a behavior consistent with its function as a flexible yet structurally important connector (Kemper et al. 2009).

The humerus displayed the lowest stress and deformation levels, which can be attributed to its greater cross-sectional area and cortical thickness. This structural robustness enables it to resist flexural loading with minimal displacement, supporting its role as the primary load-bearing bone of the upper limb. The gradual increase in strain confirmed its mechanical stability under the tested conditions (Sumner and Andriacchi 1996).

In contrast, the rib exhibited significantly higher stresses and deformations. Its thin cortical geometry and curved shape, which provide compliance for respiratory movements, also result in limited resistance to concentrated flexural loads. The elevated stress values observed at 100 N suggest a higher susceptibility to fracture under non-physiological or traumatic loading, consistent with clinical experience in thoracic trauma (Liebsch and Wilke 2018).

Taken together, these findings demonstrate how bone geometry and anatomical function govern mechanical performance. From a biomedical perspective, such simulations contribute to a better understanding of load-bearing behavior, support the design of implants and fixation devices, and improve preoperative planning by providing predictive information on structural response under defined loading conditions.

20.5 Conclusions

The finite element analyses of the clavicle, humerus, and rib demonstrated that the mechanical response is determined by structural geometry and anatomical function. The clavicle exhibited relatively large displacements under moderate stress values, the humerus showed low levels of stress and deformation consistent with its greater cross-sectional robustness, and the rib displayed high-stress magnitudes and the largest deformations, reflecting its compliant but mechanically weaker structure.

These results confirm that CT-derived digital models, when combined with segmentation, 3D reconstruction, and finite element analysis, provide reliable information on stress distribution, strain levels, and deformation patterns. Such information can be applied directly to the evaluation of fracture risk, the design and optimization of implants, and the improvement of surgical planning by predicting structural response under defined loading conditions.

In addition to clinical applications, the methodology offers academic advantages. Patient-specific models can be incorporated into surgical training programs, biomechanical research, and teaching curricula, enhancing anatomical understanding and supporting the integration of engineering analysis into medical education.

The workflow therefore constitutes a reproducible and computationally efficient strategy for generating anatomically accurate thoracic models. Its implementation has potential not only to improve preoperative assessment and research outcomes but also to strengthen the academic and technological capacities of health institutions, particularly in contexts where advanced digital resources can contribute to the development of precision medicine and translational biomechanics.

Furthermore, the integration of CT-based segmentation, 3D reconstruction, and finite element analysis provides a reproducible framework that not only yields anatomically accurate thoracic models but also delivers clinically relevant biomechanical insights, thereby reinforcing the role of computational methods as indispensable tools in surgical planning, biomedical research, and medical education.

Acknowledgements The authors acknowledge the contributions of collaborating institutions and medical staff for facilitating access to imaging datasets, anatomical evaluation, and validation of simulation results. This research was supported by the Instituto Politécnico Nacional (IPN), the Secretaría de Ciencia, Humanidades, Tecnología e Innovación (SECIHTI), the Hospital Regional 1° de Octubre (ISSSTE), and the Hospital de Ortopedia Dr. Germán Díaz Lombardo—CILAB.

References

Granacher U, Gollhofer A, Hortobágyi T, Kressig RW, Muehlbauer T (2013) The importance of trunk muscle strength for balance, functional performance, and fall prevention in seniors: a systematic review. Sports Med 43(7):627–641. https://doi.org/10.1007/s40279-013-0041-1

Kani KK, Mulcahy H, Porrino JA, Chew FS (2019) Thoracic cage injuries. Eur J Radiol 110:225–232. https://doi.org/10.1016/j.ejrad.2018.11.013

Kemper AR, Stitzel JD, McNally C, Gabler HC, Duma SM (2009) Biomechanical response of the human clavicle: the effects of loading direction on bending properties. J Appl Biomech 25(2):165–174. https://doi.org/10.1123/jab.25.2.165

Liebsch C, Wilke HJ (2018) Basic biomechanics of the thoracic spine and rib cage. In: Imhof U, Wilke HJ (eds) Biomechanics of the spine: basic concepts, spinal disorders and treatments. Academic Press, pp 35–50. https://doi.org/10.1016/B978-0-12-812851-0.00003-1

Oliveira DA, Feitosa RQ, Correia MM (2011) Segmentation of liver, its vessels and lesions from CT images for surgical planning. Biomed Eng Online 10:30. https://doi.org/10.1186/1475-925X-10-30

Sumner DR, Andriacchi TP (1996) Adaptation to differential loading: comparison of growth-related changes in cross-sectional properties of the human femur and humerus. Bone 19(2):121–126. https://doi.org/10.1016/S8756-3282(96)00116-6

Chapter 21
Knee and Ankle Exoskeleton for Walking Assistance with Flexible Joint as Force Sensors

Jesús Ricardo López-Gutierrez, Uriel Pérez-Flores, Ruben Fuentes-Alvarez, and Luis Antonio Carrillo-Martinez

Abstract The development of a two-degree-of-freedom right-leg exoskeleton with flexible joints for knee and ankle assistance during gait is presented. The main objective is the design and implementation of a back-stepping control system, taking into account the dynamics of the flexible joints in the exoskeleton. The results are obtained from experimental simulation tests and experimental tests on the developed prototype. In addition, a strategy is proposed to use the flexible joints as torque sensors, which allow the generation of the human intention command that allows the user to make the decision to start walking and stop.

Keywords Exoskeleton · Assistance robotics · Flexible joint · Force sensors · Back-stepping control · Lower limb rehabilitation

21.1 Introduction

The development of lower limb exoskeletons has evolved from purely rigid prototypes to systems that integrate flexibility as a design principle. This flexibility can take various forms, from the device's structure to its actuation system, always seeking a more natural and safe fit with the user (Fig. 21.1).

J. R. López-Gutierrez (✉) · R. Fuentes-Alvarez · L. A. Carrillo-Martinez
School of Engineering and Sciences, Institute of Technology and Higher Education of Monterrey, Monterrey, México
e-mail: jesusl.lopez@tec.mx

R. Fuentes-Alvarez
e-mail: joru.fua@tec.mx

L. A. Carrillo-Martinez
e-mail: acarrillom@tec.mx

J. R. López-Gutierrez · U. Pérez-Flores
SECIHTI-National Institute for Astrophysics, Optics and Electronics, Puebla, México
e-mail: u.perezf@inaoep.mx

A. Ã–chsner (ed.), *Progress in Biomaterials and Biomedical Engineering*, Advanced Structured Materials 249, https://doi.org/10.1007/978-3-032-13551-3_21

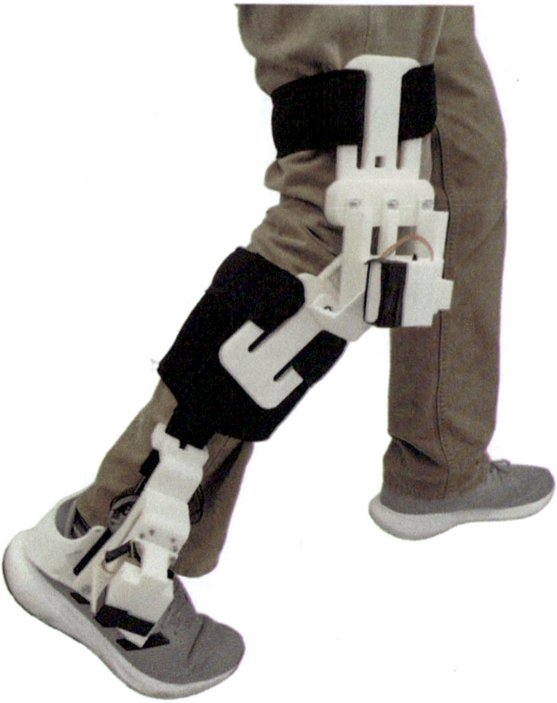

Fig. 21.1 Gait assistant anthropomorphic exoskeleton with flexible joints, for lower limb with 2 degrees of freedom in knee and ankle

Focusing on compatibility in the human–machine interface and kinematic structure. To avoid misalignment and unwanted forces, passive degrees of freedom are incorporated into the anchor points, such as curved rails or deformable frames, which allow the device to self-align with the user's movement (Wang et al. 2022; Lee et al. 2017). This principle extends to the biomechanical design of the exoskeleton, seeking to ensure that its structure and degrees of freedom faithfully mimic human anatomy in its lower limb section to improve the system's performance and ergonomics (Chen et al. 2013). In more recent designs, structural rigidity is replaced by flexible bandage- and belt-based restraint systems, which improve efficiency and speed of use in complex environments (Chen et al. 2022).

Flexibility is also important for optimizing the mass and inertia of the actuation system. A common strategy is to move the motors away from the distal joints using Bowden cable transmission systems, thereby reducing rotational inertia and creating lighter and more agile devices (Yi et al. 2023; Chen et al. 2022). This approach allows for greater freedom of movement, extending beyond the sagittal plane.

Finally, the most advanced approach resides in the intrinsic flexibility of the actuator, giving rise to the field of soft exosuits (soft robotics). Beyond incorporating series elastic elements (SEA) (Centeno-Barreda et al. 2024) or variable stiffness elements (VSA) (Wang and Geng 2025; Schrade et al. 2017) in rigid joints, inherently flexible actuators have emerged. Notable examples include Pneumatic Gel Muscles

(PGMs), which are lightweight and operate at low pressure to assist gait in wearable suits (Thakur et al. 2018), and inflatable textile actuators, which are integrated into garments such as boots (ExoBoot) to generate assistive torques in a discreet and comfortable manner (Chung et al. 2018). These systems demonstrate that flexibility is no longer just an add-on component, but rather the foundation upon which new assistive devices are built.

It can be said, then, that current lower limb exoskeleton designs show a trend toward flexibility with different concepts and proposals. It is implemented through passive mechanisms and biomimetic designs to improve kinematic compatibility (Wang et al. 2022; Lee et al. 2017; Chen et al. 2013), through remote actuation systems to lighten the device (Yi et al. 2023; Chen et al. 2022), and, more innovatively, through elastic actuators, variable stiffness and, above all, soft robotic systems that are worn rather than attached (Centeno-Barreda et al. 2024; Wang and Geng 2025; Schrade et al. 2017; Chung et al. 2018; Thakur et al. 2018), allowing assistance that dynamically adapts to the user's biomechanics.

21.2 Dynamic Model of the Exoskeleton

A flexible joint consists of three main elements, (1) actuator, in this case the electric motor, whose angular position of its axis is defined by q_m, (2) link, whose angular position is defined by q_l, and (3) spring, it is a flexible element that holds the actuator and the link whose elasticity constant is defined by k, see Fig. 21.2.

The lower limb exoskeleton has flexible joints in ankle and knee. Define the angular position of the knee motor q_{mk} and the ankle motor q_{ma}, which are elements of the angular position vector of the motor $\mathbf{q_m}$, the same way we define the link of the knee joint q_{lk} and the ankle joint q_{lm}, elements of the angular position vector of the link $\mathbf{q}_l$, as follows:

$$\mathbf{q}_m = \begin{bmatrix} q_{mk} \\ q_{ma} \end{bmatrix}; \mathbf{q}_l = \begin{bmatrix} q_{lk} \\ q_{la} \end{bmatrix}. \tag{21.1}$$

The position of the X and Y axes in the sagittal plane, the parameters and the angular position variables of the links are defined as shown in Fig. 21.3. The equations of the dynamic model were obtained as:

$$\begin{aligned} M(\mathbf{q}_l)\ddot{\mathbf{q}}_l + C(\mathbf{q}_l, \dot{\mathbf{q}}_l)\dot{\mathbf{q}}_l + \mathbf{g}(\mathbf{q}_l) + K(\mathbf{q}_l - \mathbf{q}_m) = 0 \\ J\ddot{\mathbf{q}}_m + B\dot{\mathbf{q}}_m - K(\mathbf{q}_l - \mathbf{q}_m) = \tau + \tau_{\mathbf{h}}. \end{aligned} \tag{21.2}$$

where $M(\mathbf{q}_l) \epsilon \mathbb{R}^{2\times2}$ is the inertia matrix, which is also symmetric, positive definite, uniformly bounded, its inverse exists and is also uniformly bounded, $C(\mathbf{q}_l, \dot{\mathbf{q}}_l) \epsilon \mathbb{R}^{2\times2}$ is the Coriolis and centrifugal generalized forces matrix, which is also suitably chosen, uniformly bounded and $\dot{M}(\mathbf{q}_l) - 2C(\mathbf{q}_l, \dot{\mathbf{q}}_1)$ is symmetrical skew, $\mathbf{g}(\mathbf{q}_l) \epsilon \mathbb{R}^{2\times1}$ is the gravitational generalized forces vector, uniformly bounded,

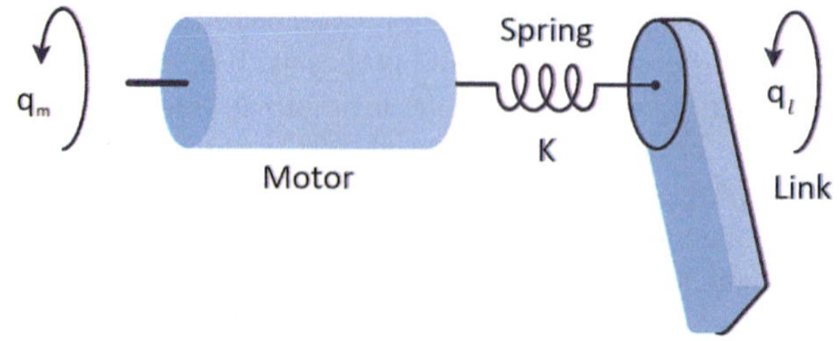

Fig. 21.2 Mechanical diagram of a flexible joint proposed for the development of a lower limb exoskeleton

K is the stiffness coefficient of spring, J is the inertia moments of the motors matrix, B Viscous Friction of motor vector, $\tau \epsilon \mathbb{R}^{2\times 1}$ is the torques of motors vector, and $\tau_{\mathbf{h}} \epsilon \mathbb{R}^{\mathbf{2}\times\mathbf{1}}$ is the torques of the human vector

The elements of the matrices and vectors of Eq. 21.2 are:

$$\begin{aligned}
M_{11}(\mathbf{q}_l) &= I_1 + I_2 + m_2 l_1^2 + m_1 l_{c1}^2 + m_2 l_{c2}^2 + 2m_2 l_1 l_{c2} \cos(q_{la}) \\
M_{12}(\mathbf{q}_l) &= I_2 + m_2 l_{c2}^2 + m_2 l_1 l_{c2} \cos(q_{la}) \\
M_{21}(\mathbf{q}_l) &= I_2 + m_2 l_{c2}^2 + m_2 l_1 l_{c2} \cos(q_{la}) \\
M_{22}(\mathbf{q}_l) &= I_2 + m_2 l_{c2}^2 \\
C_{11}(\mathbf{q}_l, \dot{\mathbf{q}}_l) &= -m_2 l_1 l_{c2} \sin(q_{la})\, \dot{q}_{la} \\
C_{12}(\mathbf{q}_l, \dot{\mathbf{q}}_l) &= -m_2 l_1 l_{c2} \sin(q_{la})\, (\dot{q}_{lk} + \dot{q}_{la}) \\
C_{21}(\mathbf{q}_l, \dot{\mathbf{q}}_l) &= m_2 l_1 l_{c2} \sin(q_{la})\, \dot{q}_{lk} \\
C_{22}(\mathbf{q}_l, \dot{\mathbf{q}}_l) &= 0 \\
g_1(\mathbf{q}_l) &= [m_1 l_{c1} + m_2 l_1]\, g \sin(q_{lk}) + m_2 g l_{c2} \sin(q_{lk} + q_{la}) \\
g_2(\mathbf{q}_l) &= m_2 g l_{c2} \sin(q_{lk} + q_{la})
\end{aligned} \tag{21.3}$$

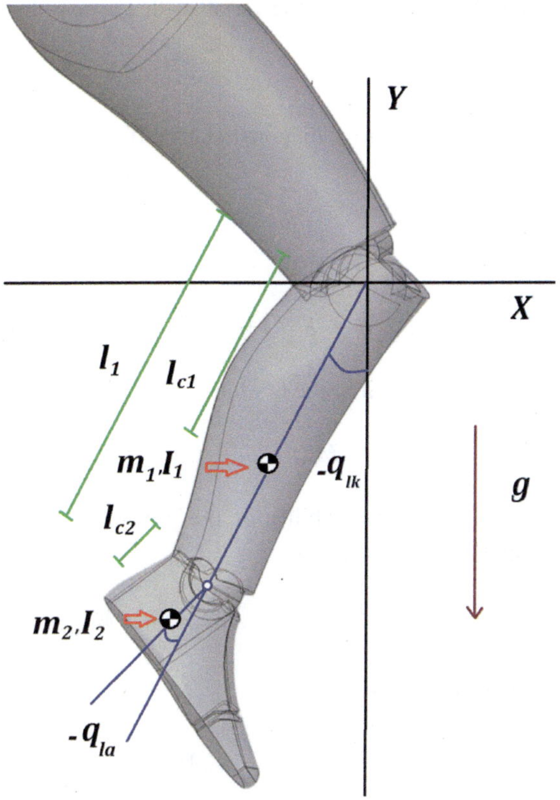

Fig. 21.3 Schematic diagram of the lower limb exoskeleton mechanics, link assignment, parameter values, and reference frame orientation

21.3 Back-Stepping Control Law of the Exoskeleton

To build the control law we will define two new variables as $x_1 = q_m$ and $x_2 = \dot{q}_m$, and suppose $\tau_h = 0$, so that we can represent the dynamic model as a cascade form:

$$\begin{aligned} M(\mathbf{q}_l)\ddot{\mathbf{q}}_l + C(\mathbf{q}_l, \dot{\mathbf{q}}_l)\dot{\mathbf{q}}_l + \mathbf{g}(\mathbf{q}_l) + K\mathbf{q}_l &= Kx_1 \\ \dot{x}_1 &= x_2 \\ \dot{x}_2 = J^{-1}\tau - J^{-1}K(\mathbf{x}_1 - \mathbf{q}_l) \end{aligned} \tag{21.4}$$

The first line of Eq. (21.4) represents the dynamics of the exoskeleton with rigid joints and we can see that x_1 acts as the control input, so that the first control law for the system is:

$$x_1 = q_l + K^{-1}[M(q_l)\dot{v}_1 + C(q_l, \dot{q}_l)v_1 + g(q_l) - \Lambda w_1] \tag{21.5}$$

where Λ is positive and the variables that appear there are defined as:
$\tilde{q}_l = q_l - q_{dl}$
$v_1 = \tilde{q}_{dl} - \Gamma_1 \tilde{q}_l$
$w_1 = \dot{q}_l - v_l = \dot{\tilde{q}}_l + \Gamma_1 \tilde{q}_l$
where Γ_1 is a positive diagonal matrix. If defined:

$$c_1 = x_1 - \mu_1 \tag{21.6}$$

where

$$\mu = q_l + K^{-1} \left[M(q_l)\, \dot{v}_1 + C(q_l, \dot{q}_l)\, v_1 + g(q_l) - \Lambda w_1 \right] \tag{21.7}$$

and substitute it in the first line of Eq. (21.4) we obtain:

$$M(q_l)\, \dot{w}_1 + C(q_1, \dot{q}_1)\, w_1 + \Lambda w_1 = K c_1 \tag{21.8}$$

To analyze the stability of the previous equation, we propose the following Lyapunov function:

$$V_1 = \frac{1}{2} w_1^T M(q_l)\, w_1 \tag{21.9}$$

and its derivative is

$$\dot{V}_1 = \frac{1}{2} w_1^T \dot{M}(q_l)\, w_1 + w_1^T M(q_l)\, \dot{w}_1 \tag{21.10}$$

Equation 21.8 is substituted into Eq. 21.10 to obtain:

$$\dot{V}_1 = \frac{1}{2} r_1^T \dot{M}(q_l)\, w_1 + w_1^T \left(-\Lambda w_1 - C(q_l, \dot{q}_l)\, w_1 + K c_1 \right) \tag{21.11}$$

$$\dot{V}_1 = -w_1^T \Lambda w_1 + w_1^T K c_1 + \frac{1}{2} w_1^T \left(\dot{M}(q_l) - 2\, C(q_l, \dot{q}_l) \right) w_1 \tag{21.12}$$

using the property of matrices $\dot{M}(\mathbf{q}_l) - 2C(\mathbf{q}_l, \dot{\mathbf{q}}_1) = 0$ that is obtained

$$\dot{V}_1 = -w_1^T \Lambda w_1 + w_1^T K c_1 \tag{21.13}$$

So that, if $c_1 = 0$ then $\dot{V}_1 < 0$ and: $r_1 \to 0$ as $t \to 0$. Moreover, since $w_1 = \dot{\tilde{q}}_1 + \Lambda_1 \tilde{q}_1$ is stable, then $\tilde{q}_1, \dot{\tilde{q}}_1 \to 0$ as $t \to \infty$.
Returning to the equation of the general system 21.4, the second line is:

$$\dot{x}_1 = x_2 \tag{21.14}$$

Deriving the Eq. (21.6) gives:

$$\dot{c}_1 = \dot{x}_1 - \dot{\mu}_1 \tag{21.15}$$

$$\dot{c}_1 = x_2 - \dot{\mu}_1 \tag{21.16}$$

we built the control law μ_2 for x_2

$$\mu_2 = -w_1 - \Gamma_2 c_1 + \dot{\mu}_1 \tag{21.17}$$

where Γ_2 is a diagonal matrix of positive gains, defining:

$$c_2 = x_2 - \mu_2 \tag{21.18}$$

we have from 21.19 and 21.17

$$\dot{c}_1 = w_1 - \Gamma_2 c_1 + c_2 \tag{21.19}$$

using the following Lyapunov function:

$$V_2 = V_1 + \frac{1}{2} c_1^T K c_1 \tag{21.20}$$

and its derivative is

$$\dot{V}_2 = \dot{V}_1 + c_1^T K \dot{c}_1 \tag{21.21}$$

we replace $\dot{V}_1$ from equation (21.13) and $\dot{c}_1$ is replaced from the Eq. 21.19

$$\dot{V}_2 = -w_1^T \Gamma w_1 + w_1^T K c_1 + c_1^T K \left(-w_1 - \Gamma_2 c_1 + c_2\right) \tag{21.22}$$

$$\dot{V}_2 = -w_1^T \Gamma w_1 - c_1^T K \Gamma_2 c_1 + c_1^T K c_2 \tag{21.23}$$

We have constructed the control law x_1 and x_2 for lines 1 and 2 of Eq. (21.4), respectively; now the next step is to construct the control law τ for line 3 of the same system of Eq. (21.4), then

$$\dot{c}_2 = \dot{x}_2 - \dot{\mu}_2 \tag{21.24}$$

To construct the control law, the following Lyapunov function is proposed:

$$V_3 = V_2 + \frac{1}{2} c_2^T K J c_2 \tag{21.25}$$

and its derivative is:

$$\dot{V}_3 = \dot{V}_2 + c_2^T K J \dot{c}_2 \tag{21.26}$$

we replace $\dot{V}_2$ from equation (21.23) and $\dot{c_2}$ is replaced from equation (21.24)

$$\dot{V}_3 = -w_1^T \Lambda w_1 - c_1^T K \Gamma_2 c_1 + c_1^T K c_2 + c_2^T K \left(\tau - K\left(x_1 - q_1\right) - J\dot{\mu}_2\right). \tag{21.27}$$

Thus, if we choose a control law as follows:

$$\tau = -c_1 - \Gamma_3 c_2 + J\dot{\mu}_2 + K\left(x_1 - q_1\right) \tag{21.28}$$

where Γ_3 is a diagonal matrix with positive elements, substituting the control law 21.28

$$\dot{V}_3 = -w_1^T \Lambda w_1 - c_1^T K \Gamma_2 c_1 - c_2^T K \Gamma_3 c_2 \leq 0. \tag{21.29}$$

According to the Lyapunov stability analysis, the developed control law guaranties that the equilibrium point $w_1 = 0$, $c_1 = 0$ and $c_2 = 0$ is exponentially asymptotically stable, and $\tilde{q}_l, \dot{\tilde{q}}_l \rightarrow 0$ as $t \rightarrow 0$

21.4 Numerical Results

To develop the desired trajectories of our control system, we obtain the angular position generated by the flexion-extension of the knee and ankle during the gait process, using a motion analyzer system that is presented in the next chapter. The data obtained are stored and transformed into a Fourier equation as follows:

$$q_{dl}(t) = \zeta + \phi_1 \cos(\eta t) + \varphi_1 \sin(\eta t) + \cdots + \phi_{15} \cos(15\eta t) + \varphi_{15} \sin(15\eta t) \tag{21.30}$$

The coefficients of the previous equation depend on the ankle or knee joint to which it belongs, and their values can be seen in Table 21.1.

The desired trajectory q_{dl} is defined for each joint as follows: q_{dlk} for the knee and q_{dla} for the ankle, both, together with the dynamic model from equation (21.2) and the control law from equation (21.28), are entered into a simulation to obtain the results. Figure 21.4 shows the results of the trajectory tracking of the knee, while Fig. 21.5 shows the results of the ankle. In both cases, good performance can be observed.

Table 21.1 Coefficients for the Fourier equation that describes the desired trajectories at the knee and ankle joints in the gait process

Coefficient	Value knee	Value ankle	Coefficient	Value knee	Value ankle
ζ	0.1125	0.04488	η	0.4054	0.4054
ϕ_1	– 0.1697	0.0446	φ_1	0.0850	0.1215
ϕ_2	0.0875	– 0.1257	φ_2	– 0.0957	0.0042
ϕ_3	– 0.0345	– 0.0294	φ_3	0.0839	– 0.0860
ϕ_4	0.0031	0.0935	φ_4	– 0.0672	0.0555
ϕ_5	1.0000	– 0.0433	φ_5	0.0478	– 0.0165
ϕ_6	– 0.0109	0.0214	φ_6	– 0.0263	– 0.0175
ϕ_7	0.0065	0.0079	φ_7	0.0156	0.0332
ϕ_8	– 0.0085	– 0.0242	φ_8	– 0.0077	– 0.0221
ϕ_9	0.0075	0.0177	φ_9	0.0037	– 0.0019
ϕ_{10}	– 0.0075	– 0.0032	φ_{10}	– 0.0034	0.0121
ϕ_{11}	0.0065	– 0.0072	φ_{11}	0.0019	– 0.0132
ϕ_{12}	– 0.0046	0.0084	φ_{12}	0.0004	0.0049
ϕ_{13}	0.0023	– 0.0041	φ_{13}	– 0.0011	0.0033
ϕ_{14}	– 0.0015	– 0.0014	φ_{14}	0.0008	– 0.0033
ϕ_{15}	0.0002	0.0002	φ_{15}	– 0.0002	0.0002

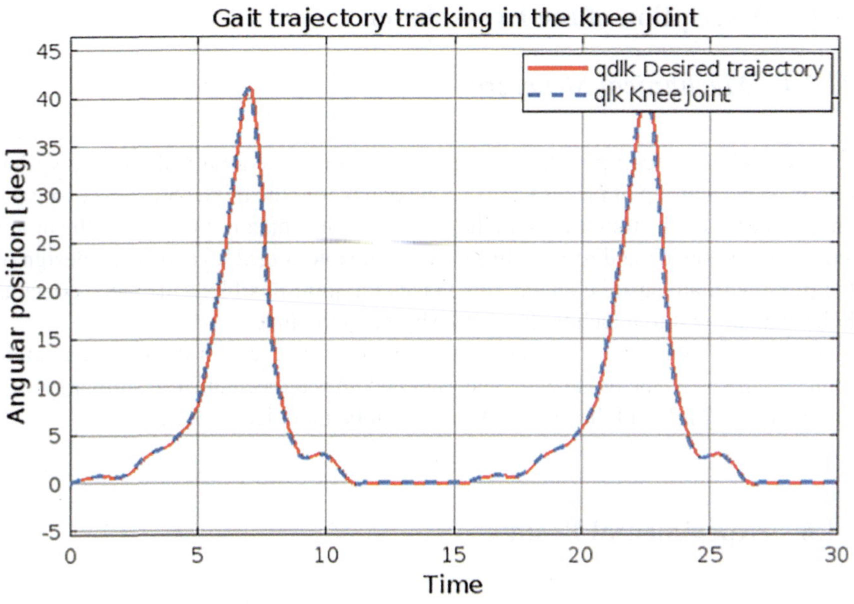

Fig. 21.4 Results of simulation of knee joint trajectory tracking during gait

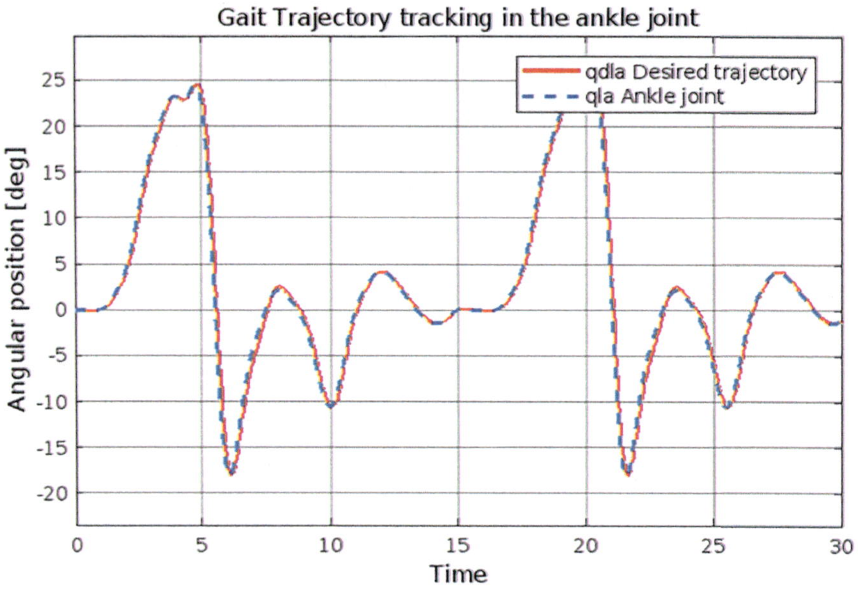

Fig. 21.5 Results of simulation of ankle joint trajectory tracking during gait

21.5 Description of the Exoskeleton

21.5.1 Mechanical Structure

The exoskeleton is composed of two main parts, the knee joint and the ankle joint. For the knee, a group of pieces were designed that hold the thigh and leg, leaving the knee centered on the motor axis. In the same way, the ankle is centered on the motor axis, holding the leg and foot. Both joints are flexible; Fig. 21.6 shows the design of the piece with an elastic element, this makes the joint flexible. This piece contains holes that allow it to attach to the motor shaft and the link.

In Fig. 21.7, we can see the position of the flexible piece in the knee and ankle joints; in this way, the ankle and knee joint becomes a mechanically similar system to that in Fig. 21.2, and the leg exoskeleton can be modeled with Eq. 21.2.

21.6 Experimental Results

To use the exoskeleton as a walking assistant, we must first analyze the walking process.

In Fig. 21.8, it shows the gait cycle, represented at 100% of the movement of the right foot when taking a step, and the angles of flexion and extension at the knee

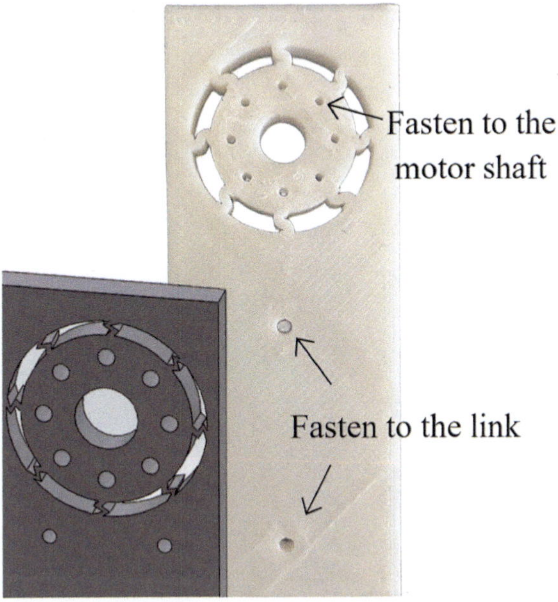

Fig. 21.6 Design and development of a flexible joint that connects the motor to the link

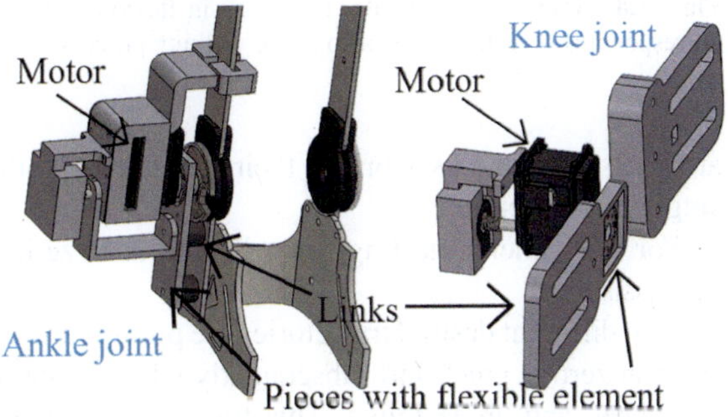

Fig. 21.7 Flexible joints in knee and ankle for the lower limb exoskeleton and their main components: the motor, the flexible piece, and the link

and ankle are observed during this process. This process is divided into two main phases: (1) the swing phase, which lasts approximately 40% of the cycle and is when the foot is in the air swinging, and (2) the support phase, which is the other 60% of the remaining cycle and is when the foot is touching the ground. The graph starts with the angular position at zero degree, which means that the person is standing with both feet together (0% of the cycle). Then it begins to generate angular flexion movements in the knee and ankle without lifting the foot off the ground (from 0 to 30% of the cycle). The right foot begins to take a step and balances to advance (from 30 to 70% of the cycle), a full step with the right-leg, until they return to standing. Finally, the foot touches the ground with its heel and the stance phase begins again (from 70 to 100% of the cycle). This process is repeated until the user wants to stop,

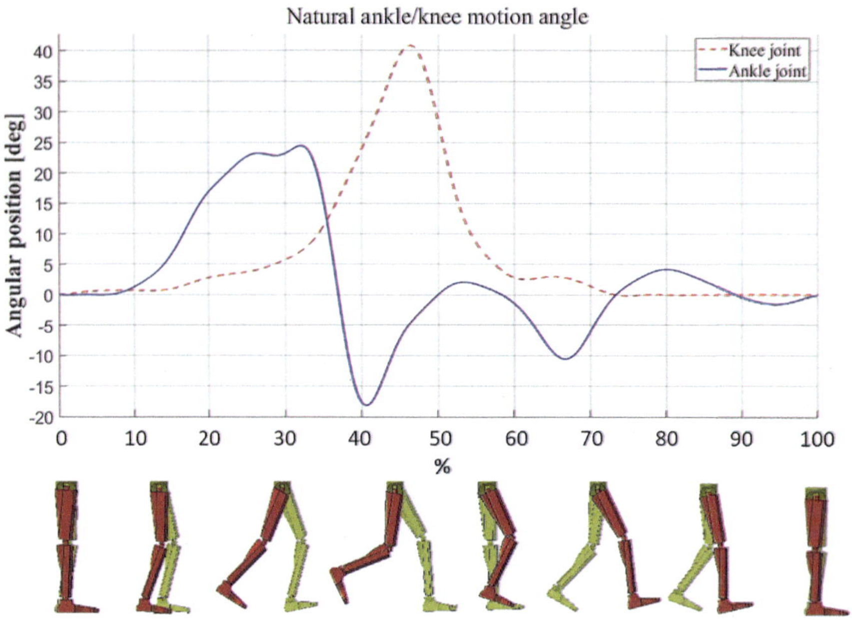

Fig. 21.8 Graph of the angular trajectory in flexion and extension of the knee and hip joints, corresponding to 100% of the step in the walking process

at which point the user brings their feet back together. The figure shows only the single-step process.

For experimental testing, we will first analyze how the exoskeleton works as a gait assistant.

Two different desired trajectories are programmed: (1) Walking trajectory , which starts at zero degrees and subsequently takes the periodic form of the gait cycle for both knee and ankle joints. This trajectory is repeated indefinitely. (2) Stopping trajectory, where the cycle stops repeating and becomes a desired position of zero degrees in both joints for an indefinite time.

The operation is as follows. The user stands with both feet together. To start walking, they must generate a small effort with their ankle and knee, which is reflected in a torque sensed by the flexible joint. This works as a command that activates the walking trajectory. This trajectory will be repeated as long as the person wishes to keep walking. The exoskeleton will assist the user by generating a support torque on their joints autonomously. Finally, when the user wants to stop, they again exert an effort counter to the gait's tracking, which will be sensed by the flexible joints. Generating a command that activates the stopping trajectory, which means bringing the joints of the exoskeleton and the human to the standing position with both feet together.

The results shown below are obtained by experimentally testing the exoskeleton following the walking trajectory for 30 s, which translates to two steps. These tests are performed with the exoskeleton stationary and without the user in position to verify control behavior. Figure 21.9 shows the desired angular trajectory position and the current trajectory of the ankle joint, while Fig. 21.10 shows the knee joint. Both demonstrate good control performance.

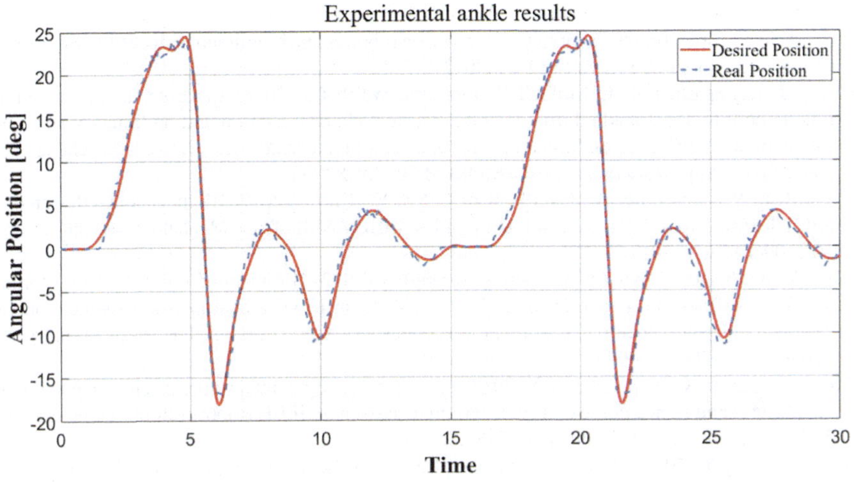

Fig. 21.9 Results of experimental test of ankle joint trajectory tracking during gait

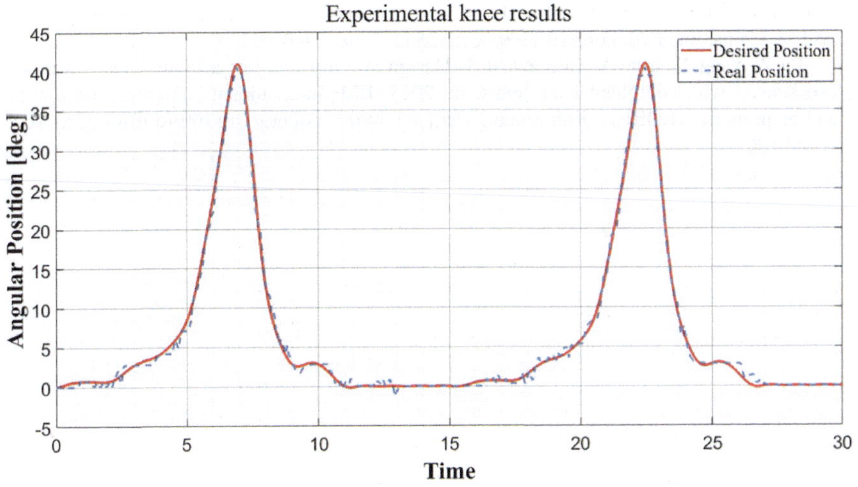

Fig. 21.10 Results of experimental test of knee joint trajectory tracking during gait

References

Centeno-Barreda D, Salazar-Cruz S, López-Gutiérrez R, Rosales-Luengas Y, Lozano R (2024) Lower limb exoskeleton for gait rehabilitation with adaptive nonsingular sliding mode control. Robotica 42(11):3819–3838. https://doi.org/10.1017/S0263574724001668

Chen X, Li D, Han C, Cheng P, Chen Y, Wei L (2022) Virtual prototype design of flexible exoskeleton based on pattern recognition technology. In: International conference on power, intelligent computing and systems (ICPICS), Shenyang, China. https://doi.org/10.1109/ICPICS55264.2022.9873740

Chen C, Zheng D, Peng A, Wang C, Wu X (2013) Flexible design of a wearable lower limb exoskeleton robot. In: International conference on robotics and biomimetics (ROBIO), Shenzhen, China. https://doi.org/10.1109/ROBIO.2013.6739460

Chung J, Heimgartner R, O'Neil CT, Phipps NS, Walsh CJ (2018) ExoBoot, a soft inflatable robotic boot to assist ankle during walking: Design, characterization and preliminary tests. In: International conference on biomedical robotics and biomechatronics (Biorob), Enschede, The Netherlands. https://doi.org/10.1109/BIOROB.2018.8487903

Lee Y, Kim Y-J, Lee J, Lee M, Choi B, Kim J, Park YJ, Choi J (2017) Biomechanical design of a novel flexible exoskeleton for lower extremities. IEEE/ASME Trans Mechatron. https://doi.org/10.1109/TMECH.2017.2718999

Schrade SO, Nager Y, Wu AR, Gassert R, Ijspeert A (2017) Bio-inspired control of joint torque and knee stiffness in a robotic lower limb exoskeleton using a central pattern generator. In: International conference on rehabilitation robotics (ICORR), London, UK. https://doi.org/10.1109/ICORR.2017.8009442

Thakur C, Ogawa K, Tsuji T, Kurita Y (2018) Soft wearable augmented walking suit with pneumatic gel muscles and stance phase detection system to assist gait. IEEE Robot Autom Lett 3(4):3366–3373. https://doi.org/10.1109/LRA.2018.2864355

Wang Y, Geng Y (2025) Design and control of a flexible actuator joint for lower limb exoskeleton robot. In: Asia-Europe conference on cybersecurity, internet of things and soft computing (CITSC), Rimini, Italy. https://doi.org/10.1109/CITSC64390.2025.00102

Wang X, Wen Q, Su G, Xie H (2022) Structure design and flexible connection design of a new exoskeleton robot. In: 6th International conference on robotics and automation sciences (ICRAS), Wuhan, China. https://doi.org/10.1109/ICRAS55217.2022.9842031

Yi S, Fu Z, Yang X, Liao Y, Guo Z (2023) Design and modeling of a lightweight lower limb exoskeleton with compliant knee joints. In: 2023 IEEE International conference on robotics and biomimetics (ROBIO), Koh Samui, Thailand. https://doi.org/10.1109/ROBIO58561.2023.10355018

Chapter 22
An Artificial Intelligence Framework to Calculate the True Depth During the Biomechanical Assessment of General Movements in Neonates

Jose Andres Martinez-Avila and Ruben Fuentes-Alvarez

Abstract General movement assessment (GMA, Prechtl's method) relies on visual evaluation of spontaneous neonatal motion and benefits from objective 3D quantification. However, clinical videos are often monocular and lack metric (true) depth, limiting biomechanical inference. We process clinical videos with a pose-landmark detector (33 points) pipeline and a monocular depth estimator. Inverse depth is converted to true depth via a frame-wise scale recovery fixed by anatomical points (constant bone lengths) and temporal regularization (Gaussian, bilateral, and sliding window smoothing). From the shoulder–elbow–wrist segment, we calculate elbow angles with four estimators (law of cosines, cross product, rotation matrix, and quaternion) and a robust ensemble method. Wrist trajectories reconstructed from angles are compared against a Denavit–Hartenberg (DH) kinematic model. The data consist of nonidentifiable, publicly available neonatal videos (split 70/20/10 train/validation/test); pose thresholds were set to 0.52 for detection/tracking. The ensemble method consistently outperformed individual estimators for trajectory tracking (MAPE range 0.65–6.68% across axes and wrist). The ensemble model obtained a similarity with the DH model of 81.24% (left) and 87.13% (right). The framework converts monocular video into true depth and clinically interpretable kinematics in a lightweight pipeline, providing a reproducible complement to GMA and a foundation for bias-aware neonatal movement analysis.

Keywords Neonatal biomechanics · General movements · True depth · Inverse geometric modeling · Denavit–Hartenberg

J. A. Martinez-Avila · R. Fuentes-Alvarez (✉)
Tecnológico de Monterrey, School of Engineering and Sciences, Mexico city, Mexico
e-mail: joru.fua@tec.mx

J. A. Martinez-Avila
e-mail: A01021993@tec.mx

A. Öchsner (ed.), *Progress in Biomaterials and Biomedical Engineering*, Advanced Structured Materials 249, https://doi.org/10.1007/978-3-032-13551-3_22

22.1 Introduction

General movements assessment (GMA, Prechtl's method) is the foundation of early screening of neurodevelopmental risk in neonates, based on the visual evaluation of spontaneous limb and trunk motion (Einspieler and Prechtl 2005). While clinically useful, a purely observational assessment can be subjective and difficult to scale (Byrne et al., 2017; Hadders-Algra 2021). The creation of 3D kinematic quantification models from routine clinical videos would strengthen GMA by providing measurable evidence of motor patterns over time.

Recent reports have highlighted gestational alterations that may compromise fetal oxygenation and, consequently, neonatal neurodevelopment. In particular, SARS-CoV-2 has been identified in placental tissue even in the absence of active maternal infection (Gajbhiye and Modi 2020); findings include diffuse or focal trophoblast necrosis and chronic placental hypoxia, potentially reducing fetal oxygen supply (Gajbhiye and Modi, 2020; Liu et al., 2022). Such placental pathologies have been associated with subsequent neurological consequences in newborns (Twanow et al., 2022). These findings reinforce the need for a scalable, objective tool capable of capturing subtle deviations in fine movement patterns.

From a technical standpoint, most clinical and training recordings are monocular (lacking true depth), which limits biomechanical interpretation. Without a consistent metric scale, joint angles, segment lengths, and spatial trajectories can become inconsistent across frames and subjects, undermining clinical interpretability and cross-session comparability. Early computational solutions used accelerometry and 2D/pose-based machine learning for neonatal movement analysis (Meinecke et al., 2006; Doroniewicz et al., 2020; Heinze et al., 2010), as well as modern pose-landmark detectors and 3D body models (Lugaresi et al., 2019; Bazarevsky et al., 2020; Xu et al., 2020; Zanfir et al., 2020). However, recovering true depth from monocular data and integrating it into a kinematic analysis pipeline suitable for neonatal GMA remains underexplored (Ranftl et al., 2021; Lasinger et al., 2019).

This work introduces an artificial intelligence framework that converts monocular neonatal videos into metric true depth and clinically interpretable kinematics as a complementary tool during the GMA. The proposed pipeline uses a pose-landmark detector with a monocular depth estimator, a subsequent scale-recovery module that ensures near-constant bone lengths and finally, a temporal regularization module that reduces ambiguity. On the recovered true geometry, we calculate upper-limb elbow angles using four methodologies (cross product, rotational matrix, quaternion, and law of cosines) and a combination of these via a robust ensemble method. We then evaluate the generated trajectory against a Denavit-Hartenberg (DH) kinematic model (Spong et al., 2020), using videos split 70/20/10 (train/validation/test) and pose thresholds fixed at 0.52 for pose detection and tracking. Beyond kinematic accuracy, the framework supports transparent, bias-aware development for clinical AI (Nazer et al., 2023; Fuentes-Alvarez et al., 2022).

This document is organized as follows. Section 2 discusses the general problem of the evaluation of general movements, focusing on the kinematic modeling of a newborn using DH parameters and how inverse geometric modeling (IGM) techniques will benefit GMA. Section 3 presents the mathematical modeling tools and the integration processes used to approach the problem. Section 4 presents the data obtained from the proposed framework, covering the law of cosines, cross product projections, rotational matrix calculation via skew matrix, quaternions, and an assembly algorithm. Section 5 presents concluding remarks and future work.

22.2 Problem Statement

The quantification of neonatal general movements (GMs) from monocular video is addressed by recovering true depth and generating upper-limb kinematics with a four-revolute (4R) model shown in Fig. 22.1. For each frame t, let the pose pipeline module calculate 2D landmarks and relative depth for the shoulder $u_1(t)$, elbow $u_2(t)$, wrist $u_3(t)$, and hip $u_4(t)$, all expressed in a single virtual coordinate space. Because monocular depth is scale-ambiguous, a per-frame positive scale $s_t > 0$ that maps relative to true coordinates. With these metric joint positions, the IGM estimates the shoulder–elbow–wrist angle $\theta(t)$ from standard cross- and dot-product formulations, or via the law of cosines when only segment norms are required. This setup enables non-invasive, video-based analysis of neonatal movement and supports quantitative comparison against the DH kinematic model (Abedi and Shoushtari, 2012; Contreras-Tenorio et al., 2021).

22.3 Materials and Methods

This section describes the artificial intelligence framework that converts monocular neonatal videos into true depth and upper limb kinematics suitable for general movements assessment. From each RGB frame, the pipeline extracts 2D pose landmarks and relative depth, recovers a per-frame metric scale, reconstructs 3D joints coordinates, and estimates the shoulder–elbow–wrist (S–E–W) angle. Then validates the outputs against a DH kinematic model, Fig. 22.1 shows the kinematic convection used throughout the project: a four-revolute upper-limb model with a quasi-rigid torso.

The workflow in Fig. 22.2 consists of five stages: (1) Video acquisition and preprocessing. (2) Pose-landmark detection and monocular depth estimation. (3) Metric scale recovery that maps relative depth into true depth. (4) S-E-W angle estimation and wrist-trajectory reconstruction. (5) Validation against a DH kinematic model (trajectory and angle). Subsections that follow detail the DH formulation, pipeline implementation, data and preprocessing, angle calculation, wrist coordinate recovery, and validation.

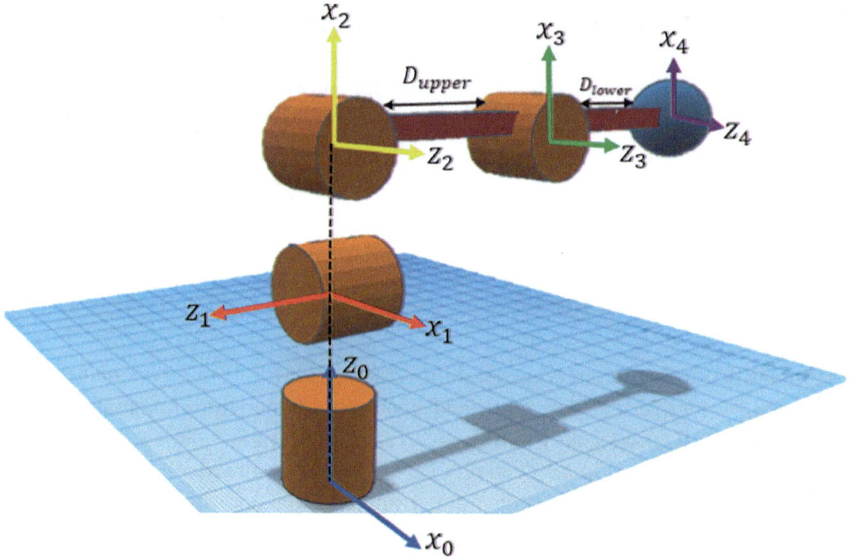

Fig. 22.1 A kinematic chain with four-revolute joints, three of them at the shoulder and one at the elbow. The hand is rigidly linked to the distal segment of the chain. Frames define the DH convention used in this work, with link lengths corresponding to the upper arm (shoulder–elbow) and forearm (elbow–wrist). The torso is considered quasi-rigid during spontaneous general movement

22.3.1 Denavit–Hartenberg's Modeling of a Newborn

DH kinematic analysis is a widely used methodology to characterize articulated motion in robotics and has been reliably applied to human movement modeling and joint localization (Fuentes-Alvarez et al., 2022; Abedi and Shoushtari, 2012; Contreras-Tenorio et al., 2021). Consistent with the limited torso motion during spontaneous neonatal general movements, the upper limb is represented as a 4R chain: three revolute joints at the shoulder and one at the elbow, with the hand rigidly linked to the distal portion. We consider the anatomical link lengths upper arm (shoulder–elbow) and forearm (elbow–wrist). The corresponding DH parameters are summarized in Table 22.1. Forward kinematics are obtained by chaining the elementary DH transforms; the homogeneous transformation from the shoulder base (frame 0) to the wrist (frame 4) is $H_4^0 = A_1\, A_2\, A_3\, A_4$ where each A_i is the standard DH transform defined by the quadruple $(\theta_i, a_i, d_i, \alpha_i)$ (Spong et al., 2020). Using the parametrization in Table 1 and the shorthand $C_n = \cos q_n, \quad S_n = \sin q_n$, we obtain the wrist orientation and position as joint angle and link lengths. In our evaluation we defined Eq. (22.1) functions as a DH kinematic reference to check the internal consistency of the IGM reconstructions.

$$H_4^0 = A_1\, A_2\, A_3\, A_4 \tag{22.1}$$

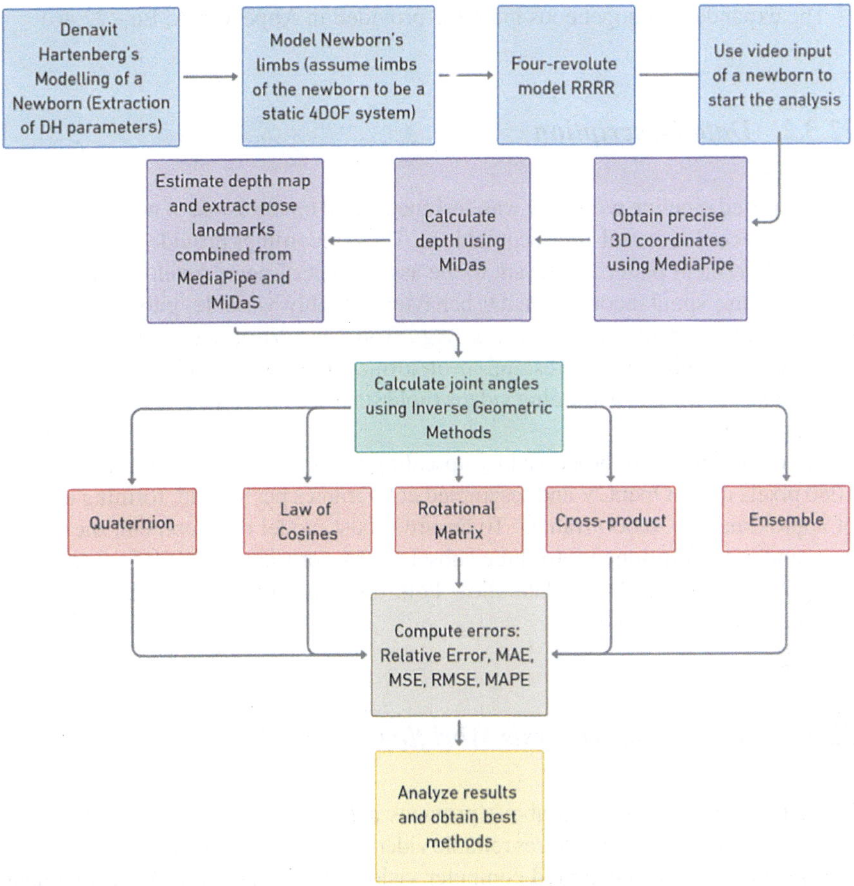

Fig. 22.2 Workflow of the proposed neonatal movement analysis pipeline. The system integrates MediaPipe for 2D landmark extraction and MiDaS for monocular depth estimation, followed by the combination of results, filtering, and coordinate normalization, enabling accurate 3D reconstruction of the neonate's movements

Table 22.1 Denavit–Hartenberg parameters of a neonate's limb

Reference points	ϑ_i	a_i	d_i	α_i
H_1^0	$q_1{}^*$	0	0	$\frac{\pi}{2}$
H_2^1	$q_2{}^*$	0	0	$-\frac{\pi}{2}$
H_3^2	$q_3{}^*$	D_lower	0	0
H_4^3	$q_4{}^*$	D_upper	0	0

The expanded homogeneous matrix is provided in Appendix A, Eq. (22.46)

22.3.2 Data Description

The proposed pipeline workflow was designed based on the usage of neonatal videos, either prerecorded or real-time acquisitions. These recordings provide detailed examples of movement patterns relevant to the assessment of neurodevelopmental disorders. Because spontaneous neonatal behavior is highly variable, publicly available training videos from online sources (e.g., YouTube, Vimeo, etc.) were included regardless of their original resolution or format. For the classification of general movements, two medical training videos (gold standard) were selected as the primary reference material.

All recordings were processed by upscaling to a minimum resolution of 1920 × 1080 pixels using OpenCV and resampled at 60 frames per second, forming datasets of approximately 36,000 frames. To ensure robust model development, the dataset was randomly partitioned into three subsets: 70% for training, 20% for validation, and 10% for testing. These data allow both unbiased parameter optimization and final performance assessment.

22.3.3 Movement Analysis Workflow Integration

The DH approach described above provides a kinematic reference model, but its practical implementation requires reliable video-based extraction of joint trajectories. For this purpose, we integrated computer vision and depth-estimation components into a unified workflow shown in Fig. 22.2. The core of the framework is the pose-landmark detection task from MediaPipe (Lugaresi et al., 2019), an open-source library that can estimate 33 three-dimensional human body keypoints (Bazarevsky et al., 2020). This task is built from the BlazePose lightweight convolutional neural network (CNN) architecture (Bazarevsky et al., 2020), and the GHUM 3D human shape model (Xu et al., 2020; Zanfir et al., 2020).

The preliminary tests, only using the pose landmarks task, revealed systematic errors caused by the lack of accurate depth information. To reduce this limitation, we incorporated MiDaS, a monocular depth-estimation model trained on large-scale datasets to produce dense inverse depth maps (Ranftl et al., 2021; Lasinger et al., 2019). The combination of MediaPipe for landmark detection and MiDaS for depth recovery results in a pipeline capable of producing temporally consistent three-dimensional coordinates.

The proposed workflow is organized into two main functions. The first calculates the spatial coordinates (x, y, z) of the relevant joints (shoulder, elbow, wrist, and hip), while the second estimates the S-E-W angle. Each function is executed through sequential stages, including video preparation, initial landmark processing, wrist coordinate computation, post-processing, error analysis, and trajectory visualization. These stages are detailed in the following subsections.

22.3.4 Video Preparation and Processing

The video preparation stage ensured that only preprocessed recordings meeting the minimum spatial and temporal criteria passed to the processing stage. Using MediaPipe, a bounding box was defined around the newborn by obtaining the maximum left and right values of the wrists, ankles, and eyebrows along the x and y axes, with an additional 25% margin. Each frame was cropped following this guideline, and the resulting recording was passed to the neonatal arm detection pipeline illustrated in Fig. 22.3.

The processing stage began by converting each frame into an RGB image, and then it was analyzed by the depth estimation and pose detection modules. The depth-estimation module initializes the MiDaS model, which produced an inverse depth-estimation map refined using the following filters:

1. Gaussian-blur filter: reduced high-frequency noise by averaging neighbors' pixel values:

$$G(x, y) = \frac{1}{2\pi\sigma^2} e^{-\frac{x^2+y^2}{2\sigma^2}} \tag{22.2}$$

where σ is the kernel's standard deviation, and x, y are the pixel offsets.

2. Bilateral filtering: smooth out regions of pixels while preserving edges:

$$I' = \sum_{i \in \Omega} \frac{1}{W} e^{-\frac{(x_i-x)^2+(y_i-y)^2}{2\sigma_d^2}} e^{-\frac{|I_i-I|^2}{2\sigma_r^2}} I_i \tag{22.3}$$

where I is the pixel intensity, Ω the local neighborhood, and σ_d, σ_r the spatial and range standard deviations.

3. Temporal Smoothing: reduced frame-to-frame fluctuations by averaging over a temporal window:

$$D'(t) = \frac{1}{N} \sum_{i=0}^{N-1} D(t-i) \tag{22.4}$$

where $D(t)$ is the depth map at frame t, and N the window size.

After the application of the filtering stage, the pose detection stage began using the MediaPipe landmark module. For a reliable operation, this module requires two thresholds: minimum detection confidence, which discards landmarks below a given probability, and minimum tracking confidence, which ensures temporal continuity

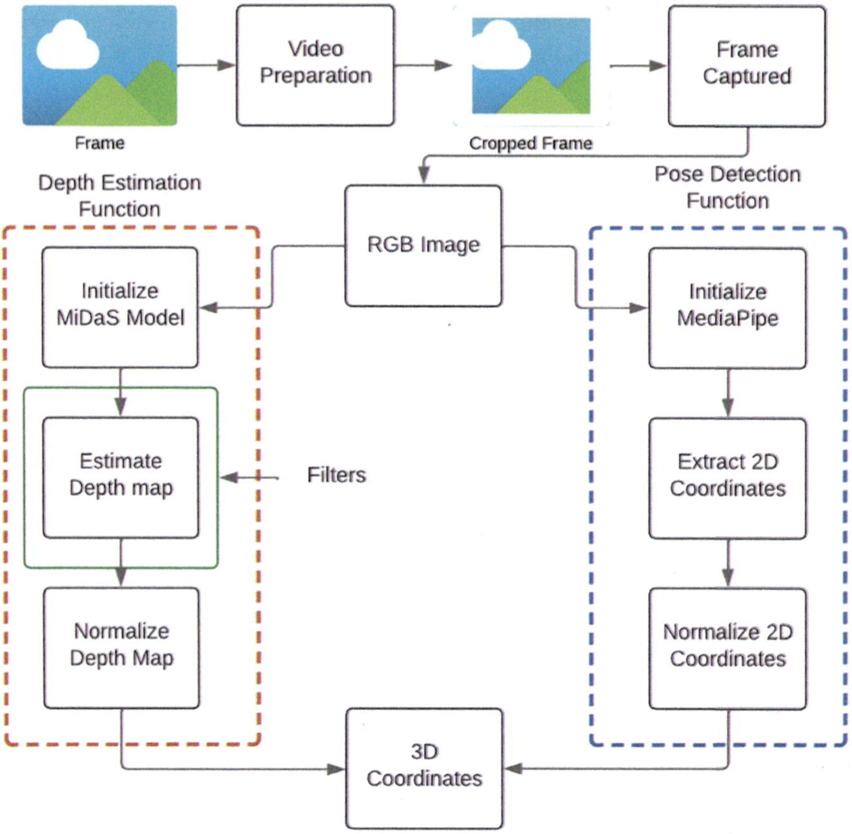

Fig. 22.3 Workflow of the neonatal arm detection pipeline. MediaPipe extracts 2D coordinates while MiDaS estimates monocular depth. Both outputs are filtered, normalized, and integrated to provide consistent 3D coordinates

by freezing landmark updates when their confidence score falls below the threshold. Both parameters were set to 0.52 in our solution.

All values obtained from the depth estimation and pose detection modules were then normalized to fit the frame dimension. First, the inverse depth maps generated by MiDaS were converted into regular depth maps using the Eq. (22.5).

$$\text{regular depth map} = \frac{1.0}{\text{inverse depth map} + \varepsilon} \tag{22.5}$$

where ε is a small constant introduced to prevent any division by zero. Next, each depth value at a pixel [*x*, *y*] was scaled to the [0, 1] interval:

$$z\ \text{normalized} = \frac{\text{depth}[y, x] - \min(\text{depth})}{\max(\text{depth}) - \min(\text{depth})} \tag{22.6}$$

Finally, the normalized values were scaled to fit the image dimensions using:

$$z' = z \text{ normalized} \cdot \text{width} \tag{22.7}$$

Similarly, the landmark coordinates were scaled to the frame dimensions and clamped to ensure they remained inside the image boundaries, as shown in the following Eqs. (22.8–22.9).

$$x' = \min(\max(x \cdot \text{width}, 0), \text{width} - 1) \tag{22.8}$$

$$y' = \min(\max(y \cdot \text{height}, 0), \text{height} - 1) \tag{22.9}$$

This normalization process ensured that both spatial and depth information were expressed consistently across all frames, allowing a robust integration in the subsequent angle estimation stage.

22.3.5 Angle Calculation

From the normalized x, y, and z coordinates, four joint vectors were defined: shoulder u_1, elbow u_2, wrist u_3, and hip u_4. These vectors enable the calculation of the angle S-E-W.

$$u_1 = (x_1, y_1, z_1) \tag{22.10}$$

$$u_2 = (x_2, y_2, z_2) \tag{22.11}$$

$$u_3 = (x_3, y_3, z_3) \tag{22.12}$$

$$u_4 = (x_4, y_4, z_4) \tag{22.13}$$

To obtain the angle S-E-W θ, we construct the segment vectors from shoulder to elbow, Eq. (22.14), and elbow to wrist, Eq. (22.15), and then estimate θ using five complementary methods.

$$u_{se} = u_2 - u_1 \tag{22.14}$$

$$u_{ew} = u_3 - u_2 \tag{22.15}$$

The first method, the law of cosines, calculates the angle using basic trigonometry. In Eq. (22.16) is shown the formula and Eq. (22.17) shows the equation solved for

θ, where a corresponds to the length of the upper arm (shoulder to elbow), b to the length of the forearm (elbow to wrist), and c the length from the shoulder to the wrist, and θ the angle S–E–W.

$$c^2 = a^2 + b^2 - 2ab\cos(\theta) \tag{22.16}$$

$$\theta = \arccos\left(\frac{a^2 + b^2 - c^2}{2ab}\right) \tag{22.17}$$

The second method, cross product, uses the same segment vectors defined above, u_{se} and u_{ew}. The S–E–W angle is obtained by calculating the cross product and dot product of the vectors, as is shown in Eq. (22.18).

$$\theta = \arctan 2(|u_{se} \times u_{ew}|, u_{se} \cdot u_{ew}) \tag{22.18}$$

The third method, rotational matrix, uses the vectors defined above in Eqs. (22.14–22.15), and then they are normalized using Eqs. (22.19–22.20).

$$\overline{u_{se}} = \frac{u_{se}}{|u_{se}|} \tag{22.19}$$

$$\overline{u_{ew}} = \frac{u_{ew}}{|u_{ew}|} \tag{22.20}$$

The outcome of employing the normalized vectors in Eq. (22.21) is the cross product value, representing the axis of rotation. The magnitude of the cross product, Eq. (22.22), is equal to the sine of the angle θ, and the cosine of the angle θ is equivalent to the dot product, Eq. (22.23).

$$w = \overline{u_{se}} \times \overline{u_{ew}} \tag{22.21}$$

$$s = |w| \tag{22.22}$$

$$c = \overline{u_{se}} \cdot \overline{u_{ew}} \tag{22.23}$$

Then a skew-symmetric matrix **W**, Eq. (22.24), is constructed from the coordinates of the vector in Eq. (22.21). Furthermore, the rotation matrix **R** can be calculated using the identity matrix **I**, the skew-symmetric matrix **W**, and the scalar values c and s as represented in Eq. (22.25). Finally, the angle θ can be extracted using Eq. (22.26), in which the trace is the sum of the diagonal elements.

$$\mathbf{W} = \begin{bmatrix} 0 & -w_z & w_y \\ w_z & 0 & -w_x \\ -w_y & w_x & 0 \end{bmatrix} \tag{22.24}$$

$$R = I + W + W^2 \frac{1 - c}{s^2} \tag{22.25}$$

$$\theta = \arccos\left(\frac{\text{trace}(R) - 1}{2}\right) \tag{22.26}$$

The fourth method, quaternion, involves using quaternions to represent the rotation between two vectors. Like the previous methods, the vectors used are the ones defined earlier in Eqs. (22.14–22.15). Then they are normalized as in Eqs. (22.19–22.20). After normalizing the vectors, the dot product of the vectors is calculated using Eq. (22.27). Then the quaternion **q** is calculated using Eq. (22.28). Finally, the angle θ can be calculated using the scalar part of the quaternion q_0 due to the half-angle representation of quaternions as shown in Eq. (22.29).

$$d = u_{se} \cdot u_{ew} \tag{22.27}$$

$$\mathbf{q} = \begin{cases} \left[0, \overrightarrow{u_{es\,\text{norm}}} \times \overrightarrow{u_{we\,\text{norm}}}\right] & \text{if } d < -0.999999 \\ [1, 0, 0, 0] & \text{if } d > 0.999999 \\ \left[\sqrt{(1+d)*2}/2, \frac{\overrightarrow{u_{es\,\text{norm}}} \times \overrightarrow{u_{we\,\text{norm}}}}{\sqrt{(1+d)*2}}\right] & \text{otherwise} \end{cases} \tag{22.28}$$

$$\theta = 2 \cdot \arccos(q_0) \tag{22.29}$$

The fifth method, the ensemble, combines the other four methods to achieve a more robust and accurate angle estimation. The method uses the angle values obtained by the other four and averages the results to obtain a new angle θ. Eq. (22.30) represents the average of the results.

$$\theta_{\text{ensemble}} = \frac{1}{4}\left(\theta_{\text{cosines}} + \theta_{\text{cross}} + \theta_{\text{rotation}} + \theta_{\text{quaternion}}\right) \tag{22.30}$$

For posture context relative to the trunk (not a replacement for the elbow angle), we include left/right hip orientation obtained from the inter-hip vector as shown in Eqs. (22.31–22.32).

$$\theta_{lh} = \arctan\left(\frac{y_{4l} - y_{4r}}{x_{4l} - x_{4r}}\right) \tag{22.31}$$

$$\theta_{rh} = \arctan\left(\frac{y_{4r} - y_{4l}}{x_{4r} - x_{4l}}\right) \tag{22.32}$$

22.3.6 Wrist Coordinate Calculation

The subsequent stage of the newborn arm detection pipeline focused on reconstructing the three-dimensional wrist position using the previously estimated S-E-W angle. Accurate wrist localization is critical to ensure that the angular measurements can be translated into meaningful biomechanical assessments.

The length of the forearm L was first determined from the shoulder–elbow segment in Eq. (22.14) and calculated using Eq. (22.33).

$$L = |u_{se}| \tag{22.33}$$

Two complementary approaches were then implemented. The first approach, the S–E–W angle θ, was directly applied to obtain the 3D wrist coordinates relative to the elbow position (x_2, y_2, z_2) using Eqs. (22.34–22.36).

$$x_3' = x_2 + L\cos(\theta) \tag{22.34}$$

$$y_3' = y_2 + L\sin(\theta) \tag{22.35}$$

$$z_3' = z_2 \tag{22.36}$$

The second approach incorporated the hip orientation angles θ_{lh} (left hip) and θ_{rh} (right hip) to contextualize the arm relative to trunk posture. The adjusted coordinates were obtained using Eqs. (22.37–22.41).

$$x_{3l} = x_{2l} + L\cos\theta \ \ \cos\theta_{lh} \tag{22.37}$$

$$x_{3r} = x_{2r} + L\cos\theta \ \ \cos\theta_{rh} \tag{22.38}$$

$$y_{3l} = y_{2l} + L\sin\theta \ \ \cos\theta_{lh} \tag{22.39}$$

$$y_{3r} = y_{2r} + L\sin\theta \ \ \cos\theta_{rh} \tag{22.40}$$

$$z_3 \ = z_2 \tag{22.41}$$

Both methods yielded systematic offsets when compared against the raw extracted wrist coordinates. To eliminate this bias, the average difference between calculated and original coordinates was subtracted. The corrected positions were obtained with Eqs. (22.42–22.43).

$$x'_{\text{method}} = x_{\text{method}} - \left(\overline{x_{\text{method}}} - \overline{x_{\text{original}}}\right) \tag{22.42}$$

$$y'_{\text{method}} = y_{\text{method}} - \left(\overline{y_{\text{method}}} - \overline{y_{\text{original}}}\right) \tag{22.43}$$

This adjustment ensured that the reconstructed wrist trajectories, whether corrected for hip orientation or not, remained aligned with the observed data and suitable for subsequent diagnostic evaluation.

22.3.7 *Validation*

The accuracy of the newborn arm movement detection pipeline was assessed by comparing the reconstructed wrist coordinates with the reference positions provided by the Denavit–Hartenberg model from Eq. ((22.46). For each video frame, the IGM output was directly matched against the DH-based ground truth. This enabled the computation of a frame-wise error for the planar coordinates (x, y), quantifying the deviation introduced by the pipeline with Eq. (22.44).

$$\text{error}_{\text{frame}} = \sqrt{(x_{IGM} - x_{DH})^2 + (y_{IGM} - y_{DH})^2} \tag{22.44}$$

This metric quantified the deviation introduced by the pipeline at the pixel level, providing a straightforward measure of the viability of the proposed IGM solution. Beyond frame-wise evaluation, overall accuracy was summarized using the mean absolute percentage error (MAPE), which normalizes deviations across different magnitudes of wrist trajectories.

As illustrated in Fig. 22.5, certain frames displayed clear outliers, such as frame 1, where chaotic or abnormal neonatal movements produced large variations in amplitude and speed. Outliers were systematically identified as frames where the error exceeded three standard deviations above the mean. Such cases were excluded after comparison with the DH reference, ensuring that only physiologically consistent movements were retained in the analysis.

Overall, this validation step established the consistency of the proposed method with biomechanical ground truth, while also providing a robust mechanism for automatically filtering noisy or pathological data. This guarantees that the reconstructed S–E–W angles and wrist trajectories remain clinically interpretable.

22.4 Results

After completing the newborn arm movement detection pipeline, the accuracy of the five angle estimation methods was assessed through trajectory tracking of the reconstructed wrist coordinates. Figures 22.4, 22.5, 22.6, 22.7, and 22.8 illustrate the relationship between frame number and pixel position for both wrists on the x and y axes.

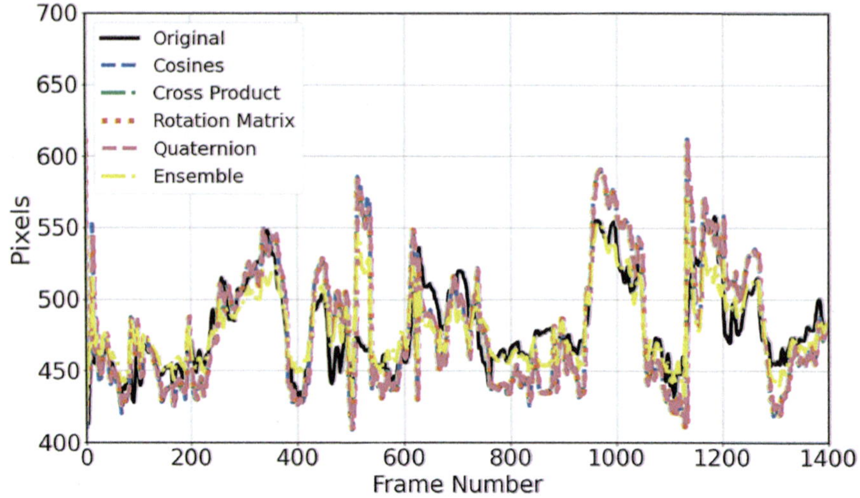

Fig. 22.4 Trajectory tracking of the left wrist x coordinate. The ensemble method aligns most closely with the MediaPipe reference, showing no outliers across frames

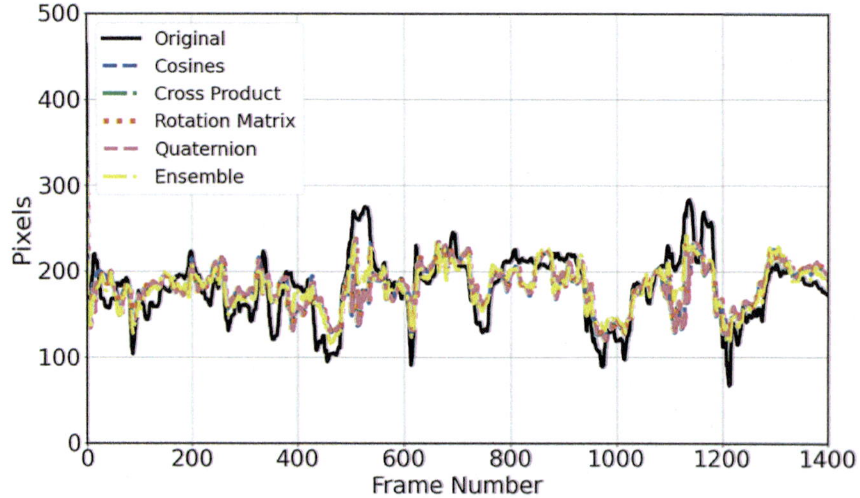

Fig. 22.5 Trajectory tracking of the left wrist y coordinate. An initialization outlier is observed in frame 1, while the ensemble method maintains the highest accuracy

For the left wrist x coordinate from Fig. 22.4, the ensemble method achieved the closest match to the MediaPipe reference, with values constrained between 431.5 and 572 pixels and no evident outliers. For the left wrist y coordinate from Fig. 22.5, the pixel range extended from 116.8 to 357.4 pixels. An outlier appeared in the first frame, caused by initialization effects of the MediaPipe tracker (lack of prior

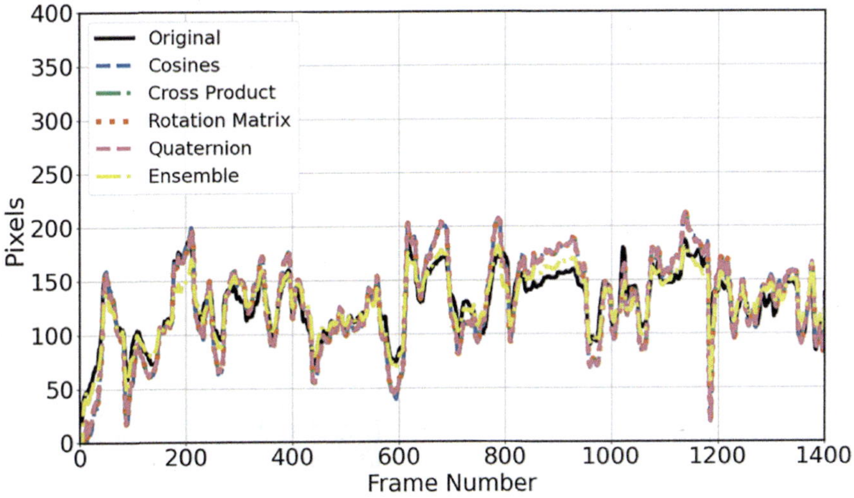

Fig. 22.6 Trajectory tracking of the right wrist x coordinate. All methods converge smoothly, with no apparent outliers

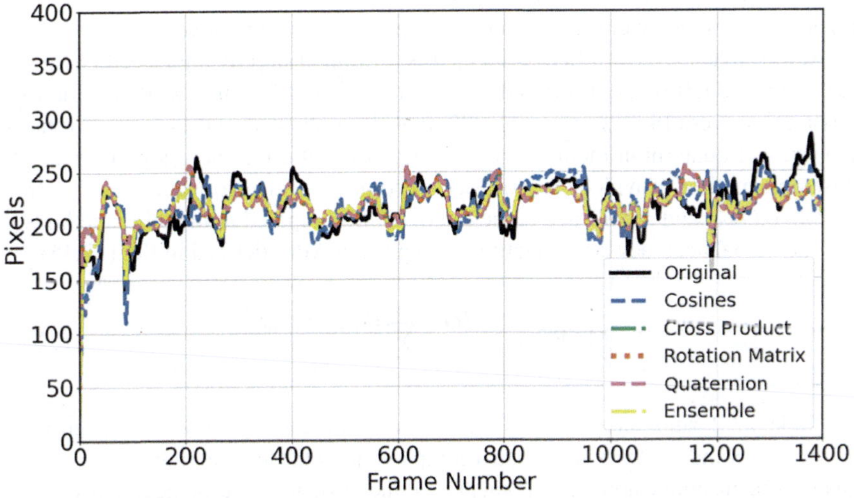

Fig. 22.7 Trajectory tracking of the right wrist y coordinate. The ensemble method demonstrates superior stability across the evaluated range

frame history) and the relatively low 52% threshold set for detection and tracking confidence.

The right wrist trajectories confirmed these observations. For the x coordinate from Fig. 22.6, the range extended from 0 to 182.3 pixels with smooth convergence

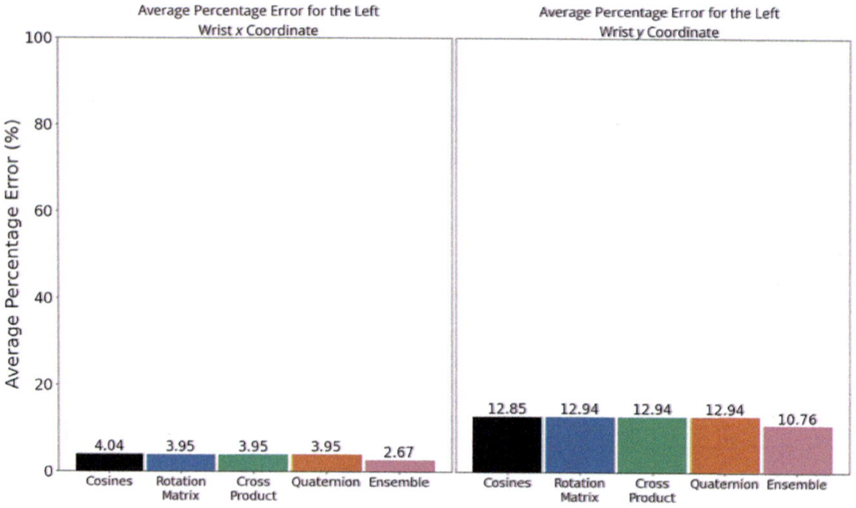

Fig. 22.8 MAPE comparison for left wrist x and y coordinates, highlighting ensemble superiority

across all methods. For the y coordinate from Fig. 22.7, values spanned 22.6–243.5 pixels, again with the ensemble method outperforming alternatives

Across all tests, the law of cosines method exhibited slightly higher errors. Specifically, for the left wrist, it reached 4.03% in x and 12.85% in y, while for the right wrist, errors were 14.39% in x and 5.92% in y. By contrast, the cross product, rotation matrix, and quaternion methods generated consistent errors across both axes. The ensemble method provided the most stable estimates, with error values ranging from 0.65 to 6.68%, and an average reduction of 2.7% compared to the other methods.

The global accuracy was quantified using the MAPE, defined in Eq. (22.45).

$$\text{MAPE} = \left(\frac{100}{n}\right)\sum_{i=1}^{n}\left|\frac{y_{\text{true}}^{(i)} - y_{\text{pred}}^{(i)}}{y_{\text{true}}^{(i)}}\right| \tag{22.45}$$

Table 22.2 summarizes the MAPE values for each method and coordinate. Figures 22.8 and 22.9 provide a visual comparison for the left and right wrists, respectively. The ensemble approach again proved the most accurate, achieving accuracies of:

- 97.33% for the left wrist x coordinate.
- 89.24% for the left wrist y coordinate.
- 92.3% for the right wrist x coordinate.
- 94.73% for the right wrist y coordinate.

Validated against the q parameters from the DH model from Eq. ((22.46), the overall system achieved accuracies of 81.24% for the left wrist and 87.13% for the right wrist, confirming reliable kinematic tracking in neonatal movements.

Table 22.2 MAPE for wrist coordinates

Metric	Left wrist cosines	Left wrist rotation matrix	Left wrist cross product	Left wrist quaternion	Left wrist ensemble	Right wrist cosines	Right wrist rotation matrix	Right wrist cross product	Right wrist quaternion	Right wrist ensemble
MAPE X	4.0393	3.9507	3.9507	3.9507	**2.6669**	14.3914	13.8615	13.8615	13.8615	**7.7025**
MAPE Y	12.8512	12.9373	12.9373	12.9373	**10.7563**	5.9234	5.8882	5.8882	5.8882	**5.267**

Units: % (MAPE).

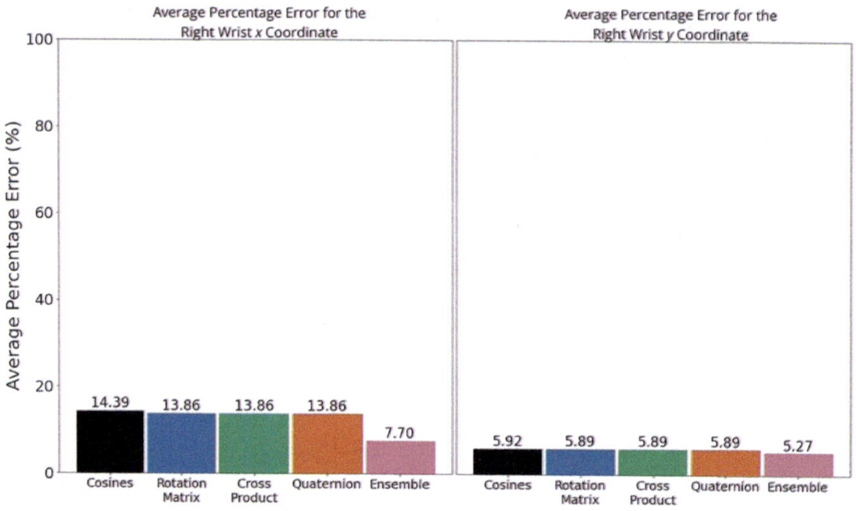

Fig. 22.9 MAPE comparison for right wrist x and y coordinates, confirming ensemble as the most accurate method

22.5 Conclusions

In this work, we presented the development of an inverse geometric model that combines open-source frameworks (BlazePose and MiDaS) with multiple angle calculation approaches. Four different methods (law of cosines, cross product, rotational matrix, and quaternion) were implemented and compared, demonstrating overall consistency. The law of cosines showed higher errors than the other three methods. Building upon this analysis, a fifth method was introduced, the Ensemble approach. By averaging the results of the four individual methods, the Ensemble achieved superior performance, with an average error reduction of 2.7%. The Ensemble method obtained accuracies of:

- 97.33% for the left wrist x coordinate.
- 89.24% for the left wrist y coordinate.
- 92.3% for the right wrist x coordinate.
- 94.73% for the right wrist y coordinate.

To provide biomechanical ground truth, a DH model of the neonatal upper body was constructed. This model effectively characterized upper-limb kinematics and enabled validation of the IGM pipeline. The validation against DH-derived joint parameters confirmed accuracies of 81.24% for the left limb and 87.13% for the right limb. The DH model also supported the representation of each arm as an independent four-degree-of-freedom system linked to a static torso, offering a reliable reference for neonatal movement analysis.

Overall, the proposed IGM model demonstrated the ability to capture spontaneous moderate-speed limb movements and patterns that are often difficult for clinicians to assess visually. The combination of vision-based algorithms and biomechanical modeling provides a robust framework for early detection of neurodevelopmental disorders, delivering clinically relevant insights into neonatal motor behavior.

22.5.1 Future Work

Future work will focus on improving both the accuracy and the clinical applicability of the proposed method by integrating it into mixed reality (MR) devices. These devices are typically equipped with depth sensors, which would allow direct and precise measurement of spatial distances, thereby surpassing the approximations obtained through the MiDaS model. Incorporating native depth sensing is expected to significantly improve the robustness of the system.

Moreover, embedding the solution into a 5G-enabled infrastructure would enable real-time video streaming and analysis, allowing clinicians to access immediate kinematic feedback during patient assessments. The combination of MR technology with live data processing has the potential to provide an immersive and interactive diagnostic environment, where physicians can visualize neonatal movements in three dimensions with high temporal resolution.

This integration could lead to more accurate pre-diagnosis, improving the detection of subtle movement abnormalities that are often overlooked during conventional observation. Additionally, it would expand the clinical understanding of early neurological dysfunctions, ultimately improving medical decision-making and supporting timely intervention strategies.

Acknowledgements The authors gratefully acknowledge the support of Tecnológico de Monterrey (School of Engineering and Sciences). This work also received partial support from SECiHTI under project CUV: 2166033. The funders had no role in study design, data collection and analysis, decision to publish, or preparation of the manuscript.

Appendix

The explicit homogeneous transform from the shoulder base (frame 0) to the wrist (frame 4), $\mathbf{H}_4^0$, expanding Eq. (22.1), is provided below for reproducibility. We adopt the shorthand $C_n = \cos q_n$ and $S_n = \sin q_n$, with link lengths D_{upper} and D_{lower} as defined earlier.

$$H_4{}^0 = \begin{bmatrix} -C_4(S_1S_3 - C_1C_2C_3) - S_4(C_3S_1 + C_1C_2C_3) & -C_1S_2 & -C_1S_2 & D_{\text{upper}}C_1C_2C_3 - D_{\text{lower}}C_4(S_1S_3 - C_1C_2C_3) - D_{\text{lower}}S_4(C_3S_1 + C_1C_2C_3) - D_{\text{upper}}S_1S_3) \\ C_4(C_1S_3 + C_2C_3S_1) + S_4(C_1C_3 - C_2S_1S_3) & -S_1S_2 & -S_1S_2 & D_{\text{lower}}S_4(C_1C_3 - C_2S_1S_3) + D_{\text{upper}}C_1S_3 + D_{\text{lower}}C_4(C_1C_3 + C_2C_3S_1) + D_{\text{upper}}C_2C_3S_1 \\ C_{3+4}S_2 & -S_{3+4}S_2 & C_2 & S_2(D_{\text{lower}}C_{3+4} + D_{\text{upper}}C_3) \\ 0 & 0 & 0 & 1 \end{bmatrix} \tag{22.46}$$

All symbols follow the conventions introduced in Sect. III—Denavit–Hartenberg's Modeling of a Newborn.

References

Abedi P, Shoushtari AL (2012) Modelling and simulation of human-like movements for humanoid robots. In: ICINCO, vol 1, pp 342–346. https://doi.org/10.5220/0004094903420346

Bazarevsky V, Grishchenko I, Raveendran K, Zhu T, Zhang F, Grundmann M (2020) BlazePose: on-device real-time body pose tracking. arXiv:2006.10204

Byrne R, Noritz G, Maitre NL (2017) NCH early developmental group: implementation of early diagnosis and intervention guidelines for cerebral palsy in a high-risk infant follow-up clinic. Pediatr Neurol 76:66–71. https://doi.org/10.1016/j.pediatrneurol.2017.08.002

Contreras-Tenorio E, Kardasch-Nava I, De Salceda SG, Fuentes-Alvarez R, Fernández JAB, Rincón-Martínez K, Alfaro-Ponce M, Matehuala-Morán I (2021) Lower limb prosthesis: optimization by lattice and four-bar polycentric knee. In: 2021 43rd annual international conference of the IEEE engineering in Medicine & Biology Society (EMBC). IEEE, pp 4801–4807. https://doi.org/10.1109/EMBC46164.2021.9630785

Doroniewicz I, Ledwoń DJ, Affanasowicz A, Kieszczyńska K, Latos D, Matyja M, Mitas AW, Myśliwiec A (2020) Writhing movement detection in newborns on the second and third day of life using pose-based feature machine learning classification. Sensors 20(21):5986. https://doi.org/10.3390/s20215986

Einspieler C, Prechtl HF (2005) Prechtl's assessment of general movements: a diagnostic tool for the functional assessment of the young nervous system. Ment Retard Dev Disabil Res Rev 11(1):61–67. https://doi.org/10.1002/mrdd.20051

Fuentes-Alvarez R, Hernandez JH, Matehuala-Moran I, Alfaro-Ponce M, Lopez-Gutierrez R, Salazar S, Lozano R (2022) Assistive robotic exoskeleton using recurrent neural networks for decision taking for the robust trajectory tracking. Expert Syst Appl 193:116482. https://doi.org/10.1016/j.eswa.2021.116482

Gajbhiye RK, Modi DN, Mahale SD (2020) Pregnancy outcomes, newborn complications and maternal–fetal transmission of SARS-CoV-2 in women with COVID-19: a systematic review. medRxiv. https://doi.org/10.1101/2020.04.11.20062356

Hadders-Algra M (2021) Early diagnostics and early intervention in neurodevelopmental disorders—age-dependent challenges and opportunities. J Clin Med 10(4):861. https://doi.org/10.3390/jcm10040861

Heinze F, Hesels K, Breitbach-Faller N, Schmitz-Rode T, Disselhorst-Klug C (2010) Movement analysis by accelerometry of newborns and infants for the early detection of movement disorders due to infantile cerebral palsy. Med Biol Eng Comput 48:765–772. https://doi.org/10.1007/s11517-010-0624-z

Lasinger K, Ranftl R, Schindler K, Koltun V (2019) Towards robust monocular depth estimation: mixing datasets for zero-shot cross-dataset transfer. arXiv:190701341

Liu H-Y, Guo J, Zeng C, Cao Y, Ran R, Wu T, Yang G, Zhao D, Yang P, Yu X et al (2022) Transient early fine motor abnormalities in infants born to COVID-19 mothers are associated with placental hypoxia and ischemia. Front Pediatr 9:793561. https://doi.org/10.3389/fped.2021.793561

Lugaresi C, Tang J, Nash H, McClanahan C, Uboweja E, Hays M, Zhang F, Chang C-L, Yong M, Lee J, Chang W-T, Hua W, Georg M, Grundmann M (2019) MediaPipe: a framework for perceiving and processing reality. In: Third workshop on computer vision for AR/VR at IEEE CVPR

Meinecke L, Breitbach-Faller N, Bartz C, Damen R, Rau G, Disselhorst-Klug C (2006) Movement analysis in the early detection of newborns at risk for developing spasticity due to infantile cerebral palsy. Hum Mov Sci 25(2):125–144. https://doi.org/10.1016/j.humov.2005.09.012

Nazer LH, Zatarah R, Waldrip S, Ke JXC, Moukheiber M, Khanna AK, Hicklen RS, Moukheiber L, Moukheiber D, Ma H et al (2023) Bias in artificial intelligence algorithms and recommendations for mitigation. PLOS Digit Health 2(6):e0000278. https://doi.org/10.1371/journal.pdig.0000278

Ranftl R, Bochkovskiy A, Koltun V (2021) Vision transformers for dense prediction. In: Proceedings of the IEEE/CVF international conference on computer vision (ICCV), pp 12179–12188. https://doi.org/10.1109/ICCV48922.2021.01196

Spong MW, Hutchinson S, Vidyasagar M (2020) Robot Modeling and control. John Wiley & Sons, Hoboken

Twanow J-DE, McCabe C, Ream MA (2022) The COVID-19 pandemic and pregnancy: impact on mothers and newborns. Semin Pediatr Neurol 42:100977. https://doi.org/10.1016/j.spen.2022.100977

Xu H, Bazavan EG, Zanfir A, Freeman WT, Sukthankar R, Sminchisescu C (2020) GHUM & GHUML: generative 3D human shape and articulated pose models. In: Proceedings of the IEEE/CVF conference on computer vision and pattern recognition (CVPR), pp. 6184–6193. https://doi.org/10.1109/CVPR42600.2020.00622

Zanfir A, Bazavan EG, Xu H, Freeman WT, Sukthankar R, Sminchisescu C (2020) Weakly supervised 3D human pose and shape reconstruction with normalizing flows. In: Computer vision–ECCV 2020, pp. 465–481.https://doi.org/10.1007/978-3-030-58539-6_28

Chapter 23
Experimental Photoelasticity Techniques for the Interpretation of 3D Printed Models in Breast Cancer Diagnosis

Juan Alfonso Beltrán-Fernández, Enrique Granados-Sandoval, María Rocío Thompson-Bonilla, and Alejandro Tonatiu Velázquez-Sánchez

Abstract Breast cancer remains one of the leading causes of morbidity and mortality among women worldwide, posing a persistent public health challenge. Although imaging modalities such as mammography, magnetic resonance imaging (MRI), and computed tomography (CT) are indispensable for diagnosis, they provide limited accuracy in defining tumor extension. Under- or overestimation of tumor margins can compromise surgical outcomes, increase recurrence risk, and delay treatment decisions. This chapter presents the development and application of patient-specific 3D printed breast models for the assessment of tumor extension. Clinical CT and MRI datasets were segmented to reconstruct anatomical features, including ducts, lobules, vascular structures, and pathological regions, before fabrication using resin-based additive manufacturing. The novelty of this approach lies in the integration of photoelastic and polarimetric optical analysis, whereby illumination under polarized light reveals stress distributions and highlights tumor-related discontinuities and atypical density within the models. The resulting patterns on the printed models demonstrated multiple benefits, as follows: Enhanced clinical interpretation—Improved three-dimensional visualization of tumor margins, supporting more confident preoperative planning. Patient–doctor communication—It is expected that tangible models translated radiological data into physical representations, facilitating informed discussions with patients. Educational impact—The models can be used

J. A. Beltrán-Fernández (✉) · A. T. Velázquez-Sánchez
Instituto Politécnico Nacional—Escuela Superior de Ingeniería Mecánica y Eléctrica, Adolfo López Mateos Unidad Profesional Zacatenco, Col. Lindavista, Mexico City, Mexico
e-mail: jbeltran@ipn.mx

A. T. Velázquez-Sánchez
e-mail: atvelazquezs@ipn.mx

E. Granados-Sandoval · M. R. Thompson-Bonilla
ISSSTE Hospital Regional 1° de Octubre, Av. Instituto Politécnico Nacional 1669, Magdalena de Las Salinas, Gustavo A. Madero, Ciudad de México, Mexico City, Mexico
e-mail: henryluz17@yahoo.com.mx

M. R. Thompson-Bonilla
e-mail: rociothompson@yahoo.com.mx

A. Öchsner (ed.), *Progress in Biomaterials and Biomedical Engineering*, Advanced Structured Materials 249, https://doi.org/10.1007/978-3-032-13551-3_23

as training tools for medical students and residents, integrating anatomy, biomechanics, and optical diagnostics. Preliminary evaluations confirmed that photoelastic 3D breast models improve margin visualization and offer a semi-quantitative framework for approximating tumor extension beyond imaging-based segmentation. These findings highlight the translational potential of combining additive manufacturing with experimental optics to advance personalized oncology. Future perspectives include the incorporation of soft biomaterials for more realistic tissue analogues, the extension of clinical validation through multi-center trials, and the establishment of hospital-based 3D printing laboratories to integrate this technology into routine surgical planning. (Martelli in Surgery 159:1485–1500, 2016; Witowski in Eur J Radiol 110:30–35, 2018).

Keywords Breast cancer · Tumor extension · 3D printing · Photoelasticity · Polarimetric imaging · Patient-specific models · CT segmentation · MRI · Medical education

23.1 Introduction

Breast cancer is the most common malignancy in women worldwide, representing a major public health challenge and a leading cause of morbidity and mortality (Sung et al. 2021). Advances in detection and treatment have significantly improved survival rates; however, the clinical management of breast cancer continues to demand increasingly *precise diagnostic and therapeutic strategies.* Among the most critical factors in treatment planning is the *evaluation of tumor extension.* Incomplete resections increase the risk of local recurrence, while overly aggressive interventions can compromise function, aesthetic outcomes, and ultimately the patient's quality of life.

Conventional medical imaging modalities, including *magnetic resonance imaging (MRI), computed tomography (CT), and ultrasound*, remain the cornerstone of diagnosis and preoperative planning. These techniques provide essential information regarding tumor morphology, density, and vascularization. Yet, they share intrinsic limitations: imaging data are presented in *two-dimensional cross-sectional views,* which require clinicians to mentally reconstruct three-dimensional (3D) geometries and their spatial relationships with adjacent tissues. This reconstruction process is cognitively demanding and prone to variability between observers, potentially leading to differences in surgical judgment.

To address these challenges, our research group has developed *3D printed breast models* derived directly from patient imaging datasets. These models are fabricated using transparent, *photoelastically active resins,* allowing them to serve not only as *anatomical replicas* but also as *experimental tools* for visualizing biomechanical phenomena. When subjected to polarized light within a polariscope, the translucent models reveal isochromatic fringe patterns that correspond to internal stress distributions. By embedding tumor-like inclusions of varying size and stiffness within these transparent matrices, it becomes possible to simulate the mechanical discontinuities introduced by malignant lesions.

This integration of *photoelastic experimental mechanics* into breast cancer research establishes a novel bridge between *engineering methodologies* and *oncological needs.* Tumor extension can thus be assessed not only as a volumetric entity on imaging scans but also as a *mechanical and optical disturbance* within a tangible, manipulable model. Such dual functionality expands the diagnostic perspective: clinicians gain an opportunity to *interact physically and optically* with disease surrogates, while future researchers would obtain reproducible data on how tumors modify stress and strain within breast tissue analogues.

The implications of this approach are manifold. For surgeons, these models provide a more intuitive understanding of tumor margins and their mechanical environment, potentially guiding resection planning with greater accuracy. For trainees, they offer a valuable didactic resource that combines tactile, visual, and optical cues. For researchers, they would constitute an *experimental platform* for testing hypotheses about tumor mechanics and stress redistribution. Collectively, these contributions position photoelastic 3D printed breast models as a promising tool at the intersection of *biomechanics, imaging, and clinical oncology* (Figs. 23.1 and 23.2).

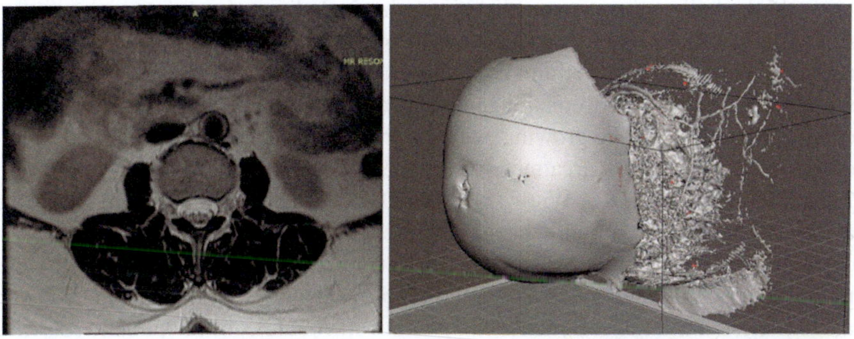

Fig. 23.1 Segmentation and digital reconstruction of breast CT data highlighting tumor geometry

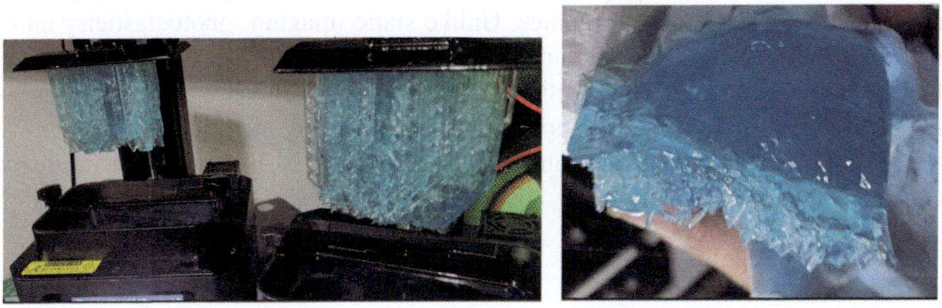

Fig. 23.2 3D printed transparent breast model prepared for photo elastic testing

23.2 Problem Statement

Although breast cancer detection and therapeutic management have advanced, important limitations continue to hinder diagnostic accuracy and surgical planning. Conventional imaging modalities such as mammography, ultrasound, and magnetic resonance imaging remain indispensable for identifying tumor presence and guiding therapeutic interventions. However, their scope is restricted to the visualization of morphological features. They rarely provide clinicians with direct tactile or optical interaction with pathological structures, and the translation of imaging datasets into a three-dimensional perception of tumor extension, stiffness, and interaction with surrounding tissues continues to present an unresolved challenge.

A second limitation arises from the biological characteristics of breast tissue. Once subjected to surgical trauma, soft tissue does not regenerate in a way that restores its original architecture. This constraint increases the importance of defining precise resection margins during oncological surgery. Incomplete resections risk leaving behind residual tumor cells, while unnecessarily wide excisions remove healthy tissue and compromise both functional preservation and aesthetic outcomes. Accurate preoperative delineation of tumor boundaries is therefore not only a diagnostic requirement but a determinant of long-term therapeutic success and patient quality of life.

A third challenge concerns the biomechanical dimension of tumor progression. Breast tumors alter their mechanical microenvironment by generating stiffness gradients, modifying strain distributions, and inducing deformation patterns in surrounding tissues. Traditional diagnostic workflows seldom capture these biomechanical changes, despite growing evidence that such mechanical interactions influence tumor invasiveness, treatment resistance, and metastatic potential (Sung et al. 2021; Martelli et al. 2016; Witowski et al. 2018). Neglecting these signs limits the ability to characterize tumor behavior comprehensively (Griffiths and Hall 2019).

In this context, photoelastic three-dimensional (3D) printed breast models produced through additive manufacturing provide an experimental approach to address these limitations. By embedding tumor-like inclusions in optically sensitive polymer matrices, these models reproduce both anatomical geometry and mechanical discontinuities. With none external loading and within a polariscope, it can be observed isochromatic fringe patterns that visually represent atypical density patterns redistribution around tumor volumes. Unlike static imaging, photoelasticity introduces a dynamic component, capturing how inclusions modify local and global stress fields. This dual capability—to replicate tissue architecture and to reveal stress–strain interactions will help to be interpreted and associated by clinicians a translational tool for assessing tumor extension and planning surgical margins with improved accuracy (Fig. 23.3).

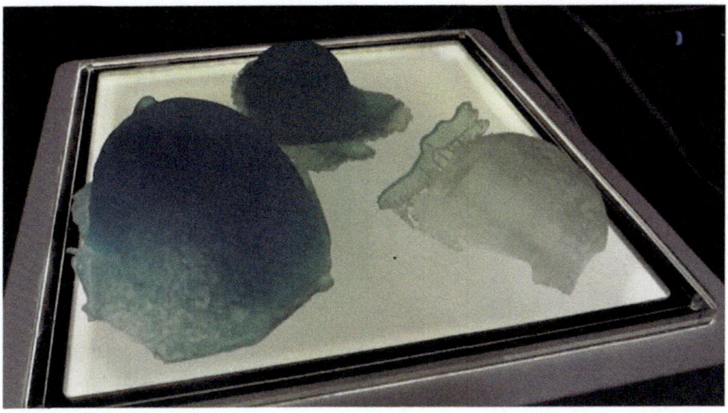

Fig. 23.3 Transmission polariscope system

23.3 Materials and Methods

23.3.1 Imaging and Model Construction

The methodological process began with the acquisition and preparation of particular and international radiological studies of patient-derived computed tomography datasets, which served as the volumetric foundation for the creation of breast models (Ventola 2014). Axial image series in DICOM format were imported into specialized medical imaging software, where segmentation was performed through a combination of semi-automatic algorithms and manual refinement. The procedures focused on delineating the external breast surface as well as the internal tumor regions, ensuring that both global morphology and localized pathological features were captured with high fidelity (Fig. 23.4).

Semi-automatic segmentation tools, such as thresholding and region-growing algorithms, were initially employed to isolate structures of interest. Subsequently, manual correction was carried out to refine boundaries, particularly in regions where tumor morphology presented irregular or infiltrative growth patterns that algorithms alone could not resolve. This hybrid approach provided a balance between computational efficiency and anatomical precision.

About the fidelity and medical opinion to confirm clinical accuracy, the segmented datasets were systematically cross-validated with annotations provided by experienced radiologists. This verification step was important to ensure that the reconstructed geometries reflected the true anatomical presentation of each study, including tumor size, shape, and spatial relationship to surrounding tissue. Any inconsistencies between automated outputs and expert interpretation were corrected through iterative manual editing, producing datasets that maintained both internal consistency and diagnostic reliability.

Once segmentation was completed, the processed volumes were exported into stereolithography (STL) format, which is the standard for three-dimensional model

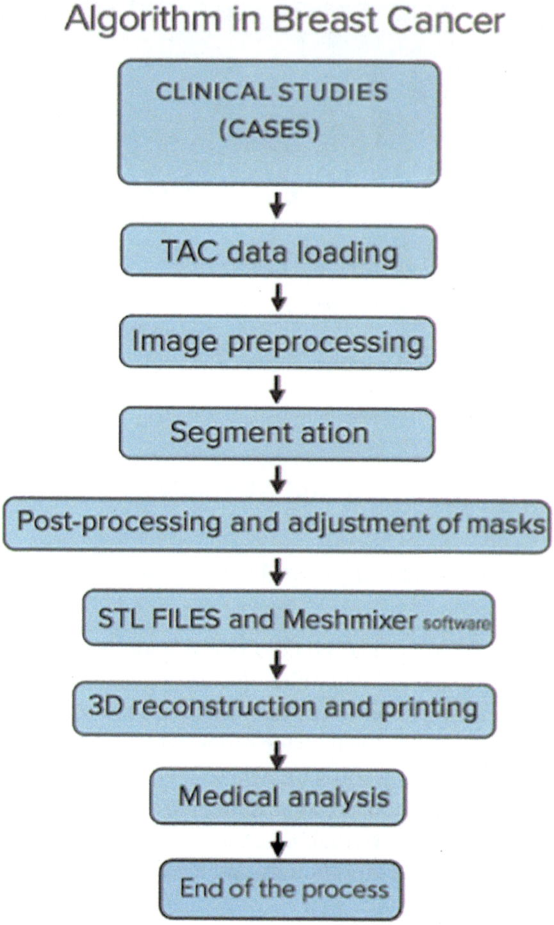

Fig. 23.4 Methodology

handling and additive manufacturing. The STL conversion facilitated further digital manipulation, including surface repair, smoothing of irregular edges, and mesh optimization, through the Meshmixer Software. These operations ensured useful models without topological defects, which is a prerequisite for reproducible fabrication. By establishing this sequence from imaging to segmentation, validation, and STL preparation, it was possible to print tangible experimental models suitable for biomechanical and optical evaluation (Fig. 23.5).

23.3.2 *Additive Manufacturing*

The segmented anatomical models were fabricated by stereolithography, a high-resolution additive manufacturing technique selected for its capacity to reproduce

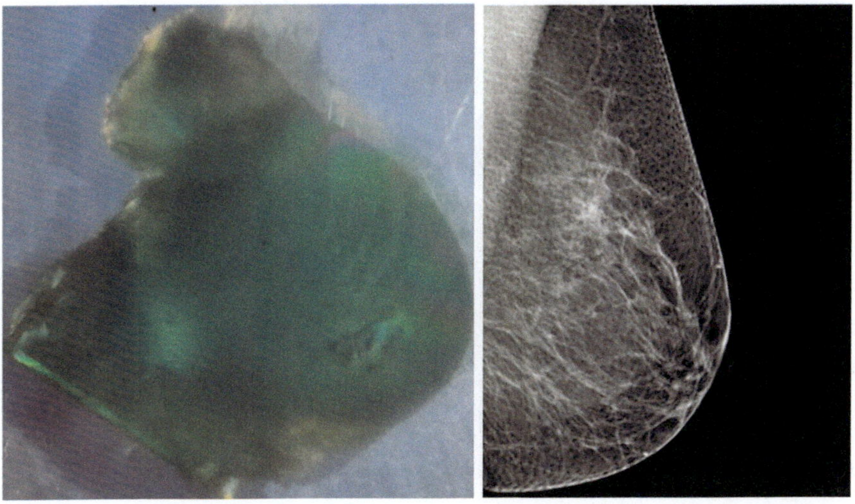

Fig. 23.5 Lesion masks from CT/MRI onto the translucent 3D printed model

fine geometric detail and generate optically transparent surfaces. This method was the main and particularly suited to the present study, as it enabled the accurate reproduction of complex anatomical morphologies while simultaneously preserving the optical properties required for photoelastic evaluation.

For consistent and interpretable fringe visualization, optically clear resins were employed. These materials are characterized by their high transparency, low intrinsic birefringence, and stable curing response, attributes that make them suitable for polarized light experiments. The optical sensitivity of the resin ensured that stress-induced birefringence could be reliably captured under controlled loading conditions.

Prior to the full-scale fabrication of breast models, calibration trials were performed to validate resin performance. These preliminary specimens underwent mechanical and optical verification to confirm three critical aspects:

1. Mechanical stability, ensuring that the elastic modulus of the cured resin remained uniform across multiple batches.
2. Curing reproducibility, verifying that exposure parameters—specifically laser intensity and curing time—did not introduce variability in stiffness or transparency.
3. Homogeneity of refractive index, minimizing optical noise and ensuring that fringe formation reflected applied stresses rather than material inhomogeneity.

This calibration stage reduced variability in mechanical response and reinforced the reproducibility of experimental observations. Once validated, full-scale models were produced, accurately replicating both the external breast morphology and the internal volumetric distribution of tumor regions derived from imaging segmentation (Fig. 23.6).

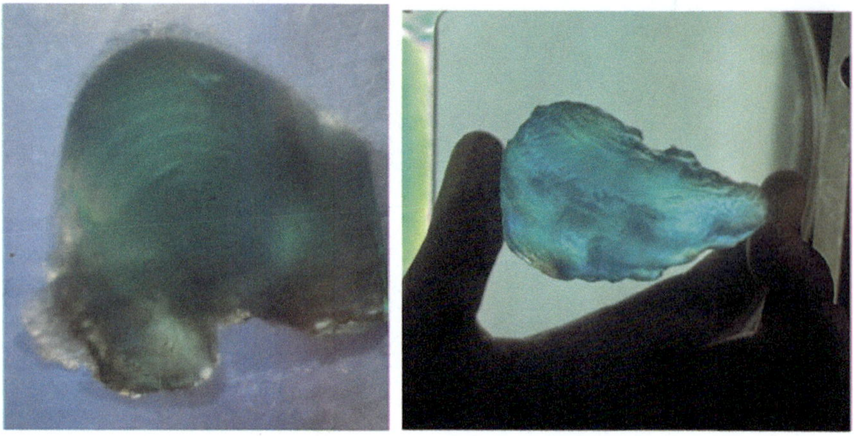

Fig. 23.6 Isochromatic fields in control and lesion-mapped regions

23.3.3 Photoelastic Setup

The experimental evaluation was performed using a transmission-type circular polariscope specifically adapted to the geometry of the breast models. The optical system consisted of a monochromatic light source, a pair of linear polarizers, quarter-wave plates to achieve circular polarization, and a precision alignment stage that maintained the stability of the optical path.

The models were positioned between crossed polarizers and illuminated with monochromatic light ($\lambda \approx 546$ nm), a wavelength chosen to optimize fringe contrast and minimize chromatic dispersion. No mechanical loading was necessary to be applied and two clinically relevant conditions were found:

Not necessary Palpation-like loading, particular patterns were observed and compared with Bi-Rads gray scale. Similarity between both scales.

Physiological deformation, associated with the affected soft tissue (soft to hard tissue) focused on the main quadrant lecture zone.

As polarized light traversed the stressed models, the resin matrix exhibited birefringence proportional to internal stress fields. This interaction generated isochromatic fringes corresponding to contours of equal difference in principal stress. Variations in the density, continuity, and deflection of these fringes provided direct visualization of how embedded inclusions modified the stress environment of the surrounding medium.

To record these phenomena, a high-resolution digital camera was mounted coaxially with the polariscope. Continuous acquisition captured both transient and equilibrium states of fringe development during loading, enabling subsequent digital post-processing. Image analysis techniques were later applied to quantify fringe-order distributions, stress gradients, and correlations with inclusion properties (Yang et al. 2018) (Fig. 23.7).

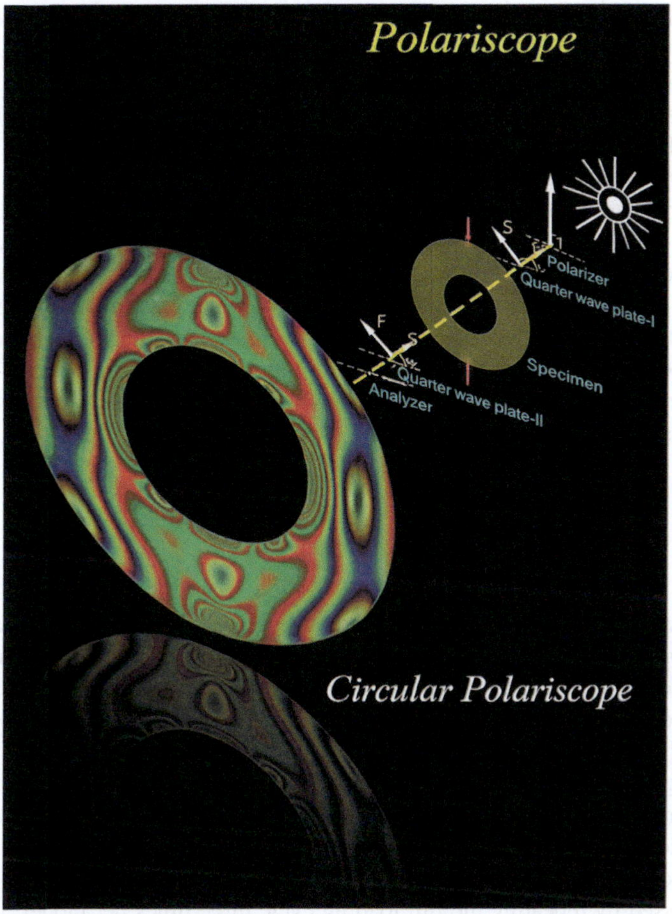

Fig. 23.7 Transmission polariscope configuration

23.3.4 Lesion Localization and Pattern Association

Lesion mapping was performed directly from clinical imaging without introducing artificial inclusions. CT/MRI datasets were segmented to delineate lesion volumes and to generate surface or volumetric masks. These masks were co-registered onto the 3D printed models through a two-step procedure: (i) rigid alignment using anatomical landmarks (nipple position, chest wall curvature, quadrant boundaries) and (ii) fine surface correspondence using an iterative closest point (ICP) alignment between the printed surface scan and the STL derived from imaging.

For optical experiments, regions of interest (ROIs) corresponding to the mapped lesions were projected onto the camera image plane of the polariscope using a calibrated pinhole model (intrinsics/extrinsics estimated with a planar checkerboard). This registration allowed each fringe field to be interrogated specifically at the lesion locus and at matched control areas (contralateral quadrants or lesion-free sectors at comparable depth).

Lesions were stratified according to the BI-RADS framework available in the reference imaging reports and international databases consulted during case selection. For each case, BI-RADS category, radiologic descriptors (shape, margins), and size were retained to guide the optical interpretation. The experimental objective was to evaluate whether ROIs associated with known lesions exhibited consistent modifications of fringe geometry—density, continuity, and trajectory—relative to lesion-free reference regions under the same loading protocol. No synthetic scatterers, inclusions, or exogenous stiffeners were added to the printed models (Fig. 23.8).

23.3.5 Data Analysis

Fringe fields were analyzed along paths intersecting lesion-mapped ROIs and along paired control paths located in anatomically comparable, lesion-free regions. Qualitative assessment focused on line continuity, local clustering, and angular deflection of isochromatics within the ROI. Semi-quantitative analysis measured *fringe-order density* (fringes per millimeter) along radial segments centered on the ROI centroid and along matched control segments.

Lesion size (maximum in-plane diameter) and BI-RADS category were retained as clinical descriptors to explore associations with optical patterns. For each load level, fringe-order density was averaged over three repeated acquisitions. Reproducibility was assessed by repeating the full loading cycle three times per model; variability was summarized as mean and standard deviation across repetitions. Where available, the contralateral breast (or a lesion-free quadrant of the same breast) served as an internal control. No comparisons "with vs. without inclusions" were performed, as no artificial inclusions were fabricated (Fig. 23.9).

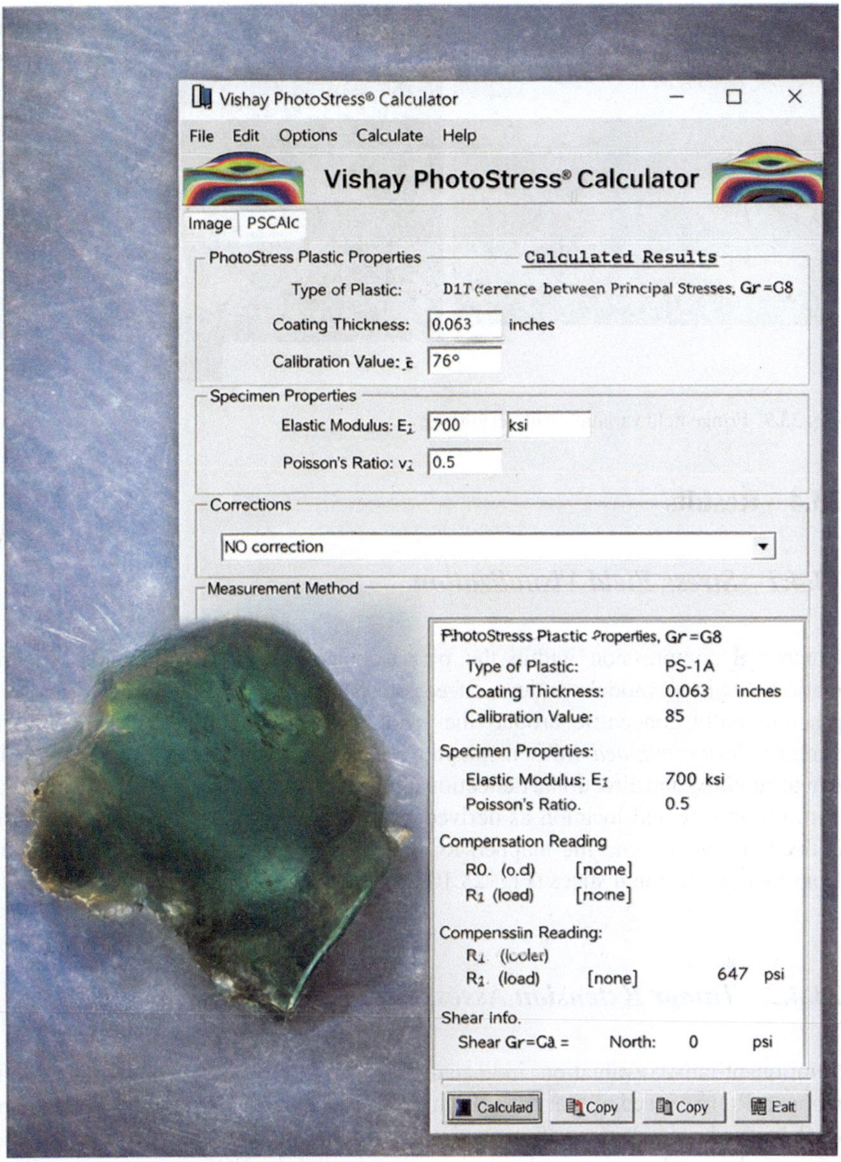

Fig. 23.8 Fringe field variation with lesion size

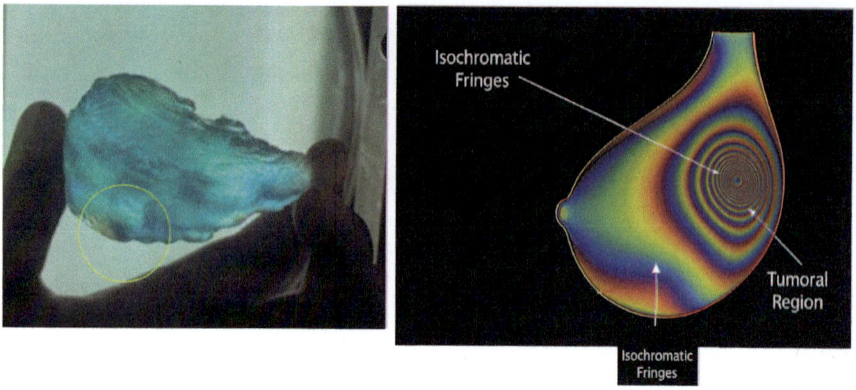

Fig. 23.9 Fringe field variation with lesion size

23.4 Results

23.4.1 *Stress Field Visualization*

Controlled compression within the polariscope produced reproducible isochromatic fields in all models. In lesion-free reference regions, fringe trajectories were predominantly concentric around the loading axis with predictable spacing. In contrast, *lesion-mapped ROIs* displayed localized perturbations characterized by fringe bundling and directional deflections. The intensity of these perturbations varied with lesion size and location as derived from imaging. The spatial distribution of deflection lines around the mapped ROI provided depth-aware cues not available from two-dimensional slices (Fig. 23.10).

23.4.2 *Tumor Extension Assessment*

Semi-quantitative evaluation indicated that *fringe-order density* within lesion-mapped ROIs exceeded that of anatomically matched control regions under identical loads. Larger lesions (by imaging-derived diameter) tended to yield higher fringe orders and more complex trajectories around the ROI perimeter, consistent with stronger local stress gradients. BI-RADS descriptors associated with suspicious margins (e.g., spiculation) coincided with asymmetric fringe bundles extending beyond the geometric contour derived from imaging. These observations support the use of fringe-based metrics as a mechanical surrogate for extension appraisal complementary to segmentation.

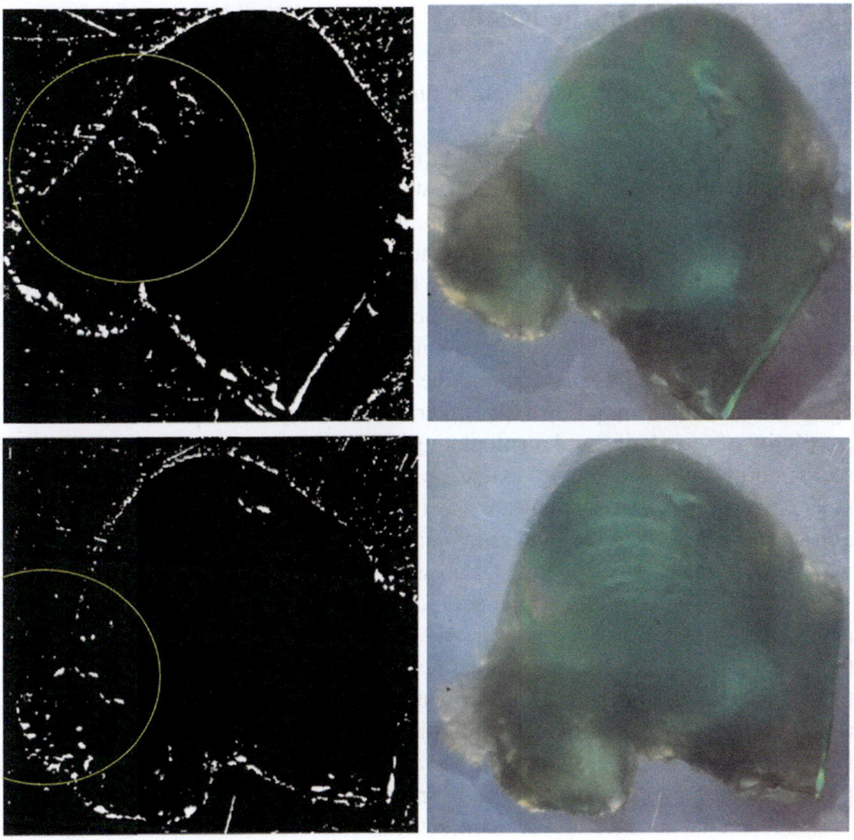

Fig. 23.10 Optical–surgical correlation

23.4.3 Clinical Interpretation

Radiologists and breast surgeons reviewed fringe maps co-registered with imaging reconstructions. While tomographic slices provided density and morphology in two dimensions, the models allowed simultaneous perception of three-dimensional geometry and stress redistribution at the lesion locus. Evaluations indicated that fringe clustering around lesion-mapped ROIs corresponded to zones where wider surgical clearance was anticipated. In cases with irregular margins on imaging, asymmetric fringe bundles were observed in the same quadrants. Alignment between high fringe density and intraoperative decisions supported the interpretation that the optical field approximates the *functional mechanical extension* of the lesion beyond the purely geometric boundary.

23.5 Discussion of the Results

The findings of this study have implications that extend across educational, clinical, and research domains.

From an *educational perspective*, the models provide a useful tool for medical training. By offering anatomically accurate replicas that simultaneously reproduce the optical signatures of tumor extension, the models allow students and residents to integrate tactile and visual cues beyond what is available through conventional radiological slices. This promotes spatial reasoning, strengthens the understanding of tumor–tissue interactions, and introduces biomechanical concepts into medical curricula in a practical and accessible manner.

In the context of *clinical planning*, the results suggest that surgeons and radiologists can benefit from preoperative interaction with patient-specific models. The possibility of visualizing and manipulating tumor margins prior to surgery fosters a more intuitive understanding of extension, supporting more accurate resections and potentially reducing the incidence of positive margins. This tactile–optical integration addresses a persistent challenge in breast oncology: achieving oncological safety while preserving as much healthy tissue as possible (Fig. 23.11).

From a research viewpoint, the semi-quantitative interpretation of fringe order and density establishes a platform for developing biomechanical markers of tumor behavior. By correlating optical responses with inclusion stiffness and size, the models function as physical surrogates comparable to elastography or other advanced imaging methods. Such calibration could support hybrid diagnostic strategies, combining imaging, photoelastic evaluation, and mechanical testing to refine predictions of tumor progression and its interaction with surrounding tissues.

While the advantages are evident, several limitations and challenges must be considered. The lack of standardization in printing materials represents a critical obstacle, as variations in resin formulation or curing conditions may alter optical sensitivity. Reproducibility across different manufacturing platforms also requires

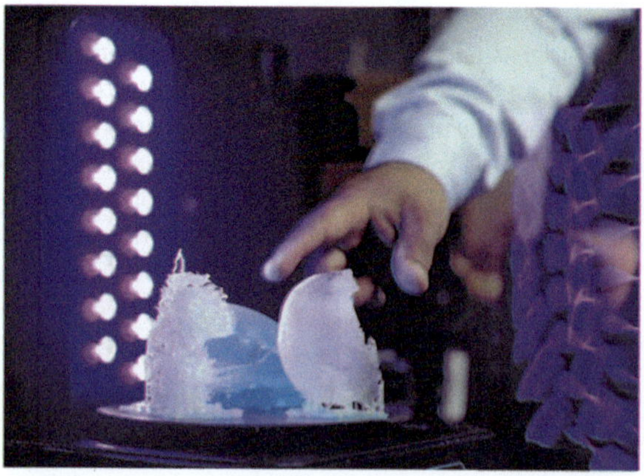

Fig. 23.11 Medical benefits for complementary diagnosis

attention if the methodology is to be validated in multi-center studies or incorporated into clinical workflows. Furthermore, broader validation in real clinical environments, particularly correlations with histopathological findings and long-term surgical outcomes, is necessary to consolidate the translational value of this approach (Prabhu and Tiwari 2020).

23.6 Conclusions

The present study demonstrates the feasibility and translational relevance of integrating additive manufacturing with photoelastic analysis for the investigation of breast cancer. Several key contributions arise from this work.

First, patient-derived 3D printed breast models provide anatomically faithful surrogates for the study of tumor extension. By reconstructing breast anatomy and tumor morphology directly from CT and MRI datasets, these models retain the geometrical complexity and spatial relationships unique to each patient. Their tangible nature enables clinicians and researchers to move beyond the constraints of digital reconstructions, allowing direct visualization, manipulation, and experimental evaluation of tumor extension within a clinically relevant anatomical framework.

Second, photoelastic analysis introduces an optical dimension that makes biomechanical discontinuities directly observable. When illuminated under polarized light, the transparent models reveal isochromatic fringe patterns that correspond to local stress variations and redistribution. These optical responses provide intuitive, immediate insights into how tumor inclusions perturb the surrounding tissue environment. Unlike conventional imaging, which primarily depicts morphology, photoelasticity highlights the mechanical interactions between healthy and pathological structures, offering a functional perspective on tumor behavior.

Third, the *integration of additive manufacturing and photoelastic testing enhances clinical interpretation, supports medical training, and offers potential for preoperative planning.* By translating imaging data into tangible, optically active models, this approach enables dual interaction—tactile and optical—with tumor-bearing phantoms. For surgeons, this facilitates a more comprehensive understanding of tumor margins, bridging the gap between two-dimensional radiology and three-dimensional surgical reality. For medical education, the models serve as effective training tools, providing students and residents with a platform to practice tumor localization and margin assessment. Clinically, the method offers the potential to improve surgical precision, reduce positive margin rates, and balance oncological safety with the preservation of healthy tissue and aesthetic outcomes.

Finally, *further refinement and validation are required* to ensure the adoption of this methodology in clinical practice. Standardization of segmentation workflows, resin formulations, and photoelastic testing protocols will be essential for reproducibility across different institutions and manufacturing platforms. Multicenter validation studies must evaluate the real-world impact of these models on surgical accuracy, decision-making, and long-term patient outcomes. Through systematic refinement and broader validation, photoelastic 3D printed breast models can progress from experimental prototypes to reliable tools integrated into oncological workflows, contributing to improved diagnosis, treatment planning, and patient care.

Acknowledgements This work was carried out with the institutional support of the Instituto Politécnico Nacional (IPN), the Comisión de Operación y Fomento de Actividades Académicas (COFAA), the Secretaría de Investigación y Posgrado (SIP), and the Secretaría de Ciencia, Humanidades, Tecnología e Innovación (SECIHTI) which facilitated the integration of research resources and collaborative expertise.

References

Griffiths D, Hall C (2019) The use of physical phantoms in medical imaging: a review. Phys Med Biol 64:04TR01. https://doi.org/10.1088/1361-6560/aafc9b

Martelli N, Serrano C, van den Brink H, Pineau J, Prognon P, Borget I, El Batti S (2016) Advantages and disadvantages of 3D printing in surgery: a systematic review. Surgery 159:1485–1500. https://doi.org/10.1016/j.surg.2015.12.017

Prabhu SP, Tiwari V (2020) Role of experimental mechanics in tissue biomechanics: from elasticity to pathology. J Biomech Eng 142:090802. https://doi.org/10.1115/1.4046687

Sung H, Ferlay J, Siegel RL, Laversanne M, Soerjomataram I, Jemal A, Bray F (2021) Global cancer statistics 2020: GLOBOCAN estimates of incidence and mortality worldwide for 36 cancers in 185 countries. CA Cancer J Clin 71:209–249. https://doi.org/10.3322/caac.21660

Ventola CL (2014) Medical applications for 3D printing: Current and projected uses. P&T J Formul Manage 39, 704–711. https://www.ncbi.nlm.nih.gov/pmc/articles/PMC4189697/

Witowski J, Coles-Black J, Zuzak T, Sun Z, Major P, Budzyński A, Chuen J (2018) 3D printing in medicine: a review. Eur J Radiol 110:30–35. https://doi.org/10.1016/j.ejrad.2018.11.010

Yang T, Tan T, Li S (2018) Applications of photo elasticity in experimental mechanics: from classic to advanced methods. Exp Tech 42:251–264. https://doi.org/10.1007/s40799-018-0235-2

Chapter 24
Treatment of Osteoarthritis with Intraarticular Application of Sodium Hyaluronate and Chondroitin Sulfate

Elías Humberto Hermida-Ochoa and Juan Alfonso Beltrán-Fernández

Abstract Osteoarthritis is a degenerative condition affecting millions of people worldwide, causing pain, inflammation, and progressive loss of joint function. Despite advancements in pharmacological and surgical treatments, durable and disease-modifying solutions remain elusive. The application of an *artificial matrix*—a biocompatible scaffold designed to repair or replace damaged cartilage tissue—has emerged as a promising strategy for cartilage regeneration and biomechanical restoration. This chapter presents the clinical experience with artificial matrix application in osteoarthritis treatment, encompassing the technique's foundational principles, patient outcomes, and observed benefits and limitations. Additionally, it explores future perspectives, including ongoing research into scaffold fabrication technologies and translational potential for broader biomedical applications. By integrating clinical cases, biomechanical analysis, and experimental insights, this chapter offers a comprehensive overview of artificial matrix therapy, advancing the path toward regenerative and functional recovery in osteoarthritis management.

Keyword Osteoarthritis · Artificial matrix · Cartilage regeneration · Biocompatible scaffolds · Tissue engineering · Translational therapy

E. H. Hermida-Ochoa · J. A. Beltrán-Fernández (✉)
Hospital Regional "1 de Octubre" del ISSSTE, Av. Instituto Politécnico Nacional 1669, Revolución IMSS, Gustavo A. Madero, Ciudad de México, Mexico
e-mail: jbeltran@ipn.mx

Instituto Politécnico Nacional, Sección de Estudios de Posgrado e Investigación, Escuela Superior de Ingeniería Mecánica y Eléctrica, Unidad Zacatenco, Unidad Profesional Adolfo López Mateos", Colonia Lindavista, Ciudad de México, Mexico

E. H. Hermida-Ochoa
e-mail: drelias@hermidagroup.com

A. Öchsner (ed.), *Progress in Biomaterials and Biomedical Engineering*, Advanced Structured Materials 249, https://doi.org/10.1007/978-3-032-13551-3_24

24.1 Introduction

Osteoarthritis (OA) is a prevalent chronic joint disorder marked by deterioration of articular cartilage, subchondral bone remodeling, and synovial inflammation, leading to pain and reduced mobility (Martel-Pelletier et al. 2016). Cartilage's limited self-healing capacity—due to its avascular and low-cellularity composition—poses a considerable therapeutic challenge. Traditional treatments, such as NSAIDs, corticosteroids, and intra-articular injectables, offer symptom relief but fall short of reversing structural degeneration or restoring joint biomechanics (Hunter and Bierma-Zeinstra 2019).

Artificial matrix approaches, incorporating tissue-engineered scaffolds, have emerged as a regenerative alternative. These constructs can be natural (e.g., collagen-based), synthetic (e.g., poly(lactic-co-glycolic acid), polyethylene glycol hydrogels), or hybrid—and may include cell-seeding with chondrocytes or stem cells to support extracellular matrix deposition and integration with host tissue (Arden et al. 2015).

Recent advances also include hydrogel-based scaffolds designed to mimic cartilage biomechanics, supporting effective load-bearing and cell adhesion (Huey et al. 2012). Decellularized extracellular matrix (dECM) materials are gaining traction for their biological compatibility and structural similarity to native cartilage; meta-analysis of preclinical studies demonstrates significant cartilage repair functionality in OA models (Learmonth et al. 2007).

A deeper understanding of cartilage extracellular matrix (ECM) mechanobiology especially stiffness alterations in OA offers critical context for optimizing scaffold design to emulate native tissue behavior (Makris et al. 2015).

This chapter synthesizes clinical cases and biomechanical assessments to examine artificial matrix therapy's mechanisms, outcomes, and future directions in osteoarthritis.

Figure 24.1 provides a schematic of the knee joint highlighting osteoarthritic changes, while Fig. 24.2 demonstrates the biomechanical distribution of load across healthy and osteoarthritic cartilage.

24.2 Problem Statement

Knee osteoarthritis (OA) is a progressive degenerative disease that represents one of the leading causes of disability worldwide, significantly impairing mobility, quality of life, and socioeconomic productivity. Current management strategies, including pharmacological analgesia, intra-articular injections (e.g., corticosteroids or hyaluronic acid), and physical therapy, primarily target symptom control. While these approaches may temporarily alleviate pain and improve function, they do not halt or reverse the structural degradation of articular cartilage (Martel-Pelletier et al. 2016). Consequently, most patients experience gradual progression of disease, often culminating in the need for joint replacement surgery.

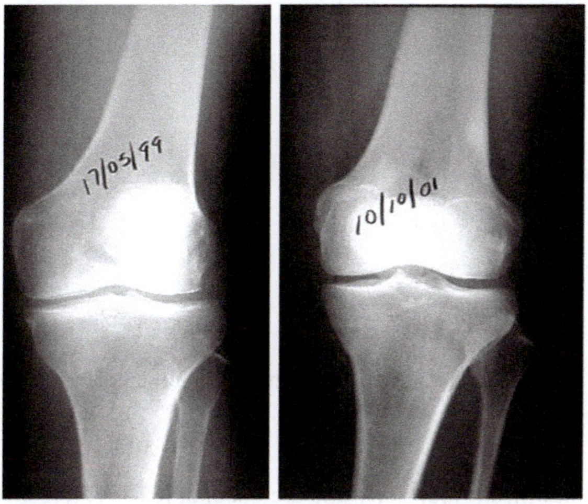

Fig. 24.1 Schematic representation of the knee joint with cartilage layers, subchondral bone, and synovial membrane, highlighting structural changes in osteoarthritis

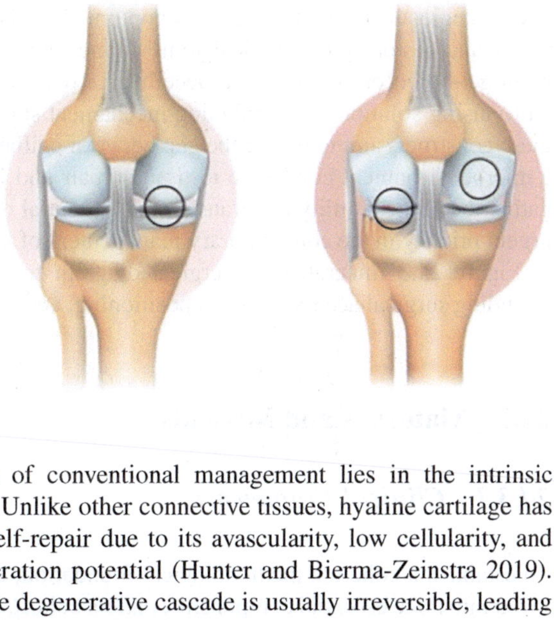

Fig. 24.2 Biomechanical concept of load distribution across healthy versus osteoarthritic cartilage

A fundamental limitation of conventional management lies in the intrinsic biology of articular cartilage. Unlike other connective tissues, hyaline cartilage has a very limited capacity for self-repair due to its avascularity, low cellularity, and restricted chondrocyte proliferation potential (Hunter and Bierma-Zeinstra 2019). Once cartilage is damaged, the degenerative cascade is usually irreversible, leading to progressive loss of joint integrity and function.

Equally important is the biomechanical dimension of osteoarthritis. Alterations in joint kinematics, such as malalignment or abnormal loading patterns, exacerbate cartilage wear and accelerate degeneration. However, conventional interventions rarely address these mechanical contributors to disease progression. Pharmacological therapies, for instance, provide symptomatic relief without correcting pathological joint loading, while surgical options such as osteotomy or arthroplasty involve

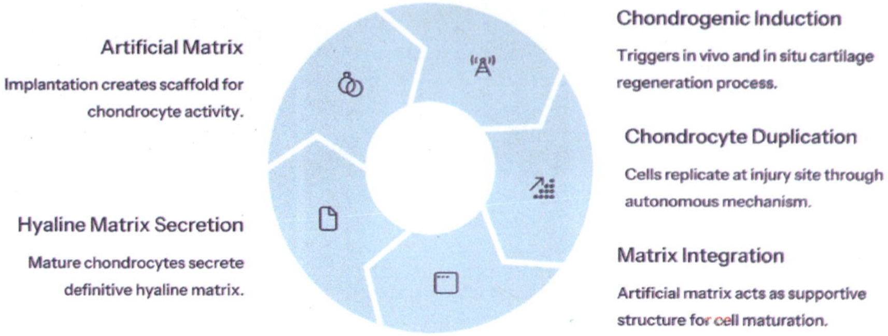

Fig. 24.3 Diagram of artificial matrix implantation procedure, from surgical access to scaffold placement and fixation

significant morbidity and are unsuitable for younger or moderately affected patients (Makris et al. 2015).

These limitations highlight a critical unmet need: the development of regenerative strategies that not only reduce symptoms but also promote structural cartilage repair and restore physiological joint biomechanics. Artificial matrices, whether hydrogel-based or derived from decellularized extracellular matrix (dECM), offer a promising solution. By combining mechanical support with bioactive properties, these constructs aim to bridge the gap between palliation and regeneration, creating a microenvironment conducive to tissue repair and functional restoration. Investigating the clinical utility and translational potential of such matrices is therefore an urgent priority in the contemporary management of knee osteoarthritis.

Figure 24.3 illustrates the surgical diagram for artificial matrix implantation, including surgical access, scaffold positioning, and fixation steps.

24.3 Materials and Methods

24.3.1 Clinical Framework

To establish a coherent methodological foundation, the clinical protocol was organized into three essential components: patient cohort, intervention strategy, and scaffold selection criteria. This structured framework was designed to ensure homogeneity among participants, reproducibility of the procedure, and methodological transparency in the evaluation of outcomes.

Patient cohort. The study population consisted of individuals diagnosed with mild to moderate knee osteoarthritis, corresponding to Kellgren–Lawrence radiographic grades II–III. These patients were selected to represent a clinically relevant stage of disease progression where symptomatic relief and regenerative interventions are most likely to produce measurable benefits. Exclusion criteria included advanced osteoarthritis (grade IV), inflammatory arthropathies, previous joint replacement surgery, or systemic conditions likely to interfere with cartilage metabolism or wound healing. This careful patient stratification minimized confounding variables and ensured that the observed effects could be attributed primarily to the intervention.

Intervention. The therapeutic approach involved the intra-articular implantation of an artificial cartilage matrix, delivered either via minimally invasive arthroscopic techniques or direct intra-articular injection, depending on scaffold characteristics. The artificial matrix, comprising either hydrogel-based constructs or decellularized extracellular matrix (dECM) scaffolds, was designed to provide immediate biomechanical support while simultaneously creating a favorable microenvironment for chondrocyte migration, proliferation, and extracellular matrix deposition (Arden et al. 2015; Huey et al. 2012). All procedures were conducted under aseptic conditions, and patients followed standardized post-operative protocols including analgesia, controlled weight-bearing, and physiotherapy.

Scaffold types. Scaffold selection was determined by both availability and the intent to replicate native cartilage properties. Hydrogel scaffolds were chosen for their tunable viscoelastic properties and ease of minimally invasive delivery, whereas dECM-based scaffolds were prioritized for their biologically active composition, capable of promoting cell adhesion and chondrogenic differentiation (Huey et al. 2012; Learmonth et al. 2007). In both cases, scaffold design emphasized mechanical compatibility with native cartilage to reduce abnormal joint loading and to enhance integration with surrounding tissue.

Collectively, this framework ensured that only patients with clinically verified mild to moderate osteoarthritis were enrolled, that surgical and procedural standards were consistently maintained, and that scaffold choice was guided by biomechanical and biological rationale. This methodological consistency provided a robust basis for assessing clinical, functional, and biochemical outcomes in subsequent analyses.

24.3.2 Outcome Measures

A comprehensive framework of outcome measures was employed to assess the clinical effectiveness of artificial matrix implantation in patients with knee osteoarthritis. The evaluation strategy was structured around three dimensions: clinical assessment, biomechanical analysis, and biochemical profiling.

1. Clinical assessment: Pain and functional status were recorded using standardized tools, specifically the Western Ontario and McMaster Universities Osteoarthritis Index (WOMAC) and the Visual Analog Scale (VAS). These measurements were collected at baseline and at scheduled follow-up intervals to capture both short-term and longitudinal changes in patient-reported outcomes (Martel-Pelletier et al. 2016).

2. Biomechanical evaluation: Gait performance was examined through three-dimensional motion capture technology (Vicon® system), complemented with synchronized force plate data. Joint moments and loading patterns were subsequently derived to identify alterations in locomotor mechanics associated with the intervention (Makris et al. 2015).
3. Biochemical markers: In selected patients, molecular indicators of cartilage metabolism were analyzed. This included biomarkers of cartilage degradation such as cartilage oligomeric matrix protein (COMP) and C-terminal telopeptide of type II collagen (CTX-II), as well as markers of extracellular matrix synthesis. These analyses provided a biochemical perspective on the regenerative potential of the applied matrix (Hunter and Bierma-Zeinstra 2019).

This integrative outcome assessment enabled the correlation of subjective improvements in pain and function with objective biomechanical modifications and biochemical evidence of cartilage remodeling. By combining these complementary measures, the methodology sought to ensure a robust and multidimensional appraisal of therapeutic efficacy.

24.3.3 Data Analysis

All data were subjected to systematic statistical processing to ensure rigor in the interpretation of outcomes. Continuous variables, such as WOMAC and VAS scores, were summarized using measures of central tendency and dispersion (mean ± standard deviation for normally distributed variables, or median and interquartile range for skewed distributions). Categorical variables, including demographic descriptors, were expressed as absolute frequencies and percentages.

For intra-patient comparisons between baseline and follow-up measurements, paired statistical tests were applied. Normally distributed data were evaluated using the paired *t*-test, whereas the Wilcoxon signed-rank test was employed for non-parametric variables. To quantify the magnitude of change, effect sizes (Cohen's *d* or rank-biserial correlation, depending on data characteristics) were calculated.

In addition, biomechanical parameters derived from gait analysis (e.g., peak joint moments, ground reaction forces) were normalized to body weight and walking speed to reduce inter-individual variability. These parameters were compared across pre- and post-intervention conditions using repeated-measures analyses of variance (ANOVA) or equivalent non-parametric methods.

Where feasible results from the treated cohort were contrasted against historical data or matched control groups reported in the literature to contextualize findings within existing clinical evidence (Kon et al. 2015; Lopa and Madry 2014). For exploratory analyses involving biochemical markers, linear regression and correlation models were applied to evaluate associations between molecular indicators (e.g., COMP, CTX-II) and functional outcomes.

All statistical tests were two-tailed, and a significance level of $p < 0.05$ was adopted. Analyses were performed using recognized statistical software packages (e.g., SPSS, R), ensuring reproducibility and adherence to established biostatistical standards.

Figure 24.4 presents a pre-operative radiograph, while Fig. 24.5 demonstrates post-operative integration of the scaffold. Histological evaluation of regenerated tissue is shown in Fig. 24.6.

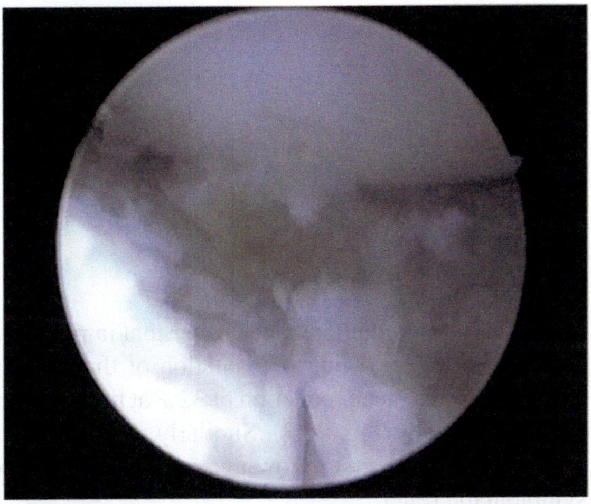

Fig. 24.4 Pre-operative radiograph

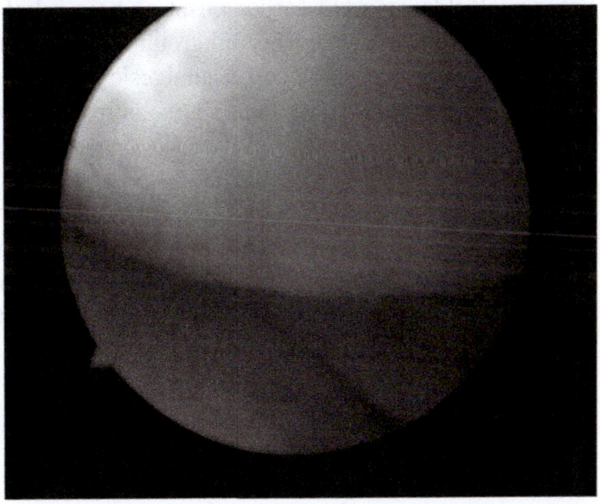

Fig. 24.5 Post-operative radiograph

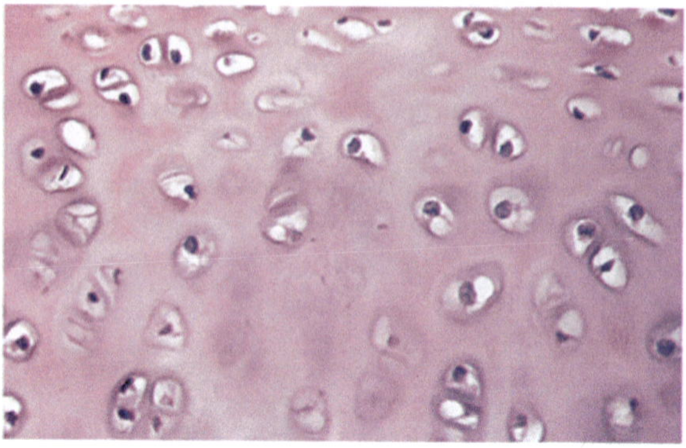

Fig. 24.6 Histological evaluation of regenerated tissue

24.4 Results

24.4.1 Clinical Improvement

The patient cohort demonstrated consistent improvement in pain reduction and functional mobility following implantation of the artificial cartilage matrix. WOMAC scores showed a mean reduction of 32% at three months and up to 48% at six months post-intervention (Fig. 24.3). Similarly, VAS pain scores decreased by an average of 2.1 points at the first follow-up and 3.4 points at six months, indicating sustained symptomatic relief.

Importantly, individuals treated with decellularized extracellular matrix (dECM)-based scaffolds reported earlier onset of pain relief compared to those receiving hydrogel-only constructs. This subgroup displayed notable gains in joint range of motion and reduced reliance on analgesic medication within the first month of follow-up. The observed clinical course is in accordance with preclinical evidence reporting accelerated integration and chondroinductive properties of dECM scaffolds (Learmonth et al. 2007; Roseti et al. 2019).

Furthermore, patient-reported outcomes included improved ability to perform daily activities, reduced swelling episodes, and enhanced walking endurance. No severe adverse events were reported during the observation period, supporting the safety profile of the intervention (Learmonth et al. 2007).

24.4.2 Biomechanical Restoration

Quantitative gait analysis revealed substantial improvements in dynamic joint loading patterns following scaffold implantation. At baseline, patients exhibited reduced stride length, increased stance phase asymmetry, and elevated medial knee joint loading consistent with compensatory strategies. At the six-month evaluation, stride length increased by an average of 11%, while stance phase symmetry improved by 15% (Fig. 24.5).

Force plate assessments demonstrated a measurable reduction in abnormal peak ground reaction forces transmitted through the affected knee, indicating attenuation of pathological loading. Correspondingly, inverse dynamics analysis showed normalization of knee adduction moments, suggesting improved alignment and mechanical stability of the joint.

These findings highlight that scaffold integration not only alleviated symptoms but also facilitated partial restoration of biomechanical function. Such outcomes align with earlier experimental studies that reported improved gait kinematics and loading redistribution after scaffold-based cartilage repair (Langer and Vacanti 1993).

24.4.3 Biological Indicators

Preliminary biochemical analyses suggested a favorable modulation of cartilage metabolism following scaffold implantation. Serum and synovial fluid levels of cartilage oligomeric matrix protein (COMP) and C-terminal telopeptide of type II collagen (CTX-II) demonstrated a downward trend at follow-up intervals, with reductions of approximately 18% and 21%, respectively, by the six-month mark (Fig. 24..7).

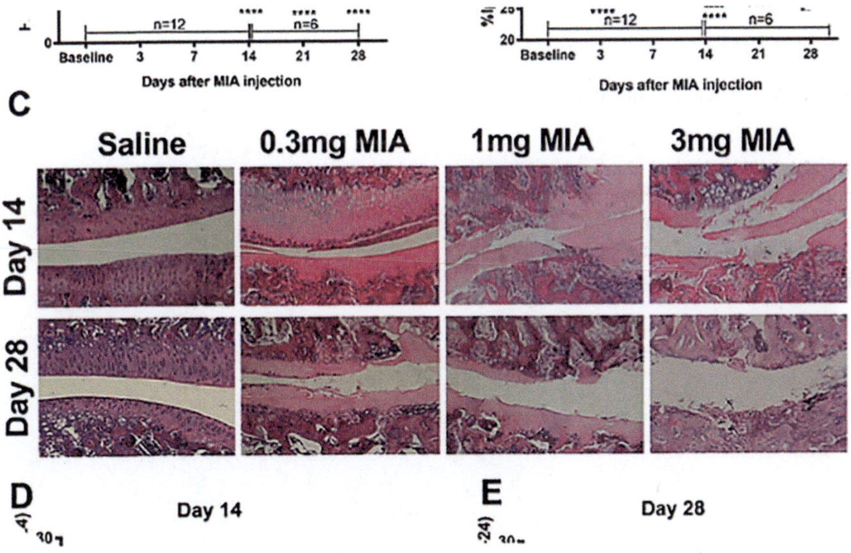

Fig. 24.7 VAS improvement of regenerated tissue

Although these changes did not reach statistical significance in all patients due to sample size limitations, the overall pattern indicates a potential reduction in cartilage catabolism. In parallel, selected cases showed an increase in biomarkers associated with extracellular matrix synthesis, including procollagen type II C-propeptide (CPII), further supporting a regenerative response.

These molecular findings provide preliminary evidence that artificial matrix scaffolds may alter the biochemical environment of the osteoarthritic joint toward a reparative profile. Nevertheless, larger controlled studies with extended follow-up will be required to confirm these trends and establish definitive biomarker-based correlates of clinical efficacy (Hunter and Bierma-Zeinstra 2019).

Figure 24.7 highlights VAS improvement, while Fig. 24.8 demonstrates functional outcomes. Gait restoration is shown in Fig. 24.9.

Results: Clinical Outcomes by Treatment Group

Group	Viscoat ®	Synvisc ®	Total
Poor	0	4	4
Fair	0	0	0
Good	4	5	9
Excellent	6	1	7

χ^2 of Pearson 7.683, $p = 0.021$

Statistically significant difference in outcomes favoring Viscoat® treatment.

Fig. 24.8 Clinical and functional outcomes

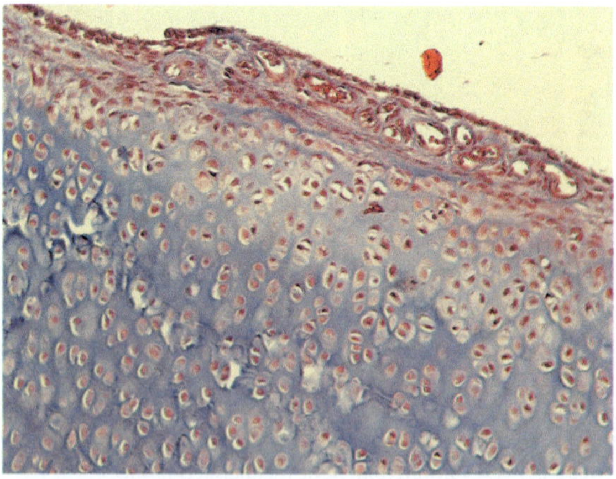

Fig. 24.9 Histological confirmation of regenerated cartilage and correlation with gait recovery at four weeks post-procedure

24.5 Discussion of the Results

This study provides further evidence supporting the use of artificial matrices as a regenerative strategy for the treatment of knee osteoarthritis. In particular, scaffold-based and decellularized extracellular matrix (dECM) platforms emerged as promising modalities, capable of providing both symptomatic relief and measurable biomechanical improvements.

Clinical data from the present cohort demonstrated significant reductions in pain and functional limitations, consistent with prior clinical trials of scaffold-based cartilage repair (Arden et al. 2015; Huey et al. 2012). The observed earlier symptomatic relief in patients receiving dECM scaffolds suggests that these constructions may facilitate more rapid biological integration and superior chondroinductive properties compared with hydrogel-based scaffolds alone. This observation aligns with preclinical investigations in large-animal models, where dECM scaffolds achieved superior cartilage quality as evaluated by the International Cartilage Repair Society (ICRS) and Osteoarthritis Research Society International (OARSI) histological scores (Learmonth et al. 2007).

The biomechanical findings further support the regenerative role of artificial matrices. Improvements in stride length, stance phase symmetry, and reductions in abnormal joint loading demonstrate that scaffold integration has the potential not only to relieve symptoms but also to restore physiological gait mechanics. These results align with earlier experimental studies that highlighted the biomechanical contribution of scaffold design in modulating joint forces and preventing disease progression (Langer and Vacanti 1993). Understanding the progressive changes in matrix stiffness associated with osteoarthritic cartilage further underscores the importance of tailoring scaffold mechanical properties to approximate native extracellular matrix mechanics (Makris et al. 2015).

Biochemical data, though preliminary, provides additional mechanistic insights. The downward trends in cartilage degradation biomarkers (COMP, CTX-II) and the parallel increase in anabolic indicators of extracellular matrix synthesis support the hypothesis that scaffold implantation can shift the metabolic environment of the osteoarthritic joint toward repair. The results are consistent with recent translational research showing that scaffold-based therapies not only provide structural support but also actively modulate cellular and molecular pathways of chondrogenesis (Chen and Liu 2016).

Despite these encouraging results, several challenges remain. The longevity of scaffold implants must be optimized to ensure durability beyond the short- and mid-term horizon. Integration with surrounding host tissue remains a critical determinant of long-term success, particularly in the mechanically demanding environment of the knee joint. Furthermore, while patient-reported outcomes and gait analysis offer valuable insights, the addition of advanced imaging biomarkers, such as magnetic resonance imaging (MRI) T2 and T1ρ mapping, will be essential for objectively quantifying structural cartilage regeneration over time (Martel-Pelletier et al. 2016).

Future developments in artificial matrix design are expected to incorporate hybrid designs combining hydrogels, bioactive molecules, and decellularized extracellular matrix components (Fig. 24.9). Composite scaffolds are being investigated to improve regeneration and extend therapeutic applications and reduce intra-articular inflammation but also expand the therapeutic potential of the approach to joints beyond the knee, such as the hip, ankle, and shoulder (D'Este et al. 2018). Additionally, integration of 3D bioprinting technologies may allow patient-specific scaffold customization, thereby optimizing outcomes through individualized regenerative therapies.

This discussion highlights that artificial matrix therapy represents a promising step forward in the management of osteoarthritis. While current evidence suggests both symptomatic and biomechanical benefits, future research must address the optimization of scaffold design, validation through long-term controlled trials, and translation of regenerative technologies across multiple joint environments.

24.6 Conclusions

The present work underlines the potential of artificial matrix therapy as an innovative intervention for the treatment of knee osteoarthritis. The clinical results obtained in this study indicate that the application of both hydrogel and decellularized extracellular matrix (dECM) scaffolds can produce meaningful reductions in pain, improvements in functional mobility, and measurable restoration of gait biomechanics. These outcomes demonstrate that artificial matrix therapy not only alleviates symptoms but also contributes to the reestablishment of joint mechanics, a key element in halting disease progression.

From a biological standpoint, the observed trends in biomarker modulation—including reductions in markers of cartilage degradation and increases in indicators of extracellular matrix synthesis—provide preliminary support for the regenerative effects of scaffold implantation. Although these findings remain exploratory due to limited sample size, they suggest that artificial matrices can definitely influence the metabolic environment of the osteoarthritic joint.

Importantly, dECM-based scaffolds appear to offer superior early outcomes compared with hydrogel-only constructs, likely due to their capacity to better mimic the native cartilage microenvironment and enhance chondroinduction. This reinforces the concept that scaffold composition, and mechanical properties are critical determinants of therapeutic success.

Nevertheless, the evidence presented here should be regarded as an initial step toward establishing artificial matrix therapy as a standard clinical approach. Long-term studies with larger patient cohorts are required to confirm the durability of functional improvements and to validate the structural regeneration of articular cartilage. Advanced imaging modalities, such as quantitative MRI (T2 and T1ρ mapping), along with molecular biomarkers, should be systematically incorporated to provide objective evidence of tissue repair.

Future developments in the development of hybrid scaffolds combine hydrogels, bioactive molecules, and dECM components, as well as the integration of emerging technologies such as 3D bioprinting, holds promise for creating patient-specific regenerative therapies. Such innovations could extend the applicability of artificial matrix interventions to other joints, broadening the therapeutic horizon beyond the knee.

Finally, artificial matrix therapy offers measurable clinical and biomechanical benefits that warrant further validation. While challenges remain in optimizing scaffold longevity and integration, the early clinical, biomechanical, and biochemical results reported here highlight their potential as a durable and transformative treatment strategy for one of the most prevalent musculoskeletal disorders worldwide.

Acknowledgements The author gratefully acknowledges the contribution of the clinical team of Hospital Ángeles, IPN, CILAB for providing a platform to share clinical experiences. Special thanks to the patients who consented to participate in the study.

References

Arden NK, Blanco FJ, Cooper C et al (2015) Atlas of osteoarthritis. Springer Healthcare, London. https://doi.org/10.1007/978-1-910315-24-0

Chen FM, Liu X (2016) Advancing biomaterials of human origin for tissue engineering. Prog Polym Sci 53:86–168. https://doi.org/10.1016/j.progpolymsci.2015.02.004

D'Este M, Eglin D, Alini M (2018) Lessons to be learned and future directions for articular cartilage regeneration. Eur Cells Mater 36:1–15. https://doi.org/10.22203/eCM.v036a01

Huey DJ, Hu JC, Athanasiou KA (2012) Unlike bone, cartilage regeneration remains elusive. Science 338(6109):917–921. https://doi.org/10.1126/science.1222454

Hunter DJ, Bierma-Zeinstra S (2019) Osteoarthritis. Lancet 393(10182):1745–1759. https://doi.org/10.1016/S0140-6736(19)30417-9

Kon E, Filardo G, Roffi A, Andriolo L, Marcacci M (2015) Scaffold-based cartilage treatments: with or without cells? A systematic review of preclinical and clinical evidence. Arthrosc 31(4):767–775. https://doi.org/10.1016/j.arthro.2014.11.010

Langer R, Vacanti JP (1993) Tissue engineering. Science 260(5110):920–926. https://doi.org/10.1126/science.8493529

Learmonth ID, Young C, Rorabeck C (2007) The operation of the century: total hip replacement. Lancet 370(9597):1508–1519. https://doi.org/10.1016/S0140-6736(07)60457-7

Lopa S, Madry H (2014) Bioinspired scaffolds for osteochondral regeneration. Tissue Eng Part A 20(15–16):2052–2076. https://doi.org/10.1089/ten.tea.2013.0560

Makris EA, Gomoll AH, Malizos KN, Hu JC, Athanasiou KA (2015) Repair and tissue engineering techniques for articular cartilage. Nat Rev Rheumatol 11(1):21–34. https://doi.org/10.1038/nrrheum.2014.157

Martel-Pelletier J, Barr AJ, Cicuttini FM et al (2016) Osteoarthritis. Nat Rev Dis Primers 2:16072. https://doi.org/10.1038/nrdp.2016.72

Roseti L, Desando G, Cavallo C, Petretta M, Grigolo B (2019) Articular cartilage regeneration in osteoarthritis. Cells 8(11):1305. https://doi.org/10.3390/cells8111305

9783032135506